Teen Health Series

Podiatry
SOURCEBOOK

Second Edition

Health Reference Series

Second Edition

Podiatry
SOURCEBOOK

*Basic Consumer Health Information about
Disorders, Diseases, Deformities, and Injuries
that Affect the Foot and Ankle, Including Sprains,
Corns, Calluses, Bunions, Plantar Warts, Plantar
Fasciitis, Neuromas, Clubfoot, Flat Feet, Achilles
Tendonitis, and Much More*

*Along with Information about Selecting a Foot
Care Specialist, Foot Fitness, Shoes and Socks,
Diagnostic Tests and Corrective Procedures, Financial
Assistance for Corrective Devices, a Glossary of
Related Terms, and a Directory of Resources for
Additional Help and Information*

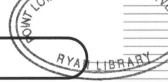

Edited by
Ivy L. Alexander

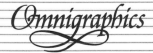

Omnigraphics

615 Griswold Street • Detroit, MI 48226

Bibliographic Note

Because this page cannot legibly accommodate all the copyright notices, the Bibliographic Note portion of the Preface constitutes an extension of the copyright notice.

Edited by Ivy L. Alexander

Health Reference Series

Karen Bellenir, *Managing Editor*
David A. Cooke, M.D., *Medical Consultant*
Elizabeth Collins, *Research and Permissions Coordinator*
Cherry Stockdale, *Permissions Assistant*
Laura Pleva Nielsen, *Index Editor*
EdIndex, Services for Publishers, *Indexers*

* * *

Omnigraphics, Inc.

Matthew P. Barbour, *Senior Vice President*
Kay Gill, *Vice President—Directories*
Kevin Hayes, *Operations Manager*
David P. Bianco, *Marketing Director*

* * *

Peter E. Ruffner, *Publisher*
Frederick G. Ruffner, Jr., *Chairman*
Copyright © 2007 Omnigraphics, Inc.
ISBN 978-0-7808-0944-4

Library of Congress Cataloging-in-Publication Data

Podiatry sourcebook : basic consumer health information about disorders, diseases, deformities, and injuries that affect the foot and ankle, including sprains, corns, calluses, bunions, plantar warts, plantar fasciitis, neuromas, clubfoot, flat feet, Achilles tendonitis, and much more; along with information about selecting a foot care specialist, foot fitness, shoes and socks, diagnostic tests and corrective procedures, financial assistance for corrective devices, a glossary of related terms, and a directory of resources for additional help and information / edited by Ivy L. Alexander. -- 2nd ed.
    p. cm.
  Summary: "Provides basic consumer health information about diagnosis and treatment of disorders, diseases, and injuries of the foot and ankle. Includes index, glossary of related terms, and other resources"--Provided by publisher.
  Includes bibliographical references and index.
  ISBN 978-0-7808-0944-4 (hardcover : alk. paper) 1. Podiatry. 2. Foot--Diseases. I. Alexander, Ivy L.
  RD563.P593 2007
  617.5'85--dc22
                                                                2006037692

Table of Contents

Visit www.healthreferenceseries.com to view *A Contents Guide to the Health Reference Series*, a listing of more than 13,000 topics and the volumes in which they are covered.

Part II: Common Foot Conditions

Part III: Foot and Ankle Injuries

Part IV: Deformities of the Foot and Ankle

Part V: Health Conditions that Affect the Feet

Preface

About This Book

The American Podiatric Medical Association estimates that people take an average of 8,000 to 10,000 steps a day. While taking a step may seem like a simple task for a healthy individual, the foot itself is a complicated structure, containing 26 bones, 33 joints, 107 ligaments, and 19 muscles. With so many components involved, there are numerous ways problems can develop. In fact, statistics suggest that three out of every four of Americans will experience a foot disorder at some point during their lives. A small percentage of foot problems are the result of congenital disorders. The vast majority, however, develop from preventable causes, such as lack of attention to foot care and poorly fitted shoes. Foot problems can also be the first sign of chronic health concerns, including diabetes, arthritis, and circulatory disorders.

Podiatry Sourcebook, Second Edition, provides basic information about the many diseases, disorders, deformities, and injuries that affect the foot and ankle. These include calluses, corns, arch problems, bunions, heel pain, neuromas, athlete's foot, plantar warts, fungal infections, ingrown toenails, sprains, and fractures. It describes common symptoms and explains how doctors of podiatric medicine (DPMs) diagnose and treat foot problems and foot-related complaints due to systemic diseases. It also discusses ways to prevent foot problems by protecting the feet, observing proper foot hygiene, and selecting appropriate footwear. A glossary of related terms and a directory of additional resources are also included.

How to Use This Book

This book is divided into parts and chapters. Parts focus on broad areas of interest. Chapters are devoted to single topics within a part.

Part I: Podiatric Medicine and Foot Health describes the roles podiatrists and their patients play in caring for the feet and ankles. It offers tips for keeping the feet healthy throughout the life span, addresses questions about proper footwear selection, and provides guidelines for injury prevention. Commonly used diagnostic, therapeutic, and surgical procedures are also explained.

Part II: Common Foot Conditions describes some of the most frequently encountered problems of the feet and nails. These include infectious conditions, such as athlete's foot and plantar warts, and pain-related concerns, such as heel pain and neuromas.

Part III: Foot and Ankle Injuries provides facts about fractures, sprains, strains, and other specific conditions and disorders associated with overuse, sports injuries, and exposure to adverse environmental conditions.

Part IV: Deformities of the Foot and Ankle pays particular attention to genetic and congenital problems of the foot and ankle. It also describes deformities associated with improper footwear, repetitive injury, or trauma.

Part V: Health Conditions that Affect the Feet focuses on diseases and other physical conditions that can have an adverse effect on the feet and ankles. These include pregnancy, diabetes, neuromuscular diseases, arthritis, lupus, and Hansen disease.

Part VI: Additional Help and Information offers a glossary of foot-care terms, information about financial assistance for podiatric-related concerns, suggestions for further reading, and a directory of resources that provide help and information to patients with foot and ankle problems.

Bibliographic Note

This volume contains documents and excerpts from publications issued by the following U.S. government agencies: Army Medical Department; Darnall Army Community Hospital, Fort Hood, Texas; Health Resources and Services Administration (HRSA); National Diabetes

Education Program (NDEP); National Institute of Arthritis and Musculoskeletal and Skin Diseases (NIAMS); National Institute on Aging (NIA); National Institute of Diabetes and Digestive and Kidney Diseases (NIDDK); National Hansen's Disease Programs (NHDP); National Institutes of Health (NIH); National Institute of Neurological Disorders and Stroke (NINDS); and U.S. Food and Drug Administration (FDA).

In addition, this volume contains copyrighted documents from the following organizations and individuals: A.D.A.M., Inc.; American Academy of Dermatology; American Academy of Family Physicians; American Academy of Orthopaedic Surgeons; American Academy of Orthotists and Prosthetists; American College of Foot and Ankle Orthopedics and Medicine (ACFAOM); American College of Rheumatology; American Orthopaedic Foot and Ankle Society; American Physical Therapy Association; American Podiatric Medical Association; Amputee Coalition of America; Association of Military Surgeons of the United States; Canadian Centre for Occupational Health and Safety (CCOHS); Cleveland Clinic Department of Orthopaedic Surgery; David A. Cooke, MD; Duke University Medical Center; Eleanor and Lou Gehrig MDA/ALS Research Center of Columbia University Medical Center; Family Foot and Ankle Centers; Foot.com; Healthcommunities.com; Lupus UK; March of Dimes Birth Defects Foundation; Massachusetts Office of Consumer Affairs and Business Regulation, Division of Professional Licensure; Medical College of Wisconsin HealthLink; Medical Multimedia Group; National Parkinson Foundation; Nemours Center for Children's Health Media; New Zealand Dermatological Society; Nicholas Institute for Sports Medicine and Athletic Trauma; Ohio State University Extension; Penton Media, Inc.; PodiatryNetwork.com; Podiatry Online; Rosalind Franklin University Gait Analysis Lab; St. Jude Children's Research Hospital; Shriners Hospitals for Children—Spokane; Texas Department of Insurance, Division of Workers' Compensation; University of Florida Cooperative Extension, Institute of Food and Agriculture Sciences; and Yale-New Haven Hospital.

Full citation information is provided on the first page of each chapter or section. Every effort has been made to secure all necessary rights to reprint the copyrighted material. If any omissions have been made, please contact Omnigraphics to make corrections for future editions.

Acknowledgements

Thanks go to the many organizations, agencies, and individuals who have contributed materials for this *Sourcebook* and to medical consultant Dr. David Cooke and document engineer Bruce Bellenir. Special thanks go to managing editor Karen Bellenir and permissions specialist Liz Collins for their help and support.

About the Health Reference Series

The *Health Reference Series* is designed to provide basic medical information for patients, families, caregivers, and the general public. Each volume takes a particular topic and provides comprehensive coverage. This is especially important for people who may be dealing with a newly diagnosed disease or a chronic disorder in themselves or in a family member. People looking for preventive guidance, information about disease warning signs, medical statistics, and risk factors for health problems will also find answers to their questions in the *Health Reference Series*. The *Series*, however, is not intended to serve as a tool for diagnosing illness, in prescribing treatments, or as a substitute for the physician/patient relationship. All people concerned about medical symptoms or the possibility of disease are encouraged to seek professional care from an appropriate health care provider.

Locating Information within the Health Reference Series

The *Health Reference Series* contains a wealth of information about a wide variety of medical topics. Ensuring easy access to all the fact sheets, research reports, in-depth discussions, and other material contained within the individual books of the *Series* remains one of our highest priorities. As the *Series* continues to grow in size and scope, however, locating the precise information needed by a reader may become more challenging.

A *Contents Guide to the Health Reference Series* was developed to direct readers to the specific volumes that address their concerns. It presents an extensive list of diseases, treatments, and other topics of general interest compiled from the Tables of Contents and major index headings. To access A *Contents Guide to the Health Reference Series*, visit www.healthreferenceseries.com.

Medical Consultant

Medical consultation services are provided to the *Health Reference Series* editors by David A. Cooke, M.D. Dr. Cooke is a graduate of Brandeis University, and he received his M.D. degree from the

University of Michigan. He completed residency training at the University of Wisconsin Hospital and Clinics. He is board-certified in Internal Medicine. Dr. Cooke currently works as part of the University of Michigan Health System and practices in Ann Arbor, MI. In his free time, he enjoys writing, science fiction, and spending time with his family.

Our Advisory Board

We would like to thank the following board members for providing guidance to the development of this *Series*:

- Dr. Lynda Baker, Associate Professor of Library and Information Science, Wayne State University, Detroit, MI

- Nancy Bulgarelli, William Beaumont Hospital Library, Royal Oak, MI

- Karen Imarisio, Bloomfield Township Public Library, Bloomfield Township, MI

- Karen Morgan, Mardigian Library, University of Michigan-Dearborn, Dearborn, MI

- Rosemary Orlando, St. Clair Shores Public Library, St. Clair Shores, MI

Health Reference Series *Update Policy*

The inaugural book in the *Health Reference Series* was the first edition of *Cancer Sourcebook* published in 1989. Since then, the *Series* has been enthusiastically received by librarians and in the medical community. In order to maintain the standard of providing high-quality health information for the layperson the editorial staff at Omnigraphics felt it was necessary to implement a policy of updating volumes when warranted.

Medical researchers have been making tremendous strides, and it is the purpose of the *Health Reference Series* to stay current with the most recent advances. Each decision to update a volume is made on an individual basis. Some of the considerations include how much new information is available and the feedback we receive from people who use the books. If there is a topic you would like to see added to the update list, or an area of medical concern you feel has not been adequately addressed, please write to:

Editor
Health Reference Series
Omnigraphics, Inc.
615 Griswold Street
Detroit, MI 48226
E-mail: editorial@omnigraphics.com

Part One

Podiatric Medicine and Foot Health

Chapter 1

Taking Care of Your Feet and Ankles

"My feet are killing me!" is one of the most enduring phrases in the English language. Like most clichés, this one is grounded in day-to-day experience: the foot and ankle region is subject to constant stresses and hazards, from the effects of ill-fitting shoes to traumatic sports injuries. The results can be painful or worse. While our feet may not literally be "killing" us, foot and ankle problems can have a significant impact on our general health and well-being.

In this chapter you will learn about the following:

- the basic anatomy of the foot and ankle
- common ailments of the foot and ankle
- ways to reduce the risk of injury
- exercises to do at home
- physical therapy treatments

In addition, we will discuss some important information that will be of special interest to people living with diabetes and other diseases. But whatever the nature of your foot/ankle problem, physical therapy can often help you recover function and keep you on the move.

Foot and Ankle Anatomy

The foot contains three main sections or functional units: the rear foot, midfoot, and forefoot. These three units work together to allow the foot to be flexible (such as accommodating an uneven surface) or to be fairly rigid (such as keeping the body upright as we go through the normal walking cycle).

Each foot contains 26 bones: 7 tarsals (ankle bones), 5 metatarsals (instep bones), and 14 phalanges (toe bones). The main arch of the foot is called the plantar arch. It runs lengthwise and touches the ground only at the heel bone and at the ball of the foot. The plantar arch is thickly padded at both ends. There is also a thick pad of fat under the heel of the foot to absorb shock. In addition to the plantar arch, the foot has two other arches: the metatarsal arch, which runs cross-wise under the instep, and the lateral arch, which runs lengthwise along the outside of the foot.

The bones and joints of the foot and ankle are held together by a strong network of muscles and ligaments. The foot is connected to the ankle where one of the tarsal bones, called the talus, meets the lower leg bones, called the tibia and the fibula.

The ankle joint is called upon to provide both great stability (keeping us standing up) and great mobility (walking, running, jumping).

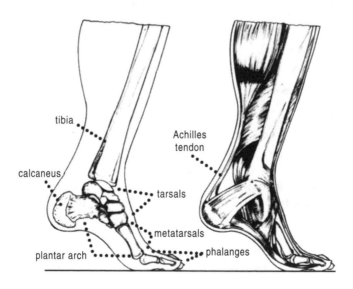

Figure 1.1. The foot and ankle.

These two functions need to be kept in balance if we're to keep our feet healthy and functioning.

The Way We Walk

Physical therapists refer to the motion of the foot during walking as a key part of the gait cycle. An individual's gait cycle consists of two phases: the stance phase and the swing phase.

In the stance phase, the foot is in contact with the ground. During the first part of the stance phase, in which the heel strikes the ground, the foot undergoes pronation; during the second part of the stance phase, in which the foot rotates forward onto the ball of the foot and the toes and recovers stability, the foot undergoes supination. The swing phase is the period during which the foot is completely off the ground.

While most of us pay little attention to this "automatic" process, problems can develop if the pronation and supination phases are not in harmony. If, for example, a person relies too heavily on the "wrong" muscles and other soft tissue to recover stability, those muscles and tissues may become stretched beyond their normal range and become inflamed.

Every person's gait cycle is somewhat different. (If you've ever noticed that the heels on your shoes wear down quickly at a particular angle, this is an indicator of your own particular style of walking.) Physical therapists sometimes videotape a patient's gait cycle to help pinpoint the source of a foot or ankle problem, particularly if the problem is not the result of injury or disease. Once the physical therapist can see exactly how a patient is walking, it's easier to design an effective therapeutic program that will improve the patient's "form." In addition, the physical therapist will usually prescribe exercises tailored to the particular needs of the patient.

The Causes of Foot and Ankle Problems

Because we are two-footed creatures, our feet and ankles are called upon to perform a remarkable achievement of biomechanics—they keep our bodies upright and stable while permitting us to run and walk. This unique capability puts great pressure on our feet and ankles. It can also turn what were initially minor problems into major ones.

Shoes are often the culprits. The legions of women who have forsaken "heels" for athletic shoes on their daily commutes to the workplace are a vivid reminder of the effect that shoes have on our daily lives. And it's not just women who suffer from the dictates of fashion: many men also feel compelled to squeeze their feet into fashionable European-style loafers or tight "executive" shoes at the expense of comfort and, ultimately, health.

It's important for all of us to know what waiters and waitresses have known for years: that if you're going to stay on your feet and keep going, your shoes have to fit right, be comfortable, and provide support—and support means maximum coverage of the surface area under the plantar arch. It's also necessary that your shoes be able to absorb shock while you walk, and that they provide stability to the heel area.

Fortunately, it's no longer necessary to sacrifice style for comfort and health—several shoe companies now specialize in making "healthy" shoes in styles that are virtually indistinguishable from "regular" shoes. When buying new shoes, remember that lace-up shoes are generally preferable. They tend to provide a snugger fit than slip-ons and more stability to the heel; lace-ups also give you more control over the fit. If you're not ready to invest in new shoes, the inexpensive shoe inserts available in drugstores can provide a degree of softness and shock absorption.

Foot and Ankle Injuries

The most commonly reported injuries in the foot/ankle region are ankle sprains. A sprained ankle simply means that the ligaments (the

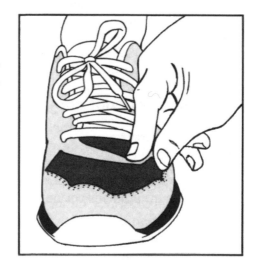

Figure 1.2. The "Pinch Test." *Poorly fitting shoes are a major source of foot problems. The "Pinch Test" can help: if you can pinch some of the shoe's material between your thumb and forefinger, there is adequate space between your toes and the side of the shoe.*

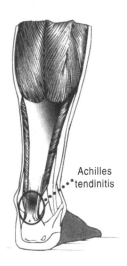

Figure 1.3. *Achilles tendonitis.*

strong bands of tissue that connect the bones of the foot) are stretched beyond their normal limits, resulting in inflammation, tearing, or rupture of the tissue.

Sprained ankles run the gamut from minor to serious. If you're in pain for more than a day or two, or if the pain is intense, you should see a physical therapist or physician. If physical therapy is required, the sprained ankle will be immobilized for a short period to prevent further damage and to give the tissue a chance to heal. After that, therapy progresses quickly with exercises designed to restore stability and strength to the muscles. It is also crucial that the patient's sense of balance be restored or enhanced through exercise.

"Shin splints" is a catch-all phrase for a number of foot and ankle problems, including overuse of the muscles and tendons of the foot and ankle. Tendons are the strong fibrous cords that attach muscles to bones. The Achilles tendon, which takes its name from ancient mythology, is easily felt at the back of the ankle. Achilles tendonitis is an inflammation of this tendon, often resulting from sports (such as basketball or aerobic dancing) that require a great deal of jumping.

Plantar fasciitis is an irritation of the plantar fascia—the tough tissue on the very bottom of the foot that begins at the heel and is attached to the toes. It can result in pain and lead to a heel spur, a bony growth on the underside, forepart of the heel bone. This kind of pain is usually at its worst in the morning, then gradually diminishes during the day. Heel spurs are caused by

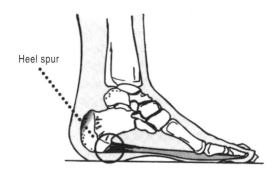

Figure 1.4. *Heel spur.*

straining the foot muscles, stretching the long band of tissue connecting the heel and the ball of the foot, and by repeated tearing of the lining of the membrane that covers the heel bone.

Metatarsalgia is pain in the forefoot, usually caused by the overprominence of one of the metatarsal heads (i.e., the heads of the bones in the ball of the foot). All of these overuse conditions can be aggravated by excessive pronation.

Most people associate repetitive motion injuries with the hand and wrist—but did you know that your feet and ankles are also vulnerable? People who are on their feet all day—salespeople, trial lawyers, teachers, nurses, athletes—are at risk for a variety of foot and ankle disorders, including tarsal tunnel syndrome. While not as well-known as its "cousin" carpal tunnel syndrome (in the wrist), tarsal tunnel syndrome can be just as painful. As with many foot problems, tarsal tunnel syndrome can often be blamed on shoes that do not provide enough arch support and heel stability. Ill-fitting shoes cause the foot to pronate excessively; when this happens, one of the thick ligaments

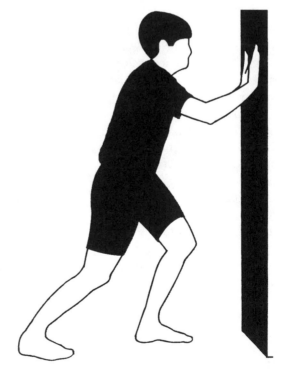

Figure 1.5. Ankle stretch. Face a wall and place both arms out in front of you, with elbows slightly bent. Keep the palms of your hands slightly above shoulder level. Lean into the wall, keeping your back leg slightly bent. Keep both feet flat on the floor. Feel the gentle stretch in the back of the ankle of the back leg. Hold and stretch for 1–20 seconds. Repeat the exercise 3–5 times on each leg.

running from the ankle to the bottom of the foot can become stretched and inflamed. This in turn can irritate a major nerve running just behind the ligament, resulting in tingling and numbness. If the standard treatments for heel pain are ineffective, a physician should be consulted about the possibility of other treatment options.

Flat feet, also called "pancake feet," is a condition in which the arch is judged to be lower than normal. There are many degrees of "flat feet," and some physical therapists will point out that curve of a "normal" arch is a subjective judgment. Nevertheless, flat feet can cause discomfort, and sometimes can lead to plantar fasciitis or other problems. High arches, as opposed to flat feet, is a condition in which the arches are higher than normal. The main concern here is to make sure that the shoes have enough surface contact and support for the arches; otherwise, the stresses put on the foot and ankle can move "up the chain" through the legs and spinal column. In some cases, high arches may require custom orthopedic shoe inserts to prevent more serious problems.

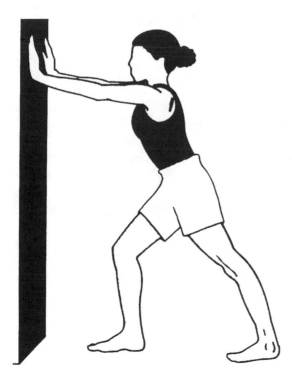

Figure 1.6. Achilles tendon stretch. Face the wall and place your arms straight out in front of you, with the palms of your hands slightly above shoulder level. Lean into the wall, bending your front leg and keeping your back leg straight. Keep both feet flat on the floor. Feel the gentle stretch in the Achilles tendon of the back leg. Hold the stretch for 10–20 seconds. Repeat the exercise 3–5 times on each leg.

Disease-Related Foot Problems

Physical therapists commonly treat foot problems associated with diseases such as diabetes or arthritis. Diabetes can lead to peripheral neuropathy, a condition in which feeling is reduced in the foot. This numbness is a serious condition that can lead to injuries and ulcers on the foot—and, in the most extreme cases, amputation. Because the patient can't feel pain or pressure, a simple blister can turn into an ulcer, infection can set in, and, in severe cases, this can be followed by gangrene and amputation of the foot or leg.

There is now a simple screening procedure that can tell you instantly if you are at high risk for peripheral neuropathy and its complications. Physical therapists and physicians use a simple device that resembles a toothbrush with a single long bristle. As the various areas of the foot are touched by the "bristle," the patient indicates if he or she can feel it. In addition, physical therapists and physicians can measure the amount of feeling in a particular area by the degree to which the bristle bends. If there are parts of your foot that are numb and at risk for injury, you'll know exactly where they are, giving you a head start in protecting the area.

Physical therapy cannot reverse peripheral neuropathy, but it can lessen its impact and ultimately help prevent amputations. While physical therapy can help improve blood flow to the feet, it is most important that the patient learn to use his or her other senses (particularly sight and touch) to detect trouble spots, and to protect the feet with the right shoes.

You should also use your mirror and ask for assistance from family members to help you detect injuries you may have overlooked. In addition to using your eyes, feel your feet with your hands—if one foot seems colder than the other, it may be getting less blood circulation and require more attention. Using this combination of professional and home care, it is now estimated that as many as 50 percent of foot amputations due to peripheral neuropathy can be avoided.

Charcot arthropathy is a very serious (and fairly rare) condition that involves a disruption or disintegration of some of the joints of the foot and ankle. Redness, swelling, and deformity of the foot may follow. The cause of Charcot arthropathy is not well understood, though (like peripheral neuropathy) it is often linked with diabetes.

Your physician must be involved in the treatment of Charcot arthropathy, which will include immobilization of the foot in a cast to prevent further trauma to the foot. A physical therapist will often be called upon to help the patient maintain mobility of the joints through exercise.

Arthritis is the inflammation and swelling of the cartilage and the lining of the joints. The foot and ankle region is especially susceptible to arthritis because of the large numbers of joints at risk (33 in each foot) coupled with the tremendous weight-bearing load on the feet.

It's difficult to generalize about the causes of arthritis. Heredity plays a role in some cases, traumatic injury or infections in others. People over 50 are most at risk. It's important that you seek professional care if you suspect that you have arthritis; left untreated, arthritis can be a debilitating or even crippling disorder. The most

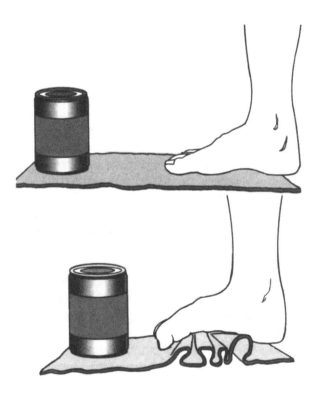

Figure 1.7. Toe-crunch exercise for strength and mobility. Lay a hand towel on the floor. Put half of your heel on the towel, half on the floor. By curling the toes, pull the towel toward you all the way to the arch. Do 10 repetitions to start and increase gradually over time. A soup can (as shown in the illustrations) can be used to make the exercise more challenging.

common form of arthritis, osteoarthritis, is a degenerative "wear-and-tear" disease associated with aging, injury, or overuse. A more serious form of the disease is rheumatoid arthritis, an autoimmune disorder that is thought to be hereditary.

Arthritis can't be cured (although rheumatoid arthritis sometimes goes through periods of remission). Your physician may suggest taking medication to reduce inflammation. And your physical therapist has many options to help you maintain function and mobility. With the right professional care, you can minimize the effects of arthritis.

If you are at risk for disease-related foot problems, try to find a multidisciplinary foot clinic for treatment. Such clinics have physicians, physical therapists, orthotists, and pedorthists (to make customized shoe inserts) on staff. Regrettably, these clinics are not yet found in all parts of the country; they are, however, an ideal setting for someone facing serious foot complications.

How Physical Therapy Can Help

While physical therapy is by definition tailored to the individual's problems and needs, certain procedures are common in dealing with foot and ankle disorders. Typically, your physical therapist will begin your rehabilitation by taking a detailed history and evaluation of your foot and ankle problem. Related problems such as diabetes, arthritis, and vascular disease are assessed during this initial phase.

The second part of your therapy is often gait analysis, in which the physical therapist observes you as you walk or, in some cases, run. The physical therapist will take detailed notes, sometimes using video cameras as a diagnostic tool.

At this point the physical therapist may assess your range of motion—how far and in what directions you can move your foot and ankle, with and without the assistance of the physical therapist. The physical therapist may also perform tests to assess the strength, sensation, and blood circulation in your foot and ankle.

Special tests may be performed as needed, including assessments of individual joints and ligaments. A biomechanical assessment can determine how the foot and ankle align with the lower extremities.

Physical therapists may choose from an array of options in treating you, including exercises for flexibility, stability, balance, strength, coordination, and restoration of range of motion, as well as massage, electrical stimulation, ultrasound, traction or mobilization, or heat or cold. These tools allow the physical therapist to create a program of rehabilitation that is custom-designed for your particular problem. In addition, the physical therapist may consult with other health care practitioners to provide special bandages, braces, supports, casts, or shoe inserts.

To avoid or overcome a foot or ankle problem you may need to learn some new habits or modify your current level of physical activity, whether it involves work, recreation, or both. Once your physical therapy goals are met, your physical therapist will help you continue therapy on your own with a home program designed to fit your needs. The goal of physical therapy is to return you to normal activity as quickly as possible, with the knowledge you need to prevent reinjury or disability.

Chapter 2

Podiatry and the Detection of Foot Problems

Podiatry deals with the medical and surgical treatment of foot disorders. [The medical professional who practices podiatry is called a podiatrist. His or her practice includes performing the following procedures.] The podiatrist:

- examines, diagnoses, and treats or prescribes course of treatment for patients with disorders, diseases, or injuries of the foot;

- interviews patients and writes case histories to determine previous ailments, complaints, and areas of investigation;

- examines footwear to determine proper fit, evidence of proper gait, and corrective care or treatment required;

- conducts physical examination of the foot, including tissue, bone, and muscular structure, with emphasis on the relationship to diabetes, peripheral vascular disease, and patho-mechanical disease;

- supplements examination by arranging for various laboratory tests, analyses, and diagnostic procedures, including x-rays;

- in consultation with the chief of the service of the health care facility, or with an individual with clinical privileges designated

"Facts for Consumers: Podiatrists" is reprinted with permission from the Massachusetts Office of Consumer Affairs and Business Regulation, Division of Professional Licensure. © Commonwealth of Massachusetts (http://www.mass .gov). Accessed December 5, 2005.

by him, interprets laboratory results and evaluates examination findings;

- refers patients to, or consults with, house physicians for further case diagnoses or treatment;

- administers treatment to eliminate pressure lesions, infections, and contagious diseases affecting the foot;

- performs appropriate therapeutic surgical procedures;

- prescribes appropriate medication; instructs nurses and other assistants in treatment and care of patients;

- prescribes and supervises construction and maintenance of orthotic foot devices and fabricates special appliances to foot or in footgear to meet the needs of individual patients;

- applies appliances to foot or in footwear;

- initiates other podiatric procedures or services and advises patients on proper care of feet and nail prophylaxis;

- reviews and studies case history and progress of patient;

- consults with surgeons and residents in establishing a therapeutic program for the patient;

- records data or case history on medical records;

- advises on kind and quality of podiatric medical supplies and equipment required.

Detecting a Foot Problem

In most cases, pain or excessive foot fatigue will alert you that you may have a foot problem. In the "normal" foot, moderate levels of activity do not cause sore or tired feet. Although overuse may cause foot fatigue, it rarely causes pain. If the foot problem persists after you have rested, consult a podiatrist. Putting even a normal foot into inappropriate shoes may cause foot problems. Painful corns, calluses, and bunions may result from improper shoes. The podiatrist can usually make you comfortable, and educate you about proper footwear. Infants and youngsters may have foot problems that cause little or no pain. These are often first noticed by alert parents, who see some abnormality of gait or foot structure. Early intervention by the podiatrist may correct the problem or prevent it from progressing.

Orthotics

Podiatrists prescribe and construct foot orthotics. These are specially designed devices that are worn inside the shoe to control abnormal foot function and/or accommodate painful areas of the foot. Properly designed foot orthotics may compensate for impaired foot function, by controlling abnormal motion across the joints of the foot. This may result in dramatic improvement in foot symptoms.

Functional foot orthotics are usually made from rigid materials, especially plastics and carbon-fiber composites. They are constructed upon a plaster impression of the feet, and modified based on the podiatrist's evaluation of your problem. They are normally quite comfortable, and do not feel hard or uncomfortable in the shoe.

Rigid orthotics normally last for years, additions such as top covers and extensions may require periodic replacement. Some patients, for example the very elderly, may not tolerate rigid functional orthotics. Under these circumstances, the podiatrist will prescribe an orthotic made from softer materials with special accommodations for painful areas. Many different materials can be utilized, such as rubber, cork, leather, and soft synthetic plastics. The podiatrist is in the unique position of being able to evaluate, diagnose, and treat your foot or leg problems. If orthotics are indicated, he or she can utilize the most advanced methods of construction.

Orthotics that are prescribed by the podiatrist and custom made for your feet, should not be confused with over-the-counter arch supports. These may help the occasional patient with minor arch discomfort, but they frequently fail because they do not properly control foot function and/or do not properly fit the patient's feet.

The consumer should beware of individuals with no or inadequate training, who hold themselves out as experts on foot problems and orthotics. Only the podiatrist, chiropodist, or medical doctor can diagnose foot problems and offer alternative treatment plans. If complications develop, the podiatrist is there to evaluate and treat those. He or she can offer the patient alternative treatments, be they medical, orthopedic, or surgical.

Common Foot Ailments

Not all feet are created equal! Some feet seem to take much abuse without complaining, many are not so lucky. Some people have sore feet in spite of wearing comfortable shoes and only moderate levels of activity. Ill-fitting or improper shoes may cause foot discomfort.

However, the foot itself may be the problem. The human foot contains about 26 bones and numerous joints, ligaments, muscles, and tendons. It is a complex structure that isn't always ideally suited to weight bearing and ambulation. We all have unique feet, and place unique demands upon them. The average person takes about 5,000 steps a day, and walks 50,000 miles in a lifetime. Our lifestyle, what shoes we wear, and how active we are, clearly affect our risk of foot problems. The young foot is more resilient, and may easily recover from minor injuries. Wear and tear eventually take their toll, and tissues lose their ability to fully recover. Hence, foot complaints become more prevalent as we age.

Your general health may adversely affect your feet. Some common examples are diabetes, arthritis, poor circulation, stroke, and osteoporosis. In fact, your podiatrist may be the first to recognize a serious health problem from an examination of your feet. Obesity may adversely affect your feet. Some types of heel and arch problems are more prevalent among overweight persons.

All feet are different, but most fall into three basic types:

- **"Normal" (rectus) foot:** Structure and alignment of the foot are well configured for the demands of daily living. Excessive wear, exceptional demands, or improper shoes can make this foot injured or painful.

- **High arched (supinated) foot:** This type of foot is poor at absorbing shock. These people are prone to problems of the entire lower extremity and back. Such feet often develop severely clawed toes and extensive plantar calluses.

- **Flat (pronated) feet:** This is one of the more common problems treated by the podiatrist. These people are prone to develop tired feet, arch strain, arthritis, and various structural deformities.

Foot pain has a multitude of causes. Your podiatrist can assess your problem, and treat it appropriately. If your foot problem has a mechanical origin, he or she may recommend functional foot orthotics. These are special supports that may compensate for structural problems, and eliminate or reduce discomfort.

Burning Feet

There are two types of burning feet, those that feel like they are burning, but are not actually hot, and those that are actually increased in temperature. Anything that increases the flow of blood to the feet will warm them. This may result from exercise, alcohol consumption, some vascular disorders, inflammation, and infection. Anything that insulates the foot can reduce heat loss and increase the temperature of the feet, for example socks, stockings, and shoes. The false perception of "hot" feet is due to changes in the nervous system. This may occur in the peripheral nerves, spinal cord, or brain. Nerve tissue may be damaged by age, impaired circulation, injury, or mechanical irritation. Conditions such as diabetes mellitus, alcohol abuse, and nutritional deficiencies may damage nerves and result in the feeling of burning feet. In some cases nerve damage is reversible. Your podiatrist may help to determine the cause of your burning feet, or direct you to the proper specialist. In spite of medical evaluation, the cause of burning feet is sometimes never determined.

Sweaty Feet

Excessive perspiration on the sole of the foot and between the toes (hyperhydrosis) is a common problem. In some cases it is related to mental stress and nervousness, especially in adolescents and young adults. Systemic diseases such as anemia and hyperthyroidism may be associated with hyperhydrosis. The excessive perspiration may be improved by the following:

- foot soaks in warm water
- wearing absorbent socks or hose (e.g., cotton or wool)
- avoiding synthetics such as nylon and Orlon®
- changing socks or hose a few times during the day
- wearing leather shoes; avoid those made of synthetics
- applying an antiperspirant preparation containing 15 to 25 percent aluminum chloride
- using an absorbent foot powder

Stubborn cases may be treated by your podiatrist with prescription medications. Substances that contain or convert into nontoxic doses of formaldehyde are often employed.

Foot Odor

Foot odor (bromhidrosis) is caused by the bacterial decomposition of normal secretions of the sweat glands. We all have a "garden" of bacteria that normally live on our skin. People with excessive foot perspiration are predisposed to this problem. Treatment is usually aimed at control of the sweating. Foot soaks in a solution containing a mild antibacterial agent (e.g., Tersaseptic®) may be helpful.

Bunions

Bunions are a common deformity of the forefoot. They may occur in either sex, and any culture, but are most common in women who wear narrow-toed dress shoes. A bunion is a displacement of the joint between the big toe and the long bone just behind it (the first metatarsal) toward the midline of the body. This joint begins to bulge on the inside of the foot and the big toe drifts in the opposite direction, sometimes coming to rest over or under the smaller toes. It seems that many factors can influence the development of a bunion deformity (hallux valgus). There may be a familial tendency to the deformity. Genetics may play an important, though not simple role. Abnormal flattening of the arch and turning out of the foot (pronation) during gait may encourage the development of a bunion. The wearing of constrictive and/or high-heeled shoes can aggravate the problem. Pain often results from shoe pressure or abnormal weight bearing due to the deformity. It is important that your bunions be properly evaluated by a podiatrist. He or she may be able to relieve pain by medications or protecting the area from pressure. Special supports, called orthotics, may help correct abnormal gait and stop further deformity. Any existing deformity can not be corrected without surgery. Many patients simply live with their bunions, taking care to wear orthotics and proper shoes. Other patients require surgery. Many procedures exist for the correction of hallux valgus. Your podiatric surgeon can recommend if surgery is right for you and, if so, select the appropriate procedure.

Corns and Calluses

Both involve excessive production of dead skin cells. This is the uppermost layer of the skin that protects it from external injury. For corns and calluses, this production is the result of intermittent pressure, from shoes or weight bearing. The skin responds to this pressure by thickening. Initially this "toughening" of the skin is helpful, but over time it builds up and becomes an irritant. Increased mass of the lesion results in increased pressure and discomfort. A vicious cycle develops which is only broken by relieving the pressure or reducing the lesion. Corns usually are on the toes, and result from shoe pressure. Calluses are usually on weight bearing areas on the bottom (plantar) surface of the foot, and result from weight bearing and/or abnormal alignment of the metatarsal bones in the ball of the foot. Both terms are expressions of the same type of lesion, which is medically termed a hyperkeratosis. Both corns and calluses may have a deeper central core, known to the podiatrist as a nucleation. This can be the site of exquisite tenderness. This core is not the "root" of the lesion, in the sense that removing this will keep the lesion from returning. It is simply the area of greatest pressure, often corresponding to a prominence of the underlining bone. Reducing this with sharp instruments and applying accommodative pads and tape, the podiatrist relieves discomfort and dissipates pressure. Unless something is done to permanently relieve pressure, the lesion will redevelop. Permanent relief is sometimes achieved by changing shoes, orthotics, or surgery to remove bony prominences and realign bones.

Toenail Problems

Toenail problems are common complaints in the podiatrist's office. They include thickening, brittleness, discoloration, and ingrown toenails. Nails, like hair, are an appendage of the skin. They are formed by layered sheets of protein with traces of other substances. Contrary to popular belief, there is very little calcium in nails. The normal toenail may be from 0.05 to 1 mm thick, and grows its full length in about six to twelve months. Nails are harder than skin, due to their high sulfur content and lack of water. The normal nail is translucent, and one can see the underlying pink nail bed.

Thickening and discoloration are often the sign of a diseased nail. With aging, the toenails thicken, grow more slowly, and become more susceptible to disease. Injury, infection, and disease may affect the toenails. The toenails and surrounding tissues are susceptible to day-to-day small repetitive injuries, for example in confining shoes. Changes in the underlying bone can cause deforming forces on the nail plate.

A common affliction of the nails is fungus infection. This may cause a thickening and degeneration of the nail plate. A microscopic examination and culture of a nail sample may help confirm the diagnosis. This is a difficult problem to treat. Your podiatrist may prescribe therapy with oral antifungal medication.

The ingrown toenail is another common problem that presents itself to the podiatrist's office. Infection may result from improper cutting of the toenails, or injury to the surrounding skin from an incurvated or deformed nail plate. Your podiatrist may simply trim the offending nail border. Some patients require regular expert nail care by the podiatrist. In many cases a simple nail surgery can permanently correct the problem.

Plantar Warts

A wart that appears on the bottom (plantar) surface of the foot may closely resemble a callus. Thick layers of dead skin may overlay a plantar wart. They may appear on non-weight bearing areas, and can usually be distinguished from calluses by the podiatrist. When a wart is reduced with a sharp blade, near the surface of the skin it appears to consist of numerous small folds packed together. These may contain a small black spot at the apex of the loop. Warts may bleed easily when pared with a sharp blade. Warts, also known as verruca, are caused by a virus. They are probably transmitted by exposure of the skin to the virus, for example on the floor of a public shower. Warts can also appear on the top surface of the foot. Here they tend to grow out from the skin, and are more easily recognized. The interval from exposure to seeing a wart may be many months. Warts on the top of the foot may be treated with various over-the-counter wart medicines. If they fail to resolve in a few weeks consult your podiatrist or physician. Plantar warts tend to be more difficult to treat. Various methods can be utilized, such as excision, freezing, burning, strong acids, laser, etc. These are often performed under local anesthesia. Unfortunately, warts have a high recurrence rate, and may require additional treatment.

Flat Feet

The human foot is a complicated structure, consisting of about 26 bones, numerous joints, ligaments, muscles, and tendons. Each set of feet is unique, but may share certain basic structural qualities. Flat feet are low arched and fairly common. Most flat feet are what podiatrists term pronated. Closer examination of the weight-bearing pronated foot reveals the following:

- turning out of the heel bone away from the center of the body
- inward rotation of the leg
- bulging of the inner aspect of the ankle
- shifting of the forefoot outward from the heel

Flat feet may be the result of abnormality in the alignment of bones, excessive elasticity of the ligaments, muscle imbalance, or some combination of these. To complicate matters further, not all pronated feet appear flat, and some feet that appear flat are not pronated. Flat feet may be severe and apparent at birth; these may require corrective treatment with plaster casts or surgery. More commonly flat (pronated) feet develop during youth, symptoms may develop any time, and some flat feet never become troublesome. They may run in families, but there is no certainty they will develop.

Pronated feet alter the alignment of the foot, ankle, leg, pelvis, and lower back. Problems may develop at any level. The pronated foot is unstable. This results in excessive and abnormal motion across joints, and may result in fatigue and strain—often described as "tired feet." Long-term consequences include: arthritis, bunions, heel spurs, Morton neuroma, and other deformities. Shin splints (pain in the muscles of the lower leg) may result from these muscles overworking in an attempt to compensate for foot instability.

This is a complex deformity that should be properly evaluated by a podiatrist. He or she may recommend functional posted foot orthotics. These are special supports that help compensate for mechanical faults, and allow your feet to function with improved efficiency. Orthotics relieve stress from compromised joints, ligaments, and muscles. Deforming forces acting on the foot are diminished.

Chapter 3

Choosing a Podiatrist

Most of us don't give much thought to our feet until something goes wrong, but your feet are one of the most important parts of your body. They support you. They get you places. And they take a lot of abuse—the average person puts about 5 million pounds of pressure on his or her feet each day, and typically walks about 115,000 miles in a lifetime! Three out of four people will experience problems with their feet at some point in their lives. But you don't have to take foot discomfort lying down. Thanks to modern podiatric procedures, there are cures for most problems.

What is a podiatrist?

A podiatrist is a highly trained medical professional who specializes in disorders of the foot and ankle. A podiatrist earns his or her Doctor of Podiatric Medicine (DPM) after completing studies at one of seven colleges of podiatric medicine in the U.S. Those specializing in foot and ankle surgery also complete up to three years of additional training through an accredited hospital residency program.

Why choose a podiatrist?

You have many choices of doctors and it's important to choose one with the most knowledge of your particular problem and one whom you trust. Your feet make up one-fourth of all the bones in your body,

---

"Educational Information" is reprinted with permission from http://www.familyfootandankle.com. © 2006 Family Foot and Ankle Centers.

and include 33 joints and 107 ligaments. Your primary care physician may be able to address many foot and ankle problems. But podiatrists focus more of their education, training, and day-to-day experience on these critical body parts than any other type of physician. They are experts in the diagnosis, treatment, and prevention of problems of the feet and ankles. Often they help patients identify serious, underlying medical conditions like diabetes and cardiovascular disease, which can inhibit circulation in the lower extremities.

How do I know if I need to see a podiatrist?

Your primary care physician should include foot examinations during routine physicals and may alert you to certain problems for follow-up by a podiatrist. You may experience a break or sprain and decide to visit a podiatrist for guidance on treatment and aftercare. And regular foot pain isn't normal. It may be a sign, for example, of a serious underlying medical condition that inhibits circulation. It may indicate a growth or tumor, a deformity from birth or one that has developed due to ill-fitting shoes, or it may result from overuse during sports or dance activities. These are just a few possibilities, but a general rule is: If it hurts, something is probably wrong.

What types of treatments can I expect from my podiatrist?

Some foot and ankle problems are resolved successfully using non-invasive treatments such as heat and massage therapy, orthotics (specially built supports that fit in your shoes), and prescribed medications. Specific treatments will be outlined by your podiatrist following a thorough examination. At other times, surgery may be the best way to eliminate long-term discomfort or correct a specific ailment. Podiatrists certified by the American College of Foot and Ankle Surgeons have passed rigorous qualification standards for performing foot and ankle surgery. In most cases, surgeries are performed on an outpatient basis and under local anesthesia. Problems that might be subject to surgical solutions range from sprains, fractures, and other types of trauma, to birth deformities, malignant and non-malignant tumors, and very common ingrown toenails, corns, bunions, or warts.

What are some preventive steps I can take to avoid foot problems in the first place?

- Examine your feet regularly and be alert to swelling, sores, changes in skin color or temperature, and unusual sensations or pain. Prompt treatment of many conditions can prevent more serious problems down the road.

- Wear properly fitted shoes with a round, fairly high toe box to avoid pressure on the toes. Heels should never be more than two inches high. Avoid shoes made of artificial leather because it doesn't stretch.

- Give the same attention to your children's feet, because they are particularly susceptible to warts, athlete's foot, arch faults, and nail problems, which should be treated.

- Children's feet grow rapidly, so check the fit of their shoes frequently and watch for uneven wear, which could indicate a foot malfunction or correctable gait problem.

- Never use "corn cures," iodine, or other harsh over-the-counter medications without consulting your doctor. Some contain acids that can cause serious damage, particularly among diabetics and those with impaired circulation.

- Cut toenails straight across.

- Warm up before exercising or participating in sports or dance. Cool down gently after a high level of activity.

Chapter 4

The Developing Foot

Chapter Contents

Section 4.1

Anatomy of the Foot and Heel

Overview

The human foot combines mechanical complexity and structural strength. The ankle serves as foundation, shock absorber, and propulsion engine. The foot can sustain enormous pressure (several tons over the course of a one-mile run) and provides flexibility and resiliency.

The foot and ankle contain:

- 26 bones (one-quarter of the bones in the human body);

- 33 joints;

- more than 100 muscles, tendons (fibrous tissues that connect muscles to bones), and ligaments (fibrous tissues that connect bones to other bones); and,

- a network of blood vessels, nerves, skin, and soft tissue.

These components work together to provide the body with support, balance, and mobility. A structural flaw or malfunction in any one part can result in the development of problems elsewhere in the body. Abnormalities in other parts of the body can lead to problems in the feet.

Parts of the Foot

Structurally, the foot has three main parts: the forefoot, the midfoot, and the hindfoot.

The forefoot is composed of the five toes (called phalanges) and their connecting long bones (metatarsals). Each toe (phalanx) is made up of several small bones. The big toe (hallux) has two phalanges, two joints (interphalangeal joints), and two tiny, round sesamoid bones that enable it to move up and down. The other four toes each have three bones and two joints. The phalanges are connected to the metatarsals

30

by five metatarsal phalangeal joints at the ball of the foot. The fore-foot bears half the body's weight and balances pressure on the ball of the foot.

The midfoot has five irregularly shaped tarsal bones, forms the foot's arch, and serves as a shock absorber. The bones of the midfoot are connected to the forefoot and the hindfoot by muscles and the plan-tar fascia (arch ligament).

The hindfoot is composed of three joints and links the midfoot to the ankle (talus). The top of the talus is connected to the two long bones of the lower leg (tibia and fibula), forming a hinge that allows the foot to move up and down. The heel bone (calcaneus) is the larg-est bone in the foot. It joins the talus to form the subtalar joint, which enables the foot to rotate at the ankle. The bottom of the heel bone is cushioned by a layer of fat.

Muscles, Tendons, and Ligaments

A network of muscles, tendons, and ligaments supports the bones and joints in the foot.

There are 20 muscles in the foot that give the foot its shape by holding the bones in position and expand and contract to impart move-ment. The main muscles of the foot are as follows:

- the anterior tibial, which enables the foot to move upward
- the posterior tibial, which supports the arch
- the peroneal tibial, which controls movement on the outside of the ankle
- the extensors, which help the ankle raise the toes to initiate the act of stepping forward
- the flexors, which help stabilize the toes against the ground

Smaller muscles enable the toes to lift and curl.

There are elastic tissues (tendons) in the foot that connect the muscles to the bones and joints. The largest and strongest tendon of the foot is the Achilles tendon, which extends from the calf muscle to the heel. Its strength and joint function facilitate running, jumping, walking up stairs, and raising the body onto the toes.

Ligaments hold the tendons in place and stabilize the joints. The longest of these, the plantar fascia, forms the arch on the sole of the foot from the heel to the toes. By stretching and contracting, it allows the arch to curve or flatten, providing balance and giving the foot strength to initiate the act of walking. Medial ligaments on the inside and lateral ligaments on the outside of the foot provide stability and enable the foot to move up and down.

Skin, blood vessels, and nerves give the foot its shape and durability, provide cell regeneration and essential muscular nourishment, and control its varied movements.

Section 4.2

The Newborn Foot

The examination of the feet is an essential component of a comprehensive evaluation of a newborn. With proper skills, this examination, which often is reassuring to new parents, can be performed quickly, yet thoroughly. Early detection of foot problems in infants allows timely corrective treatment, if required.

Examination Techniques

Despite its small size, the newborn foot is complex, consisting of 26 to 28 bones. The foot can be divided into three anatomic regions: the hindfoot or rearfoot (talus and calcaneus); the midfoot (navicular bone, cuboid bone, and three cuneiform bones); and the forefoot (metatarsals and phalanges). Differences between a newborn foot and an adult foot are summarized in Table 4.1.

Simultaneous observation of both feet can reveal many deformities. The skin should be examined for unusual creases or folds that can be formed by various foot deviations. Certain areas of the skin might be abnormally taut, indicating extra tension on the skin, while the skin on the opposite side of the foot might reveal loose, excessive skinfolds.

During the next part of the examination, various foot and ankle joints are moved through their respective ranges of motion. The joints should be assessed for flexibility or rigidity, unusual positions, lack of motion, and asymmetry.

Finally, the vascular examination consists of assessment of capillary refill and skin color, because pulses are difficult to palpate. Fortunately, the majority of newborns exhibit excellent lower extremity vascular supply, unless it is compromised by an extrinsic factor, such as an intrauterine amniotic band.

Common Foot Abnormalities

Metatarsus Adductus

Metatarsus adductus (MTA) is one of the most common foot deformities, occurring in one to two cases per 1,000 live births.[1] It is defined as a transverse plane deformity in Lisfranc (tarsometatarsal) joints in which the metatarsals are deviated medially.

On inspection, the toes angle abruptly toward the midline, creating a C-shaped lateral foot border with a prominent styloid process of the fifth metatarsal.[2] A splay can appear between the great and second toes. Skin examination frequently reveals a deep skin cleft at the medial midfoot.

A simple test that can raise the clinician's suspicions of MTA is the "V"-finger test. In this test, the heel of the foot is placed in the "V" formed by the index and middle fingers, and the lateral aspect of the foot is observed from a plantar side for medial or lateral deviation from the middle finger. Medial deviation from the middle finger at the styloid process indicates MTA.[3]

Treatment is based on the severity of the condition and is controversial. While some authors[1] advocate only observation without active

Table 4.1. Differences between the newborn and adult foot.

Feature	Newborn	Adult
Arch	Flatter, less defined	Usually well defined, except in pes planus
Typical joint range of motion	Greater range of motion	Lesser range of motion
End point of range of motion	Soft, subtle, difficult to appreciate	Firm, well defined
Amount of subcutaneous fat tissue	Greater	Lesser

intervention for mild cases, others would intervene early in all severe cases or by two months of age, if the condition is not resolved.[4] Other authors[3] recommend treatment as soon as possible, especially in moderate to severe cases. Based on the natural course of the condition, a more conservative approach seems reasonable. Of MTA cases identified at birth, 85 to 90 percent resolve by one year of age.[1,3] Another prospective study[5] confirmed these findings—87 percent of MTA cases had resolved by six years of age, with only about 4 percent remaining at age 16.

Mild (flexible, passively correctable) MTA requires only parental reassurance. Moderate (semi-flexible, reducible) MTA can be treated with stretching exercises at every diaper change. First, the heel is stabilized within the notch between the thumb and index finger. Then, the forefoot is slightly pulled distally, held between the thumb and index finger of the other hand, and gently pushed into a corrected position.[1]

For the majority of MTA cases, the prognosis is quite good. In severe cases, excessive compensation at the level of the mediotarsal joint can lead to the development of bunions, hammertoes, and other disorders.[6] Therefore, severe (rigid) MTA can be referred for serial casting and bracing. Evidence-based comparisons of splinting or casting versus manipulation alone are not yet available.[4]

Clubfoot

Clubfoot, or talipes equinovarus, is a congenital deformity that typically has four main components: inversion and adduction of the forefoot; inversion of the heel and hindfoot; equinus (limitation of extension) of the ankle and subtalar joint; and internal rotation of the leg.

Clubfoot is a complex, multifactorial deformity with genetic and intrauterine factors. One popular theory postulates that a clubfoot is a result of intrauterine maldevelopment of the talus that leads to adduction and plantarflexion of the foot.[7] Clubfoot occurs in one to two per 1,000 live births; however, the incidence is higher in Hispanics and lower in Asians.[8]

On inspection, the "down and in" appearance of the foot, which somewhat resembles that of MTA, is obvious.[3] The foot appears smaller, with a flexible, softer heel because of the hypoplastic calcaneus. The medial border of the foot is concave with a deep medial skin furrow, and the lateral border is highly convex. The heel is usually small and is internally rotated, making the soles of the feet face each other in cases of bilateral deformities.

On testing, there is pronounced tightness of the Achilles tendon with very little dorsiflexion, which differentiates clubfoot from MTA. Radiographs of clubfeet usually reveal roughly parallel axes of the talus and calcaneus.

Clubfoot can be classified into extrinsic (supple) type, which is essentially a severe positional or soft tissue deformity; and intrinsic (rigid) type, where manual reduction is impossible. The type of clubfoot determines the specific therapy. Extrinsic clubfoot can be treated by serial casting, while intrinsic clubfoot eventually may require surgery. Plaster casting should be attempted on virtually all clubfeet, supple or rigid, as soon as practical. Casts initially are changed at semiweekly to weekly intervals and are continued until the deformity responds and is corrected fully. Persistent cast treatments by experienced clinicians have been reported to be successful in most patients.[9] However, if a plateau is reached in treatment, surgery by a specialist in pediatric foot deformities should be considered, usually when the child is between six and nine months of age.[10] The goal is to obtain a stable, "platform-like" position of the foot for future ambulation.

Calcaneovalgus

The axis of calcaneovalgus deformity is in the tibiotalar joint, where the foot is positioned in extreme hyperextension, with its dorsum frequently touching the distal leg. Females are affected more often than males, and this deformity can be unilateral or bilateral.[3] It occurs in about 5 percent of all newborns[5] and is associated with external rotation of the calcaneus, an overstretched Achilles tendon, and tight anterior leg musculature, all of which warrant treatment.[11]

On inspection, the foot has an "up and out" appearance, with the dorsal forefoot practically touching the anterior aspect of the ankle and lower leg. The ankle generally can be plantarflexed to only 90 degrees or less. Radiographs can confirm clinical diagnosis.

Calcaneovalgus is a positional deformity that is highly amenable to treatment. According to some authors,[10,12] it has an excellent natural history and can spontaneously resolve on its own. Others[3] advocate a more aggressive approach because of the possibility of future complications, such as permanent muscle imbalance, peroneal tendon dislocation, and delayed ambulation. Generally, the more severe the limitation of ankle plantar flexion, the more treatment is warranted.

Treatment should begin as early as possible. Mild cases can be treated with stretching exercises performed at each diaper change. Stretching consists of gentle plantarflexion of the foot with mild inversion for a count of ten, repeated three times. In moderate cases or when stretching fails to correct the deformity, splinting or firm, high-top, lace-up shoes that prevent dorsiflexion can be used. For severe deformities with significant limitation of ankle plantarflexion, serial mobilization casting is performed until corrected, followed by nightly maintenance use of a bivalved cast or splinting of the posterior aspect of the leg for a two- to ten-week course.[3]

Congenital Vertical Talus

Congenital vertical talus is a rare deformity that must be distinguished from calcaneovalgus. Otherwise known as rocker-bottom foot, it is a rigid deformity, as opposed to a flexible calcaneovalgus foot, so it does not respond to stretching and, in most cases, requires surgery.

The hindfoot is in equinus rather than calcaneus position, with talus and calcaneus pointing downward and the forefoot dorsiflexed. This results in dislocation of the mid-tarsal bones on the head and neck of the talus.[11]

It is important to examine the entire child, looking for other abnormalities, such as arthrogryposis (multiple joint contractures present at birth) and meningomyelocele, which might be present in up to 60 percent of children with congenital vertical talus.[10,13] The foot examination usually reveals a rigid foot with a "reversed" arch, a convex plantar surface, and a deep crease on the lateral dorsal side of the foot. The ankle joint is plantarflexed, while the midfoot and forefoot are extended upward. Lateral foot radiographs are helpful in confirming the diagnosis.

Conservative therapy can assist in stretching the forefoot and hindfoot, but surgery is needed in most cases. Surgery is complex, requiring correction in all three cardinal planes, and should be performed by a specialist in pediatric foot deformities.

Digital Deformities

Polydactyly

The incidence of polydactyly (supernumerary digits of hands or feet) is the same in both sexes, with simultaneous polydactyly of the hands and feet present in about one-third of cases.[14] It is more common in blacks than whites (3.6 to 13 cases per 1,000 live births versus 0.3 to 1.3 cases per 1,000 live births, respectively).[15]

The primary cause of polydactyly is thought to be genetic. Polydactyly usually involves border digits, especially the fifth. Although some cases involve only a distal phalanx, other cases are much more complex, involving the entire digit, with duplication of nails, tendons, and vascular structures.

Treatment of complex cases involving bone requires removal of duplicated structures, whereas cases involving soft tissue can be treated with only ligation sutures applied in the nursery. Surgery generally is performed at six to nine months of age, before the child is ambulatory but able to tolerate general anesthesia.[10,15]

Syndactyly

Syndactyly (webbed toes or fingers) occurs in approximately one in 2,000 to 2,500 live births.[15] There are various levels of syndactylization, from partial to complete. The most frequent site is between the second and third toes. Syndactyly is thought to be genetic, with an autosomal dominant pattern of inheritance.

Simple syndactyly is more of a cosmetic problem than a functional one, and rarely requires treatment.[10] A radiographic evaluation is not indicated unless radical treatment is being contemplated. If the parents desire surgery, it is advisable to wait until the child is old enough to take part in the decision and participate in postoperative care. The most common complication of the surgery is skin-flap slough, leading to a recurrence of the problem.

Overlapping Toes

Overlapping toes are often familial, with the fifth toe being the most commonly affected. Frequently bilateral, the condition is distributed evenly between boys and girls. This deformity presents as adduction of the little toe with some external rotation of the digit. The metatarsophalangeal joint is dorsiflexed, and the nail plate is frequently smaller than expected.[15]

In newborns, the condition is frequently passively correctable with gentle stretching or use of various toe spacers. Nighttime paper-tape splinting to the adjacent toe has been empirically recommended, but this method lacks evidence-based outcome studies.[16] However, if a child starts to walk before the deformity is corrected, it can become rigid, causing symptoms, and can require surgical correction.[13]

Amniotic (Annular) Bands

Amniotic bands commonly involve toes and fingers. Occurring in one in 15,000 live births, they are produced by thin bands of amniotic membrane wrapping around various parts of the extremity in utero.[15] Simple bands create swelling of the distal part of the toe with concomitant lymphedema, and deeper bands can produce complete amputations.[17]

Contractions and resultant bulbous ends of the involved digits are seen easily during examination. In addition to lymphedema, it is essential to rule out vascular compromise, which is manifested by pale, cool skin with delayed capillary refill.

Simple bands are mainly cosmetic problems and do not require treatment, but complex bands, especially ones that produce neurovascular compromise, should be surgically released.[17,18]

A summary table highlighting major diagnostic findings and treatment approaches is provided online at http://www.aafp.org/afp/20040215/865.pdf.

—by Alvin I. Gore, MD, DPM, and Jeanne P. Spencer, MD

References

1. Dietz, F.R. Intoeing—fact, fiction, and opinion. *Am Fam Physician* 1994; 50:1249-59, 1262-4.

2. Mankin, K.P., Zimbler, S. Gait and leg alignment: what's normal and what's not. *Contemp Pediatr* 1997; 14:41-70.

3. Connors, J.F., Wernick, E., Lowy, L.J., Falcone, J., Volpe, R.G. Guidelines for evaluation and management of five common podopediatric conditions. *J Am Podiatr Med Assoc* 1998; 88:206-22.

4. Churgay, C.A. Diagnosis and treatment of pediatric foot deformities. *Am Fam Physician* 1993; 47:883-9.

5. Widhe, T. Foot deformities at birth: a longitudinal prospective study over a 16-year period. *J Pediatr Orthop* 1997; 17:20-4.

6. Yu, G.V., Wallace, G.F. Metatarsus adductus. In McGlamry, E.D., Banks, A.S., Downey, M.S., eds. *Comprehensive textbook of foot surgery,* 2d ed. Baltimore: Williams and Wilkins, 1992; 324-53.

7. Rodgveller, B. Talipes equinovarus. *Clin Podiatry* 1984; 1:477-99.

8. Rodgveller, B. Clubfoot. In McGlamry, E.D., Banks, A.S., Downey, M.S., eds. *Comprehensive textbook of foot surgery,* 2d ed. Baltimore: Williams and Wilkins, 1992; 354-68.

9.   Ponseti, I.V. Treatment of congenital clubfoot. *J Bone Joint Surg Am* 1992; 74:448-54.

10. Hoffinger, S.A. Evaluation and management of pediatric foot deformities. *Pediatr Clin North Am* 1996; 43:1091-111.

11. Trott, A.W. Children's foot problems. *Orthop Clin North Am* 1982; 13:641-54.

12. Wall, E.J. Practical primary pediatric orthopedics. *Nurs Clin North Am* 2000; 35:95-113.

13. Fixsen, J.A. Problem feet in children. *J R Soc Med* 1998; 91:18-22.

14. *Wheeless' Textbook of orthopaedics*. Accessed December 2, 2003, at http://www.ortho-u.net.

15. McDaniel, L., Tafuri, S.A. Congenital digital deformities. *Clin Podiatr Med Surg* 1996; 13:327-42.

16. Manusov, E.G., Lillegard, W.A., Raspa, R.F., Epperly, T.D. Evaluation of pediatric foot problems: Part I. The forefoot and the midfoot. *Am Fam Physician* 1996; 54:592-606.

17. Behrman, R.E., Kliegman, R., Jenson, H.B., eds. *Nelson Textbook of pediatrics,* 16th ed. Philadelphia: Saunders, 2000; 2062-4.

18. Canale, S.T., Campbell, W.C., eds. *Campbell's Operative orthopaedics,* 9th ed. St. Louis: Mosby, 1998; 961-2.

Section 4.3

Pediatric and Adolescent Foot and Ankle Problems

Disorders of the foot and ankle are a common cause for orthopedic referral in the infant, pediatric, and adolescent patient.

The spectrum of problems is wide and while most, fortunately, are not serious, some of the congenital abnormalities do require significant operative intervention and a prolonged period of treatment. Even many of the less serious problems are a source of major irritation to patients. They often put limitations on the routine activities required by daily living. The following are common foot and ankle disorders.

Congenital Disorders

Metatarsus adductus: Metatarsus adductus is a common congenital foot abnormality and is caused by a persistence of fetal positioning. It is one of the several congenital abnormalities known as a "packaging problem."

"Metatarsus adductus" is a frightening sounding term but means simply that the metatarsals (the long bones in the midportion of the foot) are adducted or angled toward the midline. The English have another name for this condition—they call it: "hooked forefoot." As with any medical condition, metatarsus adductus can run the gamut from mild to severe. While one classification defines the degree of metatarsus adductus based on the amount of curvature, a better classification relies on flexibility. Feet, which are very supple, typically require no treatment. Those feet that are least supple require manipulation and stretching and the use of reverse last shoes or perhaps a short period of corrective casting. Without treatment, most feet do spontaneously improve by age three. After age four surgery may be considered to correct the residual deformity.

Clubfoot: Clubfoot is a more serious disorder that is not related to the intrauterine environment, but to a growth abnormality that can be strongly influenced by genetic predisposition. The clubfoot is hooked like the adducted foot, but has true structural abnormalities that cause it to roll inward and point downward.

Untreated, this results in a major disability. Treatment begins with casting and in about 40 percent of cases, minor surgical intervention is necessary for complete correction.

Congenital vertical talus: Congenital vertical talus is a fairly rare, but serious condition. The position of the foot is a classic "rocker bottom." It must be differentiated from a hyperflexible foot, and if stiff, casting is minimally useful and surgery is required.

Developmental Disorders

Flatfoot: Flatfeet are very common and typically genetic in nature. It is due to lax ligaments and/or tendons in the foot. The most common childhood flatfoot is supple, not stiff, and usually not painful. An additional underlying cause for a stiff flatfoot must be sought. Shoe wear has not been shown to promote arch development. An arch is usually present on standing by age five. Arch supports (orthotics) are indicated for painful, supple feet and for patients with additional symptoms related to the feet (certain gait, knee, and back disorders). Arch supports are also indicated for those who wear out shoes extremely fast. Surgery can tighten the ligaments or tendons but is reserved for the most severe flatfeet.

Intoeing: Intoeing ("pigeon toed") is typically not related to the feet but to lower extremity rotation. Tibial (shin bone) torsion (twist) is the most common cause of intoeing in the child age one to two. Femoral (thigh bone) torsion is the usual culprit in ages three to 15. Bracing is controversial for tibial torsion and fully ineffective for the femur. Surgery is performed only on asymmetric limbs or those with debilitating torsional abnormalities

Knock-knees: Knock knees are typical in children age three to seven. Knock-knees come after bowlegs and usually improve by age

11. Bracing is rarely required as resolution is typically dramatic. The need for surgical intervention is rare.

Bowlegs: Bowlegs are typical in infants to age 12-14 months and may be normal to age two. Most bowlegs are symmetric, stable, and spontaneously resolve. Bracing has shown benefit to age three to four. Surgery is most often indicated for those with an abnormality of the growth plate, a condition known as Blount disease.

Overuse Injuries

Achilles tendonitis: Achilles tendonitis is an overuse injury seen rarely in children under age 14 but seen with greater frequency as skeletal maturity approaches. It is characterized by pain with activity, particularly jumping sports in the region of the Achilles tendon. Rest, activity modification, a stretching program, shoe change, icing, and the use of an antiinflammatory medication will usually promote healing and the ability to return to sports. The Achilles tendon should never be injected with cortisone as rupture due to weakening can occur.

Sever disease: Sever disease is a pre-skeletal maturity condition resulting from inflammation of the calcaneal (heel bone) growth plate near to where the Achilles tendon attaches. The treatment is similar to Achilles tendonitis with the addition of a heel pad or heel cup. Occasionally this condition will plague a youngster off and on for two to three years until growth plate closure occurs. Casting to completely immobilize the ankle joint may be required.

Plantar fasciitis: Plantar fasciitis is an inflammation of the plantar (sole of foot) fascia (a tough band of ligament type tissue which runs along the bottom of the foot). Again, treatment is directed at relieving inflammation and gently stretching the involved tissues. Arch supports also help here to support the foot and decrease pain. While injection is occasionally indicated in the adult, it is typically not done in the younger population.

Stress fractures: Stress fractures are fractures sustained as a result of repeated "micro trauma." Sudden changes in training intensity are the classic cause of these injuries that typically involve the metatarsals (the bones in the midpart of the foot). Cessation of the activity that is causing the problem and casting are the mainstays of treatment. If the activity continues prior to healing, these micro fractures can become "real fractures."

Traumatic Injuries

Ankle fractures: Ankle fractures in the skeletally immature usually involve the growth plates of the tibia or fibula (the two shin bones). They usually occur as a result of a twisting injury to the ankle. An adult with the same type of injury would have an ankle sprain (a tear in a ligament). Most of the ankle fractures seen in the pediatric population do not require operative management but do if the fracture line extends into the joint. Injury to the growth plate may, on occasion, result in a growth disturbance.

Ankle sprains: Ankle sprains in children are rare because the ligaments are stronger than the growth plate, and the growth plate fails first under the "load" of injury. When they do occur, some form of immobilization (cast or brace) is indicated in order for the ligaments to heal at their normal length. Ligaments that heal in a "lengthened" position result in long-term disability and the increased likelihood of repeated ankle sprains under even minimally vigorous loads.

Section 4.4

Aging and Your Feet

Foot Health and Aging

Medicine and health awareness have progressed so rapidly since 1900 that life expectancy of the average American has increased by about 30 years. Older persons have become an increasingly significant proportion of our total population—and their numbers are growing rapidly. In 1900, for example, there were three million Americans aged 65 or older. By 2000, older people outnumbered children for the first time in history.

If older people are to live useful, satisfying lives, they must be able to move about. Mobility is a vital ingredient in the independence that is cherished by our aging population, and foot ailments make it difficult or impossible for them to work or to participate in social activities.

According to the U.S. National Center for Health Statistics (NCHS), impairment of the lower extremities is a leading cause of activity limitation in older people. As if foot problems weren't enough of a nuisance, they can also lead to knee, hip, and lower back pain that undermine mobility just as effectively. The NCHS says one-fourth of all nursing home patients cannot walk at all and another one-sixth can walk only with assistance.

Mirror of Health

The human foot has been called the mirror of health. Foot doctors, or doctors of podiatric medicine (DPMs), are often the first doctors to see signs of such systemic conditions as diabetes, arthritis, and circulatory disease in the foot. Among these signs are dry skin, brittle nails, burning and tingling sensations, feelings of cold, numbness, and discoloration. Always seek professional care when these signs appear.

Foot Problems Can Be Prevented

For reasons that are difficult to fathom, many people, including a lot of older people, believe that it is normal for the feet to hurt and simply resign themselves to enduring foot problems that could be treated.

There are more than 300 different foot ailments. Some can be traced to heredity, but for an aging population, most of these ailments stem from the cumulative effect of years of neglect or abuse. However, even among people in their retirement years, many foot problems can be treated successfully and the pain of foot ailments relieved.

Whether due to neglect or abuse, the normal wear and tear of the years causes changes in feet. As persons age, their feet tend to spread, and lose the fatty pads that cushion the bottom of the feet. Additional weight can affect the bone and ligament structure. Older people, consequently, should have their feet measured for shoe sizes more frequently, rather than presuming that their shoe sizes remain constant. Dry skin and brittle nails are other conditions older people commonly face. Finally, it's a fact that women, young and old, have four times as many foot problems as men, and high heels are often the culprits.

Observing preventive foot health care has many benefits. Chief among them are that it can increase comfort, limit the possibility of additional medical problems, reduce the chances of hospitalization because of infection, and lessen requirements for other institutional care.

Keep Them Walking

Studies show that care for a bedridden patient costs much more than care for an ambulatory patient. In their private practices and in foot clinics, podiatric physicians are providing services designed to keep older people on their feet, and they serve in hospitals and nursing homes across the country.

Records indicate that amputations and other forms of surgery due to infections of the feet, many brought about by diabetes, have been significantly reduced in recent years because of early diagnosis and treatment. Further reduction in this area is a goal of Healthy People 2010, a U.S. Department of Health and Human Services campaign endorsed by podiatric physicians, to encourage understanding and application of preventive medical practices.

Foot Health Tips

- Properly fitted shoes are essential; an astonishing number of people wear shoes that don't fit right, and cause serious foot problems.

- A shoe with a firm sole and soft upper is best for daily activities.

- Shop for shoes in the afternoon; feet tend to swell during the day.

- Walking is the best exercise for your feet.

- Pantyhose or stockings should be of the correct size and preferably free of seams.

- Do not wear constricting garters or tie your stockings in knots.

- Never cut corns and calluses with a razor, pocket knife, or other such instrument; use over-the-counter foot products only with the advice of a podiatrist.

- Bathe your feet daily in lukewarm (not hot) water, using a mild soap, preferably one containing moisturizers, or use a moisturizer separately. Test the water temperature with your hand.

- Trim or file your toenails straight across.

- Inspect your feet every day or have someone do this for you. If you notice any redness, swelling, cracks in the skin, or sores, consult your podiatrist.

- Have your feet examined by a DPM at least twice a year.

Your podiatric physician/surgeon has been trained specifically and extensively in the diagnosis and treatment of all manner of foot conditions. This training encompasses all of the intricately related systems and structures of the foot and lower leg including neurological, circulatory, skin, and the musculoskeletal system, which includes bones, joints, ligaments, tendons, muscles, and nerves.

Chapter 5

What You Should Know about Children's Shoes

Chapter Contents

Section 5.1

Shoe Fitting for the Infant

Description

In 30 years of fitting children's shoes I have seen many changes in the shoe industry. This is especially true in the style of shoes that parents are purchasing for their babies. Hard leather soles and stiff uppers were the rule many years ago. Since that time we have progressed to rubber or PVC soles. Soft leather uppers that conform to the foot and offer greater freedom of movement are now recommended. Narrow, medium, and wide widths have since replaced the traditional B, C, D, E, EE. With all the changes in the children's shoe industry one constant remains, no matter what style of shoes you choose for your baby, they need to fit properly.

Foot problems normally found in adults are now being found among children. I have observed this more in the last ten years. In most cases this can be attributed to ill fitting or improper footwear. Often parents don't know how a shoe should fit or what areas of the shoe need to be checked for proper fitting. Hopefully this text will help insure that parents are more aware of how to fit children's shoes.

Shoes are really not required until the child starts to pull up and cruise around objects. You will notice they stand on their toes and try to edge themselves around a table, sofa, or anything else they can hold onto. Toe gripping allows them to balance themselves and learn to take steps.

Babies' feet are very soft and pliable with padding surrounding the foot. This is nature's way of protecting the underlying foot structure. This means the foot is thick, with the heel being narrower. Because of the narrower heel and the flexibility of the foot, high-tops are generally better to keep the shoe on the foot. This will also allow for the shoe to be fit a little larger than a lower top shoe.

Fitting shoes is not a science, but an art. It takes practice and experience with different types of shoes and feet. Using the following guidelines, you will be better able to fit your child with the proper shoe size.

Measuring

Both feet should be measured in a standing position if possible. Feet are flexible and will expand in length and width with body weight. There are three measurements taken from the standard Brannock device. They are length, width, and arch length. It is very important to understand that the size the foot measures is not necessarily the size shoe that the child will wear. Differences in construction, materials, last (the form the shoe is made on), and sizing systems will determine the actual shoe size. Note any differences in the sizes of the feet and be sure to fit the largest foot.

Length

How much length is necessary for growth? Generally there is one-third of an inch between sizes, and one-sixth of an inch between half sizes. Allowing one-third inch growth translates to one shoe size. This allows two to three months wear for an infant. Keep in mind the growth rate will vary with individual children. Purchasing shoes that are too large is likely to cause tripping of an already unstable walker.

Width

Judging the proper width of a shoe is not as obvious as the length. Since the length and width of a shoe are proportional, the width will increase along with the length. Width increases about one-fourth inch per full size. Many manufacturers only make mediums. Try to find brands that are made in multiple widths. Remember that the foot is three-dimensional. Two of those dimensions are width and thickness. The thicker the foot or higher the instep, the wider the shoe has to be to accommodate the foot. As we discussed earlier, infants' feet are heavily padded and thick by nature's design requiring a wider shoe. Inserting the tip of the first finger between the shoe and foot at the instep is the first gauge of how well the foot is fitting the width of the shoe. If the finger will not fit then the shoe is not wide enough. Room in the throat of the shoe is critical to allow for the forward growth of the foot into the shoe. Since the growth of the foot is three-fourths heel to ball and one-fourth toes most infants will outgrow the width of the shoe before they do the length. Parents will often check the length but not width of shoes. Using the thumb and first finger, at the ball of the foot, gently pull the leather in a lifting motion up from the foot. There should be enough room to lift the shoe material off of the foot slightly, but not in excess. Check the inside and outside of the foot for pressure points and cramped toes especially the little toe.

Heel

If you are fitting a high-top walking shoe on your baby, the heel fit is not a major concern. The heel is covered and the shoe will stay on well. On a lower shoe the heel should stay in the shoe without popping out when the baby walks. Tightness in the heel will cause more problems than if the shoe is a little loose in the heel. A little looseness is permissible, but not a large gap between the heel and the shoe.

Walk Test

If the child is not walking on their own yet, let them pull up on a chair or fitting stool. All checks on the fit of the shoe should be done with the child standing. Feet are not static but dynamic. Standing will allow the foot to expand in the length and width to the normal size it will be when walking. If the child is walking, let them take a few steps and watching their balance. Take note of the break in the shoe. It should be straight across the ball of the foot. A deep break (excess wrinkle) or breaking at an angle would indicate that the shoe is too wide. Breaking forward of the ball of the foot would indicate that the shoe is too long. Check the shoe again after the child has taken a walk in them and the foot has relaxed and set in the shoe.

Other Checks

On a low-top, shoe material should either cover the outside ankle bone or be far enough below the bone so as not to cause irritation. Always check the inside of the shoe before putting your child's shoes on. Nails, tacks, paper, plastic tags are some of the objects I have found in shoes over the years.

Fitting your child now with the proper size and style of shoe will help prevent possible foot problems in years to come. Longer life spans and more active lives mean more wear and tear on the feet. Don't let your child be like many adults that say, "I wish I had worn shoes that fit when I was a child. My feet would not be in such bad shape now." If you are able to find a local merchant that still knows how to fit shoes, then please make use of his knowledge and experience. If not, remember these tips the next time you buy shoes for your baby.

Section 5.2

Shoe Fitting for the Preschool Child

Description

We discussed fitting infants' shoes in the last section, now your child is past the infant stage and into preschool. Children have usually developed their natural gait by this time, and are running and making lateral movements. At this stage children would rather be running than walking. Being more active requires a different type of shoe and different fitting of the shoes. The growth pattern will change, depending on the child, from a steady growth about every three months, to a spurt pattern. The foot may not grow for a period of time and suddenly grow a size or more in a short period of time. Due to the fact every child is different it is impossible to predict this change in growth pattern. The parent should check, or have a shoe fitter check, the child's shoes every two or three months.

Most children of this age range are now attending a preschool, daycare, or mother's day out program. It is natural for the child to desire the popular shoes that the other children are wearing. Unfortunately because all feet are different the most popular shoe may not be the best for your child's feet. The style of children's shoes often follows the style of adult shoes, but fashion and function often do not go together. The requirements of a child's foot are quite different than that of an adult foot, so adult styles on a child's foot may be a poor choice. An example of this would be the clog style shoe that is popular now. A child who is running and climbing cannot keep this type of shoe on during normal daily activities. Another would be the slip-on style of athletic shoe that is becoming popular with adults. A slip-on

51

shoe for a child must be fit shorter than usual in order to keep the shoe from slipping off of the foot. This means that the shoe must be replaced more often than a traditional lace athletic shoe.

No two feet are alike. Some are narrow, some wide, and they vary in the overall shape. Style and shapes of shoes should match the shape of the foot. Compatibility is very important in fitting the foot. The shoe may be the proper size but the shape of the last is wrong for the foot. For example, a narrow foot would not do as well in a heavy sole, broad toe style. Wider feet would be better suited for this type of shoe. Children wear their shoes differently. Some shoes will look new after three months wear while other will look totally worn out after three weeks. How your child wears his/her shoes should be a consideration when fitting the shoes. For the child that is hard on his/her shoes, a heavier weight shoe will make a difference in how long the shoe will last.

Due to the wide variety of shoe and foot shapes, and due to the fact that right and left feet are different sizes, the perfect fit does not exist. There are some things you should check when fitting the shoes: toe room, width, throat room, heel fit, ankle bone clearance, and compatibility of shoe and foot. The following are guidelines you can use when fitting your child's shoes. Remember fitting is an art not a science, it takes practice and experience.

Toe Room

Generally there is one-third inch between sizes. Leaving one-third to one-half inch in the toes will allow for a whole size or size and one-half of growth room. Be sure that this room is allowed on the larger foot. If the shoe is too long, the break across the vamp (front of the shoe at the ball) will be at an angle instead of straight. The break or bend across the vamp may also be deeper on a shoe that is too long causing irritation across the top of the toes. As the shoe is worn, the toes will have a tendency to turn up.

Width

Shoe width is probably the most important part of fitting a shoe, but is ignored by most parents. Most parents want the shoe to fit with lots of toe room so that it can be worn for a longer period of time. However, if the shoe is not wide enough, then it will be outgrown in width long before the length becomes a factor. Foot growth is not in equal proportions; the toes are one-fourth and heel to ball is three-fourths of the total growth. If the shoe is too narrow then the foot cannot grow forward in the shoe, and length becomes less important.

You should be able to lift the leather off of the top of the foot by gently squeezing across the ball of the foot. One-sixth to one-quarter of an inch should give the child ample room for forward growth in the shoe. Be sure that the little toe is not cramped or turned under. Narrow feet are much more difficult to fit than wide feet because most manufacturers do not make narrow widths. Guidelines for fitting a narrow foot are the same, but you may have to try many more styles to find one the fits narrow enough for your child's foot. Frustrated parents will ask, "Will it hurt my child's foot to wear a shoe that is too wide?" The answer depends on the length of time the shoe is going to be worn and how wide it is. The foot will move constantly in a shoe that is too wide. The motion can cause irritations such as calluses and in some cases blisters. Sometimes insoles can be used to take up the extra space in the shoe, but it is difficult to find them in children's sizes.

Throat Room

The throat of the shoe is on the top where the foot meets the shoe. If there is not enough room between the foot and the shoe in the throat, then the foot will not be able to grow forward in the shoe. The tip of the first finger should be able to be inserted between the foot and the shoe in the throat. This will allow ample room for the forward growth of the shoe. Of course different styles of shoes will require different amounts of room. You cannot allow that much room in a slip-on shoe or loafer. If you do, the shoe will slip off as easily as it slips on. A buckle or Mary Jane style has a low cut vamp but you should still allow room on the top where the shoe and foot meet. The strap will allow for some adjustment of heel fit.

Heel Fit

Your mother always told you to make sure the heel doesn't slip when you are trying on new shoes. A little looseness in the heel is not a bad thing. If the heel is too tight however, you will be guaranteed a blister. Constant pressure on the heel will cause the body to build up a fluid to cushion the spot. Excess room will also cause problems, but just a little room will allow for more natural foot movement. Use caution on sling back shoes and clogs. These styles offer no lateral heel control. As the child runs, the heel will slip to the side, increasing the chances of twisting an ankle.

53

Ankle Bone

The ankle bone on the outside of the foot is lower on some children and can be a problem area. Athletic shoes with padded collars usually take care of this problem. On dress shoes that are harder and stiffer it can be a source of irritation. Check to see that the topline of the shoe comes above the ankle bone or well below it. Sometime a felt heel lift will help until the topline softens.

Compatibility

There are many styles of shoes on the market today, and your child will want the one that is the most popular. However, is that the best shoe for his/her foot? A shoe can be the right size but be totally wrong for the foot. Be sure the shape, or last, of the shoe matches the shape of the foot. Matching the shoe and foot shape will be more comfortable for the child and the shoe will look and wear better.

Several months ago a mother brought her daughter in with a pair of shoes that had been purchased at a specialty athletic store. Due to the fact that the child was in a school sponsored activity, the shoe was required for the uniform. The child had bunions and the beginning of hammertoes, and the shoes were very painful for her. The mother inquired about adjustment to the shoes that would allow the child to continue with her activity. After several adjustments on the shoes, they were less painful. However they still did not fit, nor were they compatible with the child's foot. Children will wear shoes that are popular or required for an activity whether they fit or not. It is the parent's job to assist the child in making correct choices. If proper fitting is started at an early age, then the foot will grow to its adult shape with few problems. Hopefully incidents like the one above will be avoided.

Chapter 6

Footwear Affects Foot Health

Chapter Contents

Section 6.1

Proper Footwear Can Reduce Foot Problems

From ancient Egyptian times down through the centuries, footwear has been designed to meet mankind's real and perceived needs—protection, support, comfort, sturdiness, and stylishness.

Feet endure tremendous pressures of daily living. An average day of walking brings a force equal to several hundred tons on them. They are subject to more injury than any other part of the body, underscoring the need to protect them with proper footwear.

Doctors of podiatric medicine are health care professionals trained for both palliative and surgical care of the foot and ankle. They also are fully qualified to recommend selection of the right pair of shoes, or address other aspects of foot health, for all members of the family.

Children's Shoes

When a child begins to walk, shoes generally are not necessary. Allowing an infant to go barefooted indoors, or to wear only a pair of socks, helps the foot grow normally and develop its muscles and strength, as well as the grasping ability of toes.

As children grow more active, and their feet develop, the need for shoes becomes apparent. It becomes necessary to change shoe sizes at a pace that frequently surprises and even dismays parents, to allow room for growth.

When purchasing shoes for children, remember these tips:

- Examine the shoe itself. It should have a firm heel counter (stiff material on either side of the heel), adequate cushioning of the insole, and a built-in arch. It should be flexible enough to bend where the foot bends—at the ball of the foot, not in the middle of the shoe.

- The child's foot should be sized while he or she is standing up and fully weight-bearing.

- There should be about one-half inch of space (or a thumb's width) between the tip of the toes and the end of the shoe. The child should be able to comfortably wiggle his or her toes in the shoe.

- Have the child walk around the store for more than just a few minutes wearing the shoe with a normal sock. Ask the child if he or she feels any pressure spots in the shoe. Feel the inside of the shoe for any staples or irregularities in the glue that could cause irritation. Examine where the inside stitching hits the foot. Look for signs of irritation on the foot after the shoe is worn.

- Shoes should not slip off at the heels. Children who tend to sprain their ankles will do better with high-top shoes or boots.

- Both feet should be measured, and if they are two different sizes, shoes should be chosen that fit the larger foot best.

Women's Shoes

Women inflict more punishment on their feet in part from improper footwear that can bring about unnecessary foot problems. Some of the problems result from high-heeled shoes (generally defined as pumps with heels of more than two inches). Doctors of podiatric medicine believe such heels are medically unsound and attribute postural and even safety problems to their use.

To relieve the abusive effects of high heels, women can limit the time they wear them, alternating with good quality sneakers or flats for part of the day.

They can also vary heel height. There are comfortable and attractive "walking" pumps (also called "comfort" or "performance" pumps) for work and social activities that blend fashion considerations and comfort. These pumps offer athletic shoe-derived construction, reinforced heels, and wider toe room.

Activity has a bearing on the considerations; wearing the right shoe for a particular activity is probably as important a factor in the choice of shoes as any.

Perhaps the best shoe for women is a walking shoe with laces (not a slip-on), a polymerized composition sole, and a relatively wider heel with a rigid and padded heel counter, no more than three-quarters of an inch in height.

Men's Shoes

The best shoes for men are good quality oxford styles, shoes ordinarily associated with wing-tip or cap toe designs. Also suitable are slip-ons, dressy loafers, and low dress boots.

Men as well as women should buy shoes for work, leisure, and special activities, matching the shoe to the activity.

Male (and female) office workers should earmark three to five pairs of shoes for business hours—general oxfords and loafers for men; pumps and oxfords for women. Cushioned-sole shoes that give good support are essential for those who spend most of their working days on their feet.

There is no question about the need for foot protection for those who work in heavy industry. Safety shoes and boots—those that are waterproof or water-resistant, with insulated steel toe caps and soles of non-conducting materials—help prevent injuries to the feet and reduce the severity of injuries that do occur. [See Chapter 9, "On Your Feet at Work," for more information on safety footwear.]

Shoes for Athletics

Different sports activities call for specific footwear to protect feet and ankles. Sports-specific athletic shoes are a wise investment for serious athletes, though perhaps a less critical consideration for the weekend or occasional athlete; nevertheless, it's a good idea to use the correct shoe for each sport. Probably a more important consideration is the condition of the shoe—don't wear any sport or other shoes beyond their useful life.

Athletic footwear should be fitted to hold the foot in the position that's most natural to the movement involved.

For example, a running shoe is built to accommodate impact, while a tennis shoe is made to give relatively more support and permit sudden stops and turns. For sports, "cross trainers" are fine for a general athletic shoe, such as for physical education classes. But if a child is involved more heavily in any single sport, he or she should have a shoe specifically designed for that sport.

Shoe Care

For longer service, keep shoes clean and in good repair. Avoid excessive wear on heels and soles. Give your shoes a chance to breathe—don't wear the same pair two days in a row (you prolong the life of shoes by rotating their use). Never wear hand-me-down shoes (this is especially important for children).

Seal of Acceptance

The American Podiatric Medical Association (APMA) awards its Seal of Acceptance to a wide variety of shoes (and shoe-related products), which have been deemed to enhance a consistently applied program of daily foot care and regular professional treatment.

The intent of such endorsements is to make a significant contribution to the foot health and foot health education of the public.

For a list of shoe companies holding the APMA Seal of Acceptance, visit the APMA's online seal information at http://www.apma.org.

Buying Tips

- Have your feet measured while you're standing.

- Always try on both shoes, and walk around the store.

- Always buy for the larger foot; feet are seldom precisely the same size.

- Don't buy shoes that need a "break-in" period; shoes should be comfortable immediately.

- Don't rely on the size of your last pair of shoes. Your feet do get larger, and lasts (shoemakers' sizing molds) also vary.

- Shop for shoes later in the day; feet tend to swell during the day, and it's best to be fitted while they are in that state.

- Be sure that shoes fit well—front, back, and sides—to distribute weight. It sounds elementary, but be sure the widest part of your foot corresponds to the widest part of the shoe.

- Select a shoe with a leather upper, stiff heel counter, appropriate cushioning, and flexibility at the ball of the foot.

- Buy shoes that don't pinch your toes, either at the tips, or across the toe box.

- Try on shoes while you're wearing the same type of socks or stockings you expect to wear with the shoes.

- If you wear prescription orthotics—biomechanical inserts prescribed by a podiatric physician—you should take them along to shoe fittings.

Your podiatric physician/surgeon has been trained specifically and extensively in the diagnosis and treatment of all manner of foot conditions. This training encompasses all of the intricately related systems and structures of the foot and lower leg including neurological, circulatory, skin, and the musculoskeletal system, which includes bones, joints, ligaments, tendons, muscles, and nerves.

Section 6.2

Lacing Techniques for Proper Shoe Fit

Certain lacing techniques for shoes can prevent injuries, alleviate pain, and relieve foot problems. The American Orthopaedic Foot and Ankle Society urges individuals to follow these general lacing tips. Individuals with specific foot problems should follow these lacing techniques to get a good fit with their shoe:

- Loosen the laces as you slip into the shoes. This prevents unnecessary stress on the eyelets (small holes for the lace) and the backs of the shoes.

- Always begin lacing shoes at the eyelets closest to your toes, and pull the laces of one set of eyelets at a time to tighten. This provides for a comfortable shoe fit.

- When buying shoes, remember that shoes with a larger number of eyelets will make it easier to adjust laces for a custom fit.

- The conventional method of lacing, crisscross to the top of the shoe, works best for the majority of people.

Narrow Feet

Use the eyelets farthest from the tongue of the shoes. It will bring up the side of the shoe.

Wide Feet

Use the eyelets closest to the tongue of the shoe. This technique gives the foot more space.

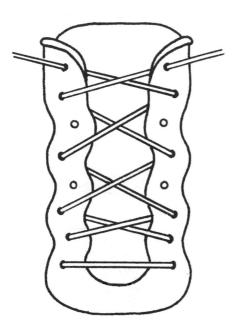

Figure 6.1. Lacing for narrow feet (image redrawn for Omnigraphics by Alison DeKleine).

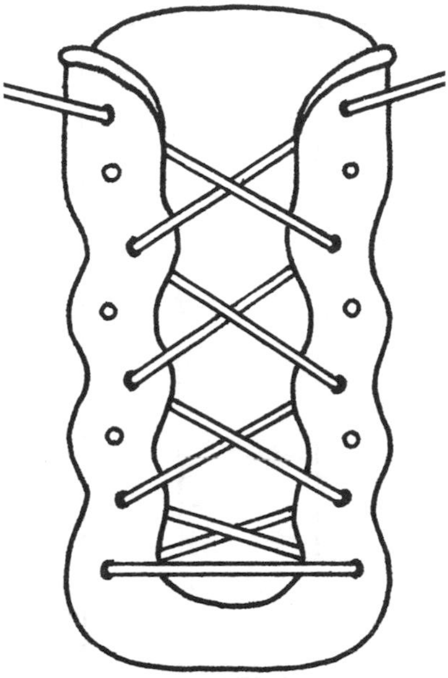

Figure 6.2. Lacing for wide feet (image redrawn for Omnigraphics by Alison DeKleine).

Heel Problems

Use every eyelet, making sure that the area closest to the heel is tied tightly while less tension is used near the toes. When you have reached the next to last eyelet on each side, thread the lace through the top eyelet, making a small loop. Then, thread the opposite lace through each loop before tying it.

Narrow Heel and Wide Forefoot

Use two laces. Thread through the top half of the eyelets and the other lace through the bottom half of the eyelets. The lace closest to the heel (top eyelets) should be tied more tightly than the other lace closest to the toes (bottom eyelets).

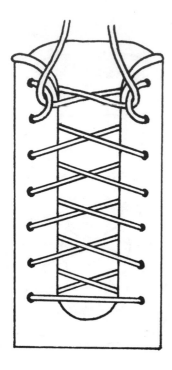

Figure 6.3. Lacing for heel problems (image re-drawn for Omnigraphics by Alison DeKleine).

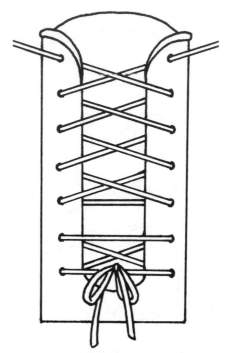

Figure 6.4. Lacing for narrow heel and wide forefoot (image redrawn for Omnigraphics by Alison DeKleine).

Section 6.3

Buying the Correct Pair of Running Shoes

"A Guide to Buying the Correct Pair of Running Shoes," Carl R. Darnall Army Medical Center, Fort Hood, TX (http://www.hood-meddac.army.mil). Accessed January 2006.

Although overtraining is a prime cause of running injuries, running in a worn-out shoe or wearing the wrong shoe are major contributing factors.

You may be wearing the wrong shoe if you have any of the following medical conditions:

- blisters
- knee pain
- ankle pain
- hip pain

- neuroma
- bruised toenails
- shin pain
- plantar fasciitis

There are a number of items to consider when buying a new pair of running shoes.

- foot type
- fit
- shoe mechanics

- body weight
- shoe life
- price

Foot Type

The most important consideration for selecting a running shoe is your foot type. Few people are lucky enough to have a biomechanically efficient foot, which distributes the person's weight perfectly from heel strike to toe off. Most of us need to rely on our running shoe to compensate for our lack of perfection.

There are three major types of foot arches: normal, flat (over-pronator), and high (over-supinator).

Determine your arch type by taking the wet test. Dunk your foot in water and then stand on any surface that will leave an imprint. Match your imprint with the most similar picture in Figure 6.5. Which arch most closely resembles your imprint?

Normal Arch

Normal feet have a normal-sized arch and leave an imprint that has a flare but shows the forefoot and heel connected by a wide band.

Biomechanics: A normal foot lands on the outside of the heel, then rolls inward (pronates) slightly to absorb shock.

Best shoes: Runners with a normal foot require stability shoes, which offer a blend of cushioning, medial support, and durability. They provide stability with a medial post or dual-density midsole, and they are built on a semi-curved last. Buy these shoes if you are a midweight runner who doesn't have any severe motion-control problems and wants a shoe with some medial support and good durability.

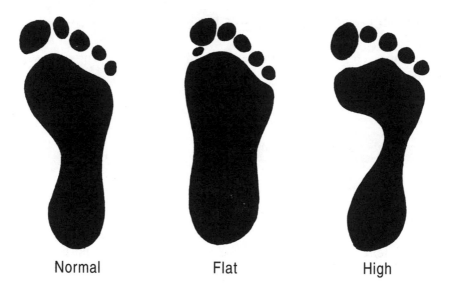

| Normal | Flat | High |

Figure 6.5. *Arches of the foot (image redrawn for Omnigraphics by Alison DeKleine).*

Flat Arch

Flat arches leave a wide and "filled in" imprint.

Biomechanics: The flat or over-pronated foot usually strikes on the outside of the heel and rolls inward (pronates) excessively. Over time, this can cause overuse injuries, such as "shin splints" and even knee pain.

Best shoes: Motion-control shoes, or stability shoes with firm midsoles and control features that reduce the degree of pronation. They may include features such as a medial post (for pronation control), a polyurethane midsole (for durability), and a carbon rubber outsole (for durability). Many are built on straight lasts, which offer stability and maximum medial support. Buy these shoes if you are an over-pronator who needs control features and places a premium on durability, if you wear orthotics and want a firm midsole and deep heel counter, or if you are a heavy runner who needs extra durability and control.

High-Arch

High-arched feet leave an imprint showing a very narrow band connecting the forefoot and heel.

Biomechanics: A curved, high-arched or over-supinator foot does not roll inward (pronate) enough, so it is not an effective shock absorber.

Best shoes: Cushioned shoes with plenty of flexibility. These generally have the softest midsoles and the least amount of medial support. They are built on a semi-curved or curved last to encourage foot motion. This is important for over-supinators who usually have a rigid, immobile foot.

Another hint to determine over-pronation versus over-supination is to look at the bottom of your old running shoes. If you are an over-pronator, your shoes will be more worn on the inside edge of your shoes than the outside edge. In severe cases, the shoe will actually slope dramatically inward. If you are a supinator, your running shoes are worn and compressed along the outside edge.

Fit

When buying a pair of shoes, try them on with the socks, inserts, or orthotic devices you plan on wearing when running.

- Try on shoes at the end of the day or after a workout when your feet are actually at their longest and widest. Feet expand up to one whole size during a workout.

- The front (toe box) of the shoe should allow your toes to move around. You should be able to fit the wide of your thumbnail between the longest toe and the end of the shoe.

- The mid-part of the shoe, when laced, should hold your foot snugly so that it doesn't slide forward and jam your toes with each step.

- The heel counter (inflexible material surrounding the heel) should fit snugly so your heel won't slip and rub, causing blisters.

Shoe Mechanics

The shoe should have some form of cushioning, and some shoes have more than others. Shoes should feel comfortable straight out of the box; there should be no break-in period.

- Be sure the sole flexes easily where your foot flexes. Buy shoes with removable insoles so you can modify or replace them with orthotics.

- The lacing area and tongue should be padded, especially if you have bony bumps on your instep.

- Try on a couple different models and sizes so you can compare. Don't rush your selection!

- Try on both shoes. Your feet may not be the same size or the shoes may not be made symmetrically.

- Walk and jog around the store for a few minutes.

Body Weight

The more you weigh, the more force you will generate. Heavier runners need a shoe that offers more shock absorption and added durability.

Shoe Life

Depending on the shoe, the surface on which you run, and your weight, running shoes should last anywhere between 300 and 500 miles before you need to replace them.

Runners logging 25 miles per week should consider replacing their shoes every three to four months. Ft. Hood soldiers running four miles each day, four days a week, log over 300 miles in 20 weeks (five months).

Shoes last longer if you run on dirt or grass. The heavier you are, the sooner you will need to replace them. If the midsole starts to show through or begins to form horizontal lines, or if you notice new aches and pains in especially your knees, shins, or ankles (since today's outsoles are so durable you may not notice any wear), you may need new shoes.

When the midsoles flatten out and the cushioning gets shot, your shoes are no longer acting as shock absorbers. Instead the shock gets passed along to your bones and joints causing leg pain.

Price

Shoes come in all price ranges, from $30 to $130+. You should plan on spending at least $65–$85. Remember, the most expensive shoe is not always the best, but many less expensive shoes are not built to help the body absorb and withstand the constant and repetitive impact from running.

Making Your Shoes Last

Store your shoes in a cool, dry place away from direct sunlight or heaters. Heat is tough on shoes, causing the glue to soften, the midsoles to flatten, and the shape to curl.

Keep your shoes dry. Moisture is also hard on running shoes. To dry, loosen the laces, open the tongue, and remove the insoles. If moist with sweat, foot powder can keep your shoes dry and free of fungus, bacteria, and odor. If completely soaked stuff them with newspaper to sop up the water.

Clean your shoes when necessary. Clean them with cold water, mild soap, and a soft brush. Let them air dry, not in a dryer.

Rotate your shoes. Buy a second pair about midway through the life of your first (when your first pair has about 200 miles on them), and alternate pairs, daily. As your first pair becomes worn out, you can use your second pair as a reference, making it easier to know when to throw out the first pair. This also lets your shoes rest and dry between runs.

Use the above information to help buy your next pair of running shoes, and run in comfort and good health.

Section 6.4

High Heels Dangerous to Your Health

The idea that high heels can be hazardous to your health isn't new—orthopedists have warned women for years that high heels can contribute to the development of a variety of conditions from corns and calluses to hammer toes, arthritis, chronic knee pain, sprained ankles, and back problems.

In 1998, a team of Harvard researchers linked high heels and knee osteoarthritis, a painful, degenerative joint disease characterized by the breakdown of the cartilage surrounding the knee. In that study, D. Casey Kerrigan, MD, associate professor of physical medicine at Harvard Medical School, and her team looked at very narrow, stiletto heels.

Wide Heels No Better

The researchers decided to look at the chunkier heels now in fashion to determine if they too are harmful to women's knees. The study, which appeared in the April 7, 2001, issue of *The Lancet*, demonstrates that wide heels increase the risk of developing osteoarthritis in the knee as much as, or more than, spindly-heeled stilettos.

"Wide-heeled shoes give you the perception of more stability when you're standing, and they feel comfortable, so women wear them all day long," Kerrigan said. "They are better for your feet than stiletto heels, but just as bad for your knees."

Study Measures Knee Torque

The study subjects were 20 healthy women with an average age of 34 and an average weight of 130 pounds. Each woman received one pair of shoes with a heel approximately 1.75 inches wide and another pair of shoes with a heel width of about half an inch. Both pairs were 2.7 inches high.

Study participants were then asked to walk 10 meters or about 32 feet, once in narrow-heeled shoes, once in wide-heeled shoes, and once barefoot. Researchers measured knee torque, how much the knee twisted during each walk.

Both types of shoes increased knee joint pressure—26 percent more for wide-heeled shoes and 22 percent for narrow-heeled shoes. This kind of repetitive stress to the knee elevates the risk for osteoarthritis, according to physicians. Low-heeled shoes or no heels, researchers conclude, are a woman's safest bet against osteoarthritic knees.

"It takes a long time to feel the effects of knee osteoarthritis, and once you do, it's too late," said Dr. Kerrigan.

Eighty percent of the 42 million Americans suffering from arthritis have osteoarthritis, in which joint cartilage and surrounding bone progressively degrade from wear and tear. Surgeons perform 300,000 artificial knee replacements in this country every year due to this condition.

The High Price of High Heels

This study confirms what orthopedists have known for a long time. High heels, whether they're thick or thin, can cause problems in women's knees, their ankles, and their feet. Shoe-related problems very frequently include ankle sprains and breaks from rolling over on high-heeled shoes. These are immediate problems, unlike osteoarthritis in the knee, which may develop after decades of wearing high heels.

What Is Osteoarthritis?

While the exact cause is unknown, we do know there are several contributing factors, including injuries, age, congenital predisposition, and obesity. It is characterized by the breakdown of the articular cartilage within the joint. Articular cartilage is a firm, rubbery material that covers the end of a bone. It acts as a cushion or shock absorber between the bones. When it breaks down, this cushion is lost, and the bones grind together. This causes the development of symptoms such as pain, swelling, and decreased motion. Osteoarthritis commonly affects weight-bearing joints such as the knee, but it may affect any joint.

Walking on high heels puts abnormal stress on both the front and the back of the knee as *The Lancet* study demonstrates. In the case of the shoes they tested, pressure on the knee was increased by 22 to 26 percent. The health of the cartilage that forms the padding between the bones in the knee is dependent on the fluid in the knee. It absorbs the nutrients it needs from this liquid to repair itself, but stress on the knee restricts the absorption of the fluid, and the cartilage begins to dry out and shred. Over time, it wears out and arthritis sets in. There are also genetic components of arthritis and there may be nutritional aspects as well, but we know high heels don't help.

Treatment Approaches

Treatment depends on the stage of the disease. If we catch it in its earlier stages, glucosamine and chondroitin sulfate supplements may be helpful. There is a lot of anecdotal evidence that taking these natural substances, which dissipate as we age, helps to rebuild cartilage.

We also give injections of Synvisc®, a substance produced from chicken cartilage that is in the same chemical family as glucosamine. The injections can be helpful for up to six months and then additional injections are necessary.

If the arthritis is more advanced, we can do arthroscopic surgery to clean the joint of debris and repair any torn cartilage. If the arthritis is well advanced, total knee replacement surgery may be necessary.

High Heels Also Cause Foot Problems

High heels can also result in a variety of foot problems, including metatarsalgia, which is pain in the ball of the foot. Another condition, called Morton neuroma, which is ten times more common in women than men, is caused by a thickening of tissue around a nerve between the third and fourth toes. It usually develops in response to irritation and excessive pressure such as the weight burden high heels place on the ball of the foot. It is often treated with orthotics, cortisone injections, and in stubborn cases, surgery.

Pointed toe shoes and shoes that pinch lead to other foot problems such as bunions, calluses, and hammer toe.

The Most Healthy Shoe

Surprisingly, flat shoes are not the ideal for overall foot and leg health. Low heels of one-half to three-quarters of an inch are good for both the front and back of the foot. Square-toed shoes with a roomy toe box help prevent the pinching and scrunching of the foot that can lead to lots of painful problems.

—by Enzo J. Sella, MD

Section 6.5

Selecting Socks

Ohio State University Extension Fact Sheet HYG-5544-0, 2001. Reprinted with permission from Ohio State University Extension. References to commercial trade names is for information purposes only. No discrimination is intended nor endorsement implied of products omitted or identified.

Buying socks may appear simple, but some day while shopping, just stop and look at the variety. Dozens of types of socks exist. Many are interchangeable in terms of quality and appearance. Others are designed to meet specific needs. So let's take a closer look at socks, so purchases can match the needs of individual wearers and their activities.

Fiber Content

Socks come in a variety of fibers and fiber combinations. Commonly used fibers include cotton, wool, nylon, acrylic, polyester, olefin, and spandex. Occasionally, luxury fibers such as silk, linen, cashmere, or mohair will be blended for softness, but this adds to the cost.

Natural fibers are absorbent. The presence of cotton and wool helps absorb perspiration. Wool absorbs up to 30 percent of its weight in moisture before feeling "wet," making it a desirable choice in winter—but once the fabric becomes saturated and moist, it feels cold to the wearer.

The term "natural blend cotton" is used on the label of many socks. These socks have a high content of cotton (60 percent) with smaller amounts of synthetics, usually nylon or spandex, for reinforcement or support. Occasionally, linen, a natural fiber, is knitted into the toe of socks for reinforcement. Linen is a relatively strong fiber and adds durability as well as absorbency and comfort. Silk socks are usually quite smooth and absorbent. They make a good layer next to the skin, but are not very durable.

Synthetic fibers, particularly nylon, are strong and make an excellent choice for socks which commonly receive hard wear. Besides durability, synthetic fibers add shrink resistance. Socks may be 100 percent nylon or reinforced at the toe and heel with this durable fiber.

71

Acrylic fibers are long wearing but also add a cushiony softness and bulk to socks made from them. Acrylic fibers are commonly found in socks for casual wear. Olefin fiber has become important for outdoor sport socks. Olefin fibers do not absorb moisture; however, both olefin and acrylic have wicking ability. This means that moisture travels along the fiber away from the skin. Acrylic and olefin socks are often worn next to the skin, with a wool or cotton sock over them to absorb moisture. Some blends of socks are made so the fibers with wicking ability are next to the skin and the absorbent fiber forms an outer layer. This accomplishes the same result as wearing two socks, but is less bulky.

Stretch fibers, including spandex, elastic, or rubber, are present in many socks. They help socks stay up and hug the leg and foot. Spandex is used extensively to provide support in the ankle, calf, and arch areas, especially in sport socks. These socks stay in place and increase blood circulation. While elastic or rubber yarns sometimes are used, they deteriorate from body oils and do not last as long as spandex stretch yarns. Also, elastic in sock tops binds more than spandex.

Construction

Socks are knitted, giving them stretch and the ability to conform to the foot and leg. Generally, a stockinette or plain knit stitch is used in the foot area and a rib stitch is used in the leg area (though some socks are made totally of rib stitch). The rib stitch is very stretchy, with the ability to return to shape. As both the stockinette and rib stitches are simple knit constructions, the stitch can ravel out if a yarn is broken. Look carefully at socks for loose threads, broken yarns, or holes that could start to run or ravel with wear. Also, look for evenly knitted stitches on socks and a flat seam at the toe. Toe seams placed high over the toe are usually more comfortable than those at the end of the toe. Both the toe and heel areas should be smooth, otherwise irritation could occur during wear.

Tube socks are circular knits and have no shaped heel area. The socks can be put on several ways and will stretch enough on any side to fit the heel area. Sometimes the tube sock has one seam at the end of the toe. Be certain this is very flat and smooth as it is in a critical area for wearing comfort.

Check also the ribbing at the top of the sock. Socks that keep falling down are annoying. Spandex yarns in the calf area will help prevent this. Generally, the wider the band of ribbing, the better the sock will stay up. Also, a narrow band of stretch yarn (often made of elastic) tends to roll over or curl at the top, causing discomfort to the wearer.

Heel shape in a sock is equally important to comfort. A square heel gives the best fit. A small, curved heel tends to slip under the foot easily and bunch in the shoe.

Another feature of construction to check is the amount of stretch in the sock. Be certain both the body and the ankle areas of the sock will slide over the foot easily. People with high insteps especially need to check this.

Toe and heel reinforcements are important features. Nylon thread is often knitted into these areas to prolong wear. Occasionally, linen yarns are knitted into the toe area for the same purpose. While linen is a strong fiber, it does not equal the durability of nylon reinforcements. In any case, four- or six-ply yarns should be used in these areas. They form thicker yarns which give longer wear.

The reinforcement should be wide enough to cover all joints on the toes. This area may be double knit for increased durability. Check for an extra high heel guard or reinforcement above the location where the back of the shoe rubs against the sock. On adult men's socks, this will be three to three and one-half inches (3–3½") from the bottom of the sock.

Concerning general construction, some socks feature cotton lisle yarns. These yarns are made from high quality, long staple cotton ply yarns. The amount of twist on these yarns is specified by Federal Trade Commission regulations. The combination of twist with heavier-ply yarns gives durability, while the soft, good quality cotton yarns add strength and comfort. Usually, socks from cotton lisle are made into plain- or stockinette-stitch socks.

One final but important point to consider is the decoration of socks. This can be knitted in or applied. Patterns knitted in, especially those involving contrasting colors, should be sharp and clear. Poorly made socks will have uneven borders and overlapping stripes in the body of the sock. Look for loose threads with knitted designs. Threads can pull out and cause raveling. Loose threads can also form loops and catch toes. Applied designs should be smooth, secure, and non-irritating to the skin. Applied designs which are stamped or painted on are less durable. The color may crack and flake off over time. Decorations like buttons, bells, lace, and bows can be sewn on. These need to be sewn on securely, but over time, may not hold up.

Finishes

Few finishes are applied to socks. However, those that are perform important functions. Antistatic finishes are desirable on socks made from synthetic fibers. They help prevent trousers from clinging to the socks and lint from collecting on them during wear and laundering.

A more common finish for socks is one that resists the buildup of odor and bacteria. The feet are among the three areas of the body that contain large sweat glands (the other two are the armpits and the palms of the hands). Feet wrapped in a layer of socks and shoes for long periods become warm and perspire. Although perspiration is odorless and 99 percent water, it provides a perfect medium for bacteria to grow. The bacteria cause foot odor. Antibacterial agents in the fiber reduce bacteria growth and resulting odor. Most antibacterial finishes used today are durable and remain after repeated launderings.

New Technology and Performance Fabrics

Special engineered polyester fibers have been developed for specific sports activities. For warmer weather, Dupont developed Coolmax® fabric. The fiber cross-section looks like a double scallop shape which gives the fiber 20 percent more surface area than regular fibers. This allows water to spread over a greater area in the fabric, so it can evaporate faster. The fiber enhances comfort and breathability by wicking away moisture so it can evaporate. Coolmax® claims to possess superior wicking and evaporation of perspiration moisture.

Coolmax® is just one brand-name in the growing category of high-technology wicking fabrics. Other brand names in this market include Dryline, Dryfit, Dryskin, Powerdry, Hydrofil, Capeline, BiPolar, and Stretch Supplex.

For colder weather, fabrics like Thermolite® contain hollow core fibers with a convoluted or twisted surface. The hollow center holds air, resulting in additional thermal insulation as well as a 20 percent reduction in fiber weight and space which enables freedom of movement. The surface and convolutions enhance wicking properties. Additional crimp in the fibers creates bulk which traps air. This fiber is designed for use in thermal underwear, gloves, socks, and turtleneck T-shirts.

Other new technologies include the development of socks which reduce abrasion. Blisters form through abrasion or rubbing of the foot, usually toes, against the sock and shoe. Breeze® socks are designed so there is greater abrasion between the sock and foot than between the sock and shoe. The sock then sticks to the foot, but slides against the shoe and protects the foot. The result is less abrasion and fewer blisters.

Types

For men, four major types of socks exist—dress, casual, sport, and work. Dress socks may be worn with business suits during the day or for special occasions. Usually, they are a flat, lightweight knit and may even have sheer panels, especially for warm-weather use. They come in calf and over-the-calf lengths.

Casual socks are worn with sports wear and in less formal situations. They are made from bulky yarns, usually wool or acrylic, or from cotton for softness and comfort. They may be blended with nylon or spandex for improved fit and durability, or olefin for comfort to wick away moisture. Casual socks, regardless of construction, normally are calf length.

Support socks have become more popular and acceptable in recent years. Generally, in men's socks they are in over-the-calf lengths. Support socks contain higher percentages of spandex to help support muscles and relieve fatigue and strain.

Work socks are designed for durability and hard wear. They use cotton fiber for absorbency and often feature nylon reinforcement in the heel and toe. Winter work socks will have wool or acrylic yarns for warmth. Traditionally, work socks have been white or natural colors, but steel blue, darker colors, and "ragg" wool socks with dark and light flecks are available now.

Socks for women are usually for casual or sports activities. They may be ankle length, calf length (crew), or knee length. Bulky yarns in wool or acrylic fibers are most common. They often have knitted-in designs in one or more contrasting colors, but lightweight nylon knits are also available and become more fashionable at times.

Trouser socks are choices available for women. These are knee high and are designed to be worn with slacks. Trouser socks may be tube style or shaped in the heel, and frequently feature either subtle or brightly colored knitted-in motifs. Trouser socks are usually nylon and are similar to heavier weight or opaque panty hose or tights. As with nylon stockings, they can and do get runs.

As emphasis on physical fitness has increased for both men and women, so have the types of socks designed for active sports. Spandex panels and ribbed construction through the ankle, arch, and calf offer support to these areas during active periods. Also, the panels hold socks in place so they do not slide down and cause discomfort. Cushioned soles constructed from stretch terry pile lining reduce shock and resist abrasion. Reinforced toe and heel areas provide durability. Toe seams are placed high on the toe for additional comfort.

Many sport socks feature a stretch terry knit stitch with looped terry throughout the sock or in selected locations. Increasingly, terry is placed on the outside and smooth knit construction next to the foot. This construction reduces rubbing and so reduces blisters and calluses.

Socks made with stitched terry yarn provide more cushion and comfort to the wearer. Tennis and racquetball players need cushioning at the ball, heel, and toe areas to absorb shock, but also at the arch and over the toes to protect the feet during heavy, fast, quick movements. Runners also need cushioning at the ball, heel, and toes to reduce shock abrasion and blisters; however, a flat knit over the instep and less bulk overall is best for socks used with this sport. Basketball players usually prefer high, cushioned socks to protect feet and legs, but also need socks which will stay up during play. Cyclists, on the other hand, prefer thin, lightweight socks so they can feel the pedals and experience more agile movement. When special socks are needed, they should be worn when buying sports shoes, since these socks can affect the fit of the shoe.

Another concern for individuals involved in active sports such as tennis, running, basketball, and, to a lesser extent, walking, is perspiration. Socks with wicking action or absorbency help keep feet dry. This reduces the potential for foot odor and athlete's foot. Both acrylic and olefin fibers feature wicking action that carries moisture away from the skin to an outside absorbent layer. Also, wool absorbs 30 percent of its weight in moisture without feeling moist. The presence of these fibers helps control moisture and increases comfort for the wearer.

Some individuals prefer short or quarter top socks that cover only the foot area, especially for warm weather activities. These socks often feature similar sport specific cushioning available in the standard length socks mentioned above. Some short styles have a tendency to slip down into the back of the shoe. Look for construction features such as pompons at the back heel, knit ribbing, or an edge roll over the heel to counteract this problem.

Thermal socks are good choices for outdoor sportswear. Individuals who ski, hunt, or work outside during cold weather will find that these socks keep the feet and toes quite warm. Thermal socks may be a textured knit featuring tiny air pockets in a waffle or popcorn design. These air pockets trap body heat to provide insulation and warmth. Neoprene socks feature a microporous core to seal in heat and keep feet dry, yet prevent perspiration buildup through the breathable structure.

The stretch terry knit in the foot area of some casual socks provides insulative properties. Also, socks made from bulky yarns that include wool and acrylic will do the same thing but to a lesser degree. Cold-weather protection can also be achieved by wearing a combination of olefin socks next to the skin and bulky, more absorbent socks over them. The wicking ability of olefin carries moisture away from the foot to the more absorbent outer layer.

One last specialty sock is the boot sock. These extra-high socks extend beyond the tops of hunting, work, and western-style boots. They usually contain some wool and nylon and may be blended with other fibers to meet specific needs.

Care

Laundering of socks requires few special precautions other than concern for color. As colors used in socks may run during laundering, wash with other dark colored items. Also, wash in warm, not hot, water to reduce color bleeding.

Always check labels for colorfastness. This is especially important with white sport socks that feature colorful stripes or designs. Colors may run into the white area if dyes are not colorfast or if water temperatures are too hot.

Finally, avoid using chlorine bleach when washing socks containing wool, silk, spandex, or elastic. Chlorine bleach will damage these fibers.

Also, check the care label of socks containing wool and/or olefin. Most wool or wool/blend socks can be machine washed and dryer dried, but some may specify hand washing. Socks made from 100 percent olefin should be air dried, since this fiber is very heat sensitive; however, socks containing blends of olefin with other fibers can usually be dryer dried at low temperatures.

— by Joyce Smith, PhD, and Norma Pitts

Reference

Gulbrandson, Ruth. *Buying Socks.* Fargo, ND: North Dakota Cooperative Extension Service, 1992.

Chapter 7

Preventing Foot Trouble

When we are in love we may be "swept off our feet." When we don't want to do something, we are said to have "cold feet." A sensible person "has both feet on the ground." Sometimes we even "vote with our feet."

Years of wear and tear can be hard on our feet. So can disease, poor circulation, improperly trimmed toenails, and wearing shoes that don't fit properly. Problems with our feet can be the first sign of more serious medical conditions such as arthritis, diabetes, and nerve and circulatory disorders.

Preventing Foot Trouble

Practice good foot care. Check your feet regularly, or have a member of your family check them. Podiatrists and primary care doctors (internists and family practitioners) are qualified to treat most foot problems. Sometimes the special skills of an orthopedic surgeon or dermatologist are needed.

It also helps to keep blood circulating to your feet as much as possible. Do this by putting your feet up when you are sitting or lying down, stretching if you've had to sit for a long while, walking, having a gentle foot massage, or taking a warm foot bath. Try to avoid pressure from shoes that don't fit right. Try not to expose your feet to cold

"Foot Care," National Institute on Aging (http://www.niapublications.org), National Institutes of Health, May 2000. Accessed September 2006.

temperatures. Don't sit for long periods of time (especially with your legs crossed). Don't smoke.

Wearing comfortable shoes that fit well can prevent many foot ailments. Here are some tips for getting a proper shoe fit:

- The size of your feet changes as you grow older so always have your feet measured before buying shoes. The best time to measure your feet is at the end of the day when your feet are largest.

- Most of us have one foot that is larger than the other, so fit your shoe to your larger foot.

- Don't select shoes by the size marked inside the shoe but by how the shoe fits your foot.

- Select a shoe that is shaped like your foot.

- During the fitting process, make sure there is enough space (3/8" to 1/2") for your longest toe at the end of each shoe when you are standing up.

- Make sure the ball of your foot fits comfortably into the widest part of the shoe.

- Don't buy shoes that feel too tight and expect them to stretch to fit.

- Your heel should fit comfortably in the shoe with a minimum amount of slipping—the shoes should not ride up and down on your heel when you walk.

- Walk in the shoes to make sure they fit and feel right. Then take them home and spend some time walking on carpet to make sure the fit is a good one.

The upper part of the shoes should be made of a soft, flexible material to match the shape of your foot. Shoes made of leather can reduce the possibility of skin irritations. Soles should provide solid footing and not be slippery. Thick soles cushion your feet when walking on hard surfaces. Low-heeled shoes are more comfortable, safer, and less damaging than high-heeled shoes.

Common Foot Problems

Fungal and bacterial conditions, including athlete's foot, occur because our feet spend a lot of time in shoes—a warm, dark, humid place that is perfect for fungus to grow. Fungal and bacterial conditions can cause dry skin, redness, blisters, itching, and peeling. If not treated right away, an infection may be hard to cure. If not treated properly, the infection may reoccur. To prevent infections, keep your feet—especially the area between your toes—clean and dry. Change your shoes and socks or stockings often to help keep your feet dry. Try dusting your feet daily with foot powder. If your foot condition does not get better within two weeks, talk to your doctor.

Dry skin can cause itching and burning feet. Use mild soap in small amounts and a moisturizing cream or lotion on your legs and feet every day. Be careful about adding oils to bath water since they can make your feet and bathtub very slippery.

Corns and calluses are caused by friction and pressure when the bony parts of your feet rub against your shoes. If you have corns or calluses, see your doctor. Sometimes wearing shoes that fit better or using special pads solves the problem. Treating corns and calluses yourself may be harmful, especially if you have diabetes or poor circulation. Over-the-counter medicines contain acids that destroy the tissue but do not treat the cause. Sometimes these medicines reduce the need for surgery, but check with your doctor before using them.

Warts are skin growths caused by viruses. They are sometimes painful and, if untreated, may spread. Since over-the-counter preparations rarely cure warts, see your doctor. A doctor can apply medicines, burn or freeze the wart off, or take the wart off with surgery.

Bunions develop when the joints in your big toe no longer fit together as they should and become swollen and tender. Bunions tend to run in families. If a bunion is not severe, wearing shoes cut wide at the instep and toes, taping the foot, or wearing pads that cushion the bunion may help the pain. Other treatments include physical therapy and wearing orthotic devices or shoe inserts. A doctor can also prescribe anti-inflammatory drugs and cortisone injections for pain. Sometimes surgery is needed to relieve the pressure and repair the toe joint.

Ingrown toenails occur when a piece of the nail breaks the skin—which can happen if you don't cut your nails properly. Ingrown toenails are very common in the large toes. A doctor can remove the part of the nail that is cutting into the skin. This allows the area to heal.

Ingrown toenails can often be avoided by cutting the toenail straight across and level with the top of the toe.

Hammer toe is caused by a shortening of the tendons that control toe movements. The toe knuckle is usually enlarged, drawing the toe back. Over time, the joint enlarges and stiffens as it rubs against shoes. Your balance may be affected. Wearing shoes and stockings with plenty of toe room is a treatment for hammer toe. In very serious cases, surgery may be needed.

Spurs are calcium growths that develop on bones of your feet. They are caused by muscle strain in the feet. Standing for long periods of time, wearing badly fitting shoes, or being overweight can make spurs worse. Sometimes spurs are completely painless—at other times they can be very painful. Treatments for spurs include using foot supports, heel pads, and heel cups. Sometimes surgery is needed.

Chapter 8

Foot Facts for Athletes

Chapter Contents

Section 8.1

Preventing Sports Injuries

"Fast Facts about Sports Injuries," National Institute of Arthritis
and Musculoskeletal and Skin Diseases, National Institutes of Health,
June 2005.

What are sports injuries?

"Sports injuries" are injuries that happen when playing sports or
exercising. Some are from accidents. Others can result from poor training practices or improper gear. Some people get injured when they
are not in proper condition. Not warming up or stretching enough
before you play or exercise can also lead to injuries. The most common sports injuries are as follows:

- sprains and strains
- knee injuries
- swollen muscles
- Achilles tendon injuries
- pain along the shin bone
- fractures
- dislocations

What's the difference between an acute and a chronic injury?

There are two kinds of sports injuries: acute and chronic. Acute
injuries occur suddenly when playing or exercising. Sprained ankles,
strained backs, and fractured hands are acute injuries. Signs of an
acute injury include the following:

- sudden, severe pain
- swelling
- not being able to place weight on a leg, knee, ankle, or foot

- an arm, elbow, wrist, hand, or finger that is very tender
- not being able to move a joint as normal
- extreme leg or arm weakness
- a bone or joint that is visibly out of place

Chronic injuries happen after you play a sport or exercise for a long time. Signs of a chronic injury include the following:

- pain when you play
- pain when you exercise
- a dull ache when you rest
- swelling

What should I do if I get injured?

Never try to "work through" the pain of a sports injury. Stop playing or exercising when you feel pain. Playing or exercising more only causes more harm. Some injuries should be seen by a doctor right away. Others you can treat yourself.

Call a doctor when the following occur:

- the injury causes severe pain, swelling, or numbness
- you can't put any weight on the area
- an old injury hurts or aches
- an old injury swells
- the joint doesn't feel normal or feels unstable

If you don't have any of these signs, it may be safe to treat the injury at home. If the pain or other symptoms get worse, you should call your doctor. Use the RICE (Rest, Ice, Compression, and Elevation) method to relieve pain, reduce swelling, and speed healing. Follow these four steps right after the injury occurs and do so for at least 48 hours:

Rest: Reduce your regular activities. If you've injured your foot, ankle, or knee, take weight off of it. A crutch can help. If your right foot or ankle is injured, use the crutch on the left side. If your left foot or ankle is injured, use the crutch on the right side.

Ice: Put an ice pack to the injured area for 20 minutes, four to eight times a day. You can use a cold pack or ice bag. You can also use a plastic bag filled with crushed ice and wrapped in a towel. Take the ice off after 20 minutes to avoid cold injury.

Compression: Put even pressure (compression) on the injured area to help reduce swelling. You can use an elastic wrap, special boot, air cast, or splint. Ask your doctor which one is best for your injury.

Elevation: Put the injured area on a pillow, at a level above your heart, to help reduce swelling.

How are sports injuries treated?

Treatment often begins with the RICE method. Here are some other things your doctor may do to treat your sports injury.

Nonsteroidal anti-inflammatory drugs (NSAIDs): Your doctor will suggest that you take a nonsteroidal anti-inflammatory drug (NSAID) such as aspirin, ibuprofen, ketoprofen, or naproxen sodium. These drugs reduce swelling and pain. You can buy them at a drug store. Another common drug is acetaminophen. It may relieve pain, but it will not reduce swelling.

Immobilization: Immobilization is a common treatment for sports injuries. It keeps the injured area from moving and prevents more damage. Slings, splints, casts, and leg immobilizers are used to immobilize sports injuries.

Surgery: In some cases, surgery is needed to fix sports injuries. Surgery can fix torn tendons and ligaments or put broken bones back in place. Most sports injuries don't need surgery.

Rehabilitation (exercise): Rehabilitation is a key part of treatment. It involves exercises that step by step get the injured area back to normal. Moving the injured area helps it to heal. The sooner this is done, the better. Exercises start by gently moving the injured body part through a range of motions. The next step is to stretch. After a while, weights may be used to strengthen the injured area.

As injury heals, scar tissue forms. After a while, the scar tissue shrinks. This shrinking brings the injured tissues back together. When this happens, the injured area becomes tight or stiff. This is when you are at greatest risk of injuring the area again. You should stretch the muscles every day. You should always stretch as a warm-up before you play or exercise.

Don't play your sport until you are sure you can stretch the injured area without pain, swelling, or stiffness. When you start playing again, start slowly. Build up step by step to full speed.

Rest: Although it is good to start moving the injured area as soon as possible, you must also take time to rest after an injury. All injuries need time to heal; proper rest helps the process. Your doctor can guide you on the proper balance between rest and rehabilitation.

Other therapies: Other common therapies that help with the healing process include mild electrical currents (electrostimulation), cold packs (cryotherapy), heat packs (thermotherapy), sound waves (ultrasound), and massage.

What can people do to prevent sports injuries?

These tips can help you avoid sports injuries.

- Don't bend your knees more than half way when doing knee bends.
- Don't twist your knees when you stretch. Keep your feet as flat as you can.
- When jumping, land with your knees bent.
- Do warm-up exercises before you play any sport.
- Always stretch before you play or exercise.
- Don't overdo it.
- Cool down after hard sports or workouts.
- Wear shoes that fit properly, are stable, and absorb shock.
- Use the softest exercise surface you can find; don't run on asphalt or concrete.
- Run on flat surfaces.

For adults:

- Don't be a "weekend warrior." Don't try to do a week's worth of activity in a day or two.
- Learn to do your sport right. Use proper form to reduce your risk of "overuse" injuries.
- Use safety gear.

- Know your body's limits.
- Build up your exercise level gradually.
- Strive for a total body workout of cardiovascular, strength-training, and flexibility exercises.

For parents and coaches:

- Group children by their skill level and body size, not by their age, especially for contact sports.
- Match the child to the sport. Don't push the child too hard to play a sport that she or he may not like or be able to do.
- Try to find sports programs that have certified athletic trainers.
- See that all children get a physical exam before playing.
- Don't play a child who is injured.
- Get the child to a doctor, if needed.
- Provide a safe environment for sports.

For children:

- Be in proper condition to play the sport.
- Get a physical exam before you start playing sports.
- Follow the rules of the game.
- Wear gear that protects, fits well, and is right for the sport.
- Know how to use athletic gear.
- Don't play when you are very tired or in pain.
- Always warm up before you play.
- Always cool down after you play.

What research is being done on treating sports injuries?

Today, treating a sports injury is much better than in the past. Most people who get sports injuries play sports and exercise again. Doctors have many new ways to treat sports injuries. Some of these new ways include the following:

- arthroscopy (fiber optic scopes put through small cuts in the skin to see inside joints)

- tissue engineering (using a person's own tissues or cells to help heal injuries)

- targeted pain relief (pain-reducing drug patches put directly on the injured area)

For Your Information

This publication contains information about medications used to treat the health condition discussed here. When this publication was printed, the National Institute of Arthritis and Musculoskeletal and Skin Diseases (NIAMS) included the most up-to-date (accurate) information available. Occasionally, new information on medication is released. For updates and for any questions about any medications you are taking, please contact the U.S. Food and Drug Administration at 888-INFO-FDA (888-463-6332, a toll-free call) or visit their website at http://www.fda.gov.

Section 8.2

Scientists Study Stress Fractures to Prevent Injuries

"Bone Scanned: Lab Research Tackles Problem of Stress Fractures in Military" and "Studies Planned to Discover Ways to Strengthen Bones," by Curt Biberdorf, *The Warrior*, U.S. Army Soldier Systems Center (Natick, MA), May-June 2004.

[Editor's note: While this text specifically relates to research being done by the Department of Defense relating to injuries soldiers acquire in the field, the program's director believes the information they learn can apply to any population of physically active people to help prevent stress fractures.]

Stress fractures caused by repetitive pounding activities of physical training take a toll on enough of the military population, specifically recruits, that a major research program called "Bone Health and

Medical Military Readiness" was started in 1997 to solve the problem.

With a collection of the latest research tools acquired since 2003, the Bone Health and Metabolic Laboratory at the U. S. Army Research Institute of Environmental Medicine (USARIEM) located at the U.S. Army Soldier Systems Center at Natick, MA, is ready to examine its piece of the puzzle.

"The goal of the whole program is to ultimately eliminate stress fractures," said Maj. Rachel Evans, a research physical therapist and director of bone health research. "Stress-fracture cases have been reported since the late 1800s and today are one of the most common and potentially debilitating overuse injuries seen in military recruits, particularly in women."

Stress fractures are overuse injuries that occur when muscles transfer the overload of strain to the bone, most commonly in the lower leg, and cause a tiny crack. They're tricky to see on x-ray and disrupt physical training, sidelining troops while costing the Defense Department as much as $100 million annually in medical costs and lost duty time, according to Evans.

Funded in part by Congress through the advocacy efforts of the National Coalition for Osteoporosis and Related Bone Diseases and the American Society for Bone and Mineral Research, and managed by USARIEM, overall research is multifaceted, examining factors such as gait mechanics, impact attenuation, and genetics. USARIEM research physiologists are studying specifically how exercise and nutrition influence stress fractures.

"A systematic approach to the study of stress fracture was needed, but hadn't been done," Evans said. "With this focused effort, and recent breakthroughs in technology, we're hoping to come up with science-based strategies to identify individuals at risk for stress fracture, and then prevent their occurrence through innovative training interventions."

Col. Karl Friedl, USARIEM commander, earlier in his career led a study on bone health at Fort Lewis, WA, and said the understanding of bone physiology is significantly advancing and has widespread ramifications on health. "There has been no program in the Department of Defense (DOD) that paid attention to bone health in the past," Friedl said. "Anything we can provide has the potential to save millions of dollars and enhance readiness through reduction in lost duty time, attrition from the military, and medical cost avoidance. We want to avoid occupationally induced stress fractures now, and osteoporosis and osteoarthritis later."

Noninvasive methods of studying bone health at USARIEM started in the early 1990s with the dual energy x-ray absorptiometry (DEXA) machine to measure bone density. Still in the lab, the older DEXA machines have been superseded by the superior software and scanning times in a new Prodigy fanbeam bone densitometer, according to Robert Mello, a research physiologist and the lab director.

The Prodigy scans total body bone density in 5-inch (instead of 1-inch) increments, increasing precision and cutting scan time from 30 minutes to six minutes. Improved software provides a clearer picture of total body composition and bone mineral density.

"We can look at regional areas of interest, such as sections of the tibia, forearm, or hip," Mello said. "Before, you had to scan an entire area. Just to have that capability is a major advance."

The Prodigy also allows researchers to scan small animals for studies on bone health, Evans said.

While the Prodigy gives a front-to-back, two-dimensional view, the peripheral quantitative computerized tomography machine allows researchers to analyze 3-D cross sections of spongy and outer bone. It's designed to reconstruct a volumetric model of bone, from which bone density, and for the first time, bone geometry, can be determined, Evans said.

"We can now look at cross-sectional images where stress fractures are most common," she said. "There's also software to quantify muscle mass at that point."

Another scanning instrument is the handheld ultrasound bone sonometer, which examines bone quality by measuring the speed of sound of ultrasonic waves axially transmitted along the bone. The results can then be used as an aid in the assessment of bone strength. "We can identify bones that may be at risk," Mello said. "The big thing is the portability so that it can easily be taken to the field."

To help understand the relationship between muscle mass and bone strength, the lab purchased an isokinetic dynamometer to assess muscle strength and endurance for the major joints of the body, except the neck.

Although research is focused on preventing stress fractures in the military, Evans said the information they learn can apply to any population of physically active people to help prevent stress fractures.

Four studies by USARIEM are planned in the next year [2005] to try to answer how muscle structure and function relate to bone quality. Researchers will examine whether differences in bone density and geometry exist between the right and left tibia, and then look at how that changes through physical training.

One objective is to find out the proper training balance, to see where bone strengthening ends and weakening begins. A third study will look at the effect of three 12-week exercise programs—aerobic training, strength training, and a combination of the two—against a sedentary control group.

"We want to look at what factors might build up bone," Evans said. "Maybe we can give [recruits] a program before going to basic training to ward off problems." Building on what they've learned in the experimental study, the plan is to transfer that information to actual basic combat training units to examine what risk factors, such as slender bones or low bone density, predispose trainees to injury.

Evans and Friedl gave examples of expected outcomes from current projects that USARIEM is managing. Soldiers with high risk for fracture may simply stand on a platform for 15-minute daily treatments of low-frequency vibration to stimulate bone development.

Recruits might benefit from specific guidance on physical training, and calcium and vitamin D supplementation resulting from studies now with navy basic trainees.

Various studies at USARIEM could lead to new recommendations on zinc and protein content in operational rations to optimize bone health. Even basic biology studies, such as one that demonstrated a refractory period in response of bone cells after mechanical stimulation, may affect military training with science-based advice to break up physical training into more than one session per day to maximize the benefit of bone health.

Section 8.3

New Insights into Devastating Basketball Foot Injury

From Duke University Medical Center News Office, March 13, 2004.
© 2004 Duke University Medical Center. Reprinted with permission.

After conducting a detailed analysis of the forces at work during commonly performed maneuvers by elite basketball players, Duke University Medical Center researchers believe they now better understand the causes of season-ending and potentially career-threatening stress fractures of the foot.

The solution, they continued, may be as simple as adding additional arch support to athletic shoes. This preventative action appears to relieve the constant stresses and pressures suffered by the fifth metatarsal, a bone on the outside of the mid-foot between the ankle bone and the small toe.

The results of the Duke study were presented March 13, 2004, at the annual meeting of the American Academy of Orthopedic Surgery by orthopedic surgeon Joseph Guettler, MD, of William Beaumont Hospital, Royal Oak, MI. Guettler conducted the research while a sports medicine fellow at Duke in the Michael W. Krzyzewski Human Performance Laboratory (K Lab) at Duke.

"These stress fractures of the fifth metatarsal are a prevalent and potentially devastating injuries suffered by elite basketball players, and they appear to occur as a result of the repetitive stresses placed on the bone," Guettler said. "The fractures are tiny, but over time they can coalesce into one large fracture. It is the equivalent in the foot of what happens in shin splints."

Since there have been few studies of stress fractures of the fifth metatarsal under "real-world" conditions, the Duke researchers wanted to characterize the stresses acting upon the bone, when they were most likely to occur, and if anything could be done to lessen the pressures.

For their analysis, the researchers recruited 11 male college basketball players. Electronic pressure sensors capable of continuous readings were inserted into the soles of their shoes. The researchers also placed electromyography (EMG) sensors on two of the muscles of the foot to measure the electrical activity of the muscles.

The players were then asked to perform three of the most common maneuvers experienced during a typical basketball game: landing on one foot following a jump during a simulated lay-up, changing direction 180 degrees during a side-to-side shuffle, and pivoting 180 degrees during a forward sprint.

Detailed measurements of maximum forces, work, and time elapsed were taken while players wore their normal shoes and also in shoes with accentuated arch support.

"The greatest elapsed time and greatest average work beneath the fifth metatarsal occurred during pivot moves," Guettler explained. "And the greatest forces were experienced when players landed after lay-ups. The forces under the fifth metatarsal were consistently greater when the maneuvers were performed in shoes without an enhanced medial arch."

"The added arch caused a statistically significant reduction in the maximum forces encountered under the fifth metatarsal during the pivot and lay-up maneuvers," he said. "Additionally, peak EMG measurements were higher for all the maneuvers for players with the arch. It appears that supporting the arch may reduce the stresses encountered beneath the fifth metatarsal and help prevent these injuries in the future."

The researchers said that muscles within the foot and how they respond also play an important role in determining whether or not a specific action has a negative effect on the fifth metatarsal. The finding that EMG activity was elevated when arch support was used is an interesting one, Guettler said, adding that this phenomenon is a future avenue of research.

"This study is a perfect example of the type of work conducted in the K Lab," said Claude T. Moorman, MD, director of sports medicine at Duke and senior member of the research team. "We identify a problem, conduct research to better understand the issues, and then come up with solutions—all with the goal of preventing injury and improving performance."

Moorman said that the Duke findings run counter to what had been assumed by shoe manufacturers—namely that high arch support was the cause of fifth metatarsal stress fractures. No one, however, had conducted the research to determine the answer, Moorman said.

Moorman and his K Lab colleagues are taking this research one step further. "We plan to use magnetic resonance imaging (MRI) techniques to image basketball players over time to hopefully gain a better understanding of the sequence of events leading up to the injury," Moorman continued. "The MRI is ideal for capturing the tiny fractures that are the hallmark of the condition."

Both Guettler and Moorman said that while the current study looked at elite athletes, the findings are also applicable to all types of athletes who participate in sports requiring similar maneuvers.

The study was supported by the K Lab and the Piedmont Society, a group founded by orthopedic surgeons who trained at Duke. Other members of the Duke were Gregory Riskan, Jeffrey Bytomski, DO, Christopher Brown, MD, and Jan Richardson, PhD.

Chapter 9

On Your Feet at Work

Chapter Contents

Section 9.1

Preventing Foot Pain in the Work Force

"Preventing Foot Pain in the Work Force" by Carolyn Neuhoff, November 17, 2003. Reprinted with permission from http://www.OccupationalHazards.com, November 2003. © 2003 Penton Media, Inc. All rights reserved.

Dr. William Scholl, designer of the Dr. Scholl's foot product line, often commented, "When your feet hurt, you hurt all over." An employee's efficiency level, concentration, willingness to work, and attitude greatly decrease when he is experiencing foot pain. This can lead to inattention on the part of employees, and, possibly, more injuries.

Detecting foot problems and resolving them quickly can also prevent injury to the knees, hips, or back caused by "favoring" a painful foot, which is potentially more expensive, more severe, and more difficult to relieve. In 1983, the American Podiatric Medical Association reported that 83 percent of the U.S. industrial work force had foot or lower leg problems resulting in discomfort, pain, or orthopedic deformities.

Most businesses have replaced the wood floors from 50 years ago with concrete, which is damaging to the lower extremities because it provides minimal resistance and no shock absorbency. It is becoming obvious that the percentage of employees that have foot and lower leg pain is increasing because of the longer standing requirements on the cement flooring.

Causes of Foot Pain

The most influential activity or foot position that affects foot pain is the stance. When a person is standing, the feet are dealing with two strong forces, one coming from the heel-to-ground contact and one from the vertical weight of the person. The three movements that are termed the "gait cycle" are also important in causing foot problems. The longest phase of the gait cycle is the contact. This accounts for 27 percent of the entire cycle and is where most of the damage takes place. A common problem is pronation, which is when a person turns the foot towards the inside so the sole bears most of the body weight,

98

and is constantly making unbalanced contact with the ground. This causes the person to re-adjust his knees, hips, pelvic region, and back to align himself enough to walk. When there is an onset of foot pain, notes the American Podiatric Medical Association (APMA), an employee should be examined by a podiatrist in order to prevent complications with the knee, hips, back, etc.

Standing all day at a workstation can be especially detrimental to a person's body, according to the Canadian Centre for Occupational Health and Safety (CCOHS). Standing for long periods of time causes a decrease in the blood supply to the lower extremities and therefore increases fatigue and soreness in the muscles. Also, prolonged standing creates an accumulation of blood in certain areas of the feet and legs, which leads to irritated and inflamed veins, otherwise known as varicose veins. In addition, the continuous pressure on a person's feet causes bone misalignment and joint degeneration.

Working in a mobile, rotating station is still bad for the lower extremities, but is better than stationary positions. When a person is in a rotating position, he or she is able to stretch and exercise different muscle groups and can avoid excessive stress from prolonged standing. However, at a stationary workstation, the feet and legs are under unrelenting gravity pressure, causing localized pressure points in the heels and the balls of the feet.

Eventually, this pressure can lead to stretching and straining of the plantar fascia, known as plantar fasciitis. It is estimated that 2 million people require treatment for plantar fasciitis in the United States every year. Plantar fasciitis is often associated with heel pain, but it involves more than the heel, notes APMA. There are many different causes of this diagnosis including: prolonged standing, structural biomechanical imbalance, irregular movement, and too much stress on the heel bone and attached tissues. Employees that stand on their feet all day are susceptible to this problem because of the amount of stress that is placed on the heel bone and the constant wear and tear of the connective tissues that comprise the plantar fascia.

The age of workers is gradually increasing as baby boomers (over 50 years old) keep their positions in factories and industries where standing all day is a job requirement. The age increase leads to more lower extremity injuries because when a person ages, all the tissues in the body, including ligaments, tendons, and fascia, lose their elasticity. The fascia and tendons decrease their shock absorbency and become more susceptible to tearing. The aging person also loses the fat pads on the bottom of the feet that helped absorb shock. Lastly, there is a decrease in the range of motion in elder employees due to the arthritic changes that occur. The decrease in range of motion leads to more shock transmitted up the leg, knee, and back because the foot joint no longer moves properly to absorb the shock.

Preventing Plantar Fasciitis

There are three basic ways that employers can attempt to prevent inflammation of the plantar fascia and minimize the occupational injury costs. Employers can add anti-fatigue matting to standing workstations, employees can wear anti-fatigue insoles in their shoes, and employees can perform preventative stretching, icing, and elevation before and after work.

Anti-fatigue mats are designed to decrease the stress on the feet and legs by providing a cushioning surface for people to stand on over prolonged periods of time, according to CCOHS. These mats can be made of rubber, carpet, vinyl, or even wood.

A customized "Lower Extremity Symptoms Survey" was developed for evaluating lower extremity limb discomfort at manufacturing facilities where workers stand all day to perform their tasks. In recent pilot studies at an aluminum manufacturing plant and a large engine plant, employees in standing positions were either interviewed or asked to complete the survey themselves. The results indicated that the use of wooden bricks in the assembly line floor greatly decreased their foot, ankle, knee, and back pain.

Both companies originally used wooden brick flooring. However, the aluminum plant is slowly replacing all the wooden bricks with cement as the bricks break. After speaking to employees, it was discovered that there was a significant degree of difference between their lower extremity discomfort when the old wooden bricks were in place and when the new cement was poured.

In order to compensate for the reported discomfort, the aluminum company provided rubber anti-fatigue matting at almost all standing workstations. This decreased some of the discomfort that began with the new cement floors. The anti-fatigue mats are most useful in stationary positions, because a mat may cause a tripping hazard to a mobile employee who is constantly moving on and off the mat.

Shoe insoles are ideal for mobile workstations. At the engine plant, there were numerous stations that required moving supplies repeatedly from one area to another area 20 feet away, which may be hazardous if mats are covering the floor. Insoles also provide relief by absorbing shock and preventing the degeneration of bone joints and bone structure.

The type of insole that will be most beneficial differs for each person. If an employee has pronated, or flat feet, then an arch support insole that has an arch build-up on the inside portion of the insole would be ideal. However, an employee who has high arches does not need an insole with arch support. Too much arch support for people who already have high arches could be more detrimental than beneficial. Instead, these workers should use flat, cushiony insoles.

Prepare for Work

A third part of the solution is to stress the importance of proper foot care and proper daily stretching of the plantar fascia. A person that is going to be standing, stationary or mobile, for an entire shift needs to properly prepare his or her feet daily.

There are certain stretching exercises that can be done in the morning, at lunch, and after work that will keep the muscles and ligaments warmed up and prepared to handle the physical stress of the day.

- Rolling an ordinary 12-ounce can under the arch of each foot for five minutes a foot is very useful in stretching the plantar fascia that runs along the arch of the foot.

- Picking up a towel off the ground using only the toes 30 times a foot stretches the forefoot muscles and the plantar muscles and tendons in the feet. These are the supporting muscles in the foot and are therefore the most important to warm up each day in order to prevent excessive strain and inflammation that result in serious pain and damage.

- Stretching the calf muscles by leaning against a wall with one knee bent and the other leg straight out behind you with both feet flat on the floor can be extremely beneficial. The plantar fascia attaches at the calcaneal and cuboidal bones and is stretched during these calf exercises.

Stretching, resting, elevating, and icing both feet for an hour after work will decrease swelling and help rejuvenate the feet for the following day.

Foot problems, especially plantar fasciitis, are a large problem in the standing work force. This diagnosis can lead to weeks of strapping and therapy (at up to $150 every visit) followed by functional orthotics (at approximately $400 per pair), and possibly surgery (approximately $5,000). Every person that works in a standing position is susceptible to these problems. Essentially, the cost may range between $2,000 and $5,000 (at minimum) per standing employee if this problem is not addressed and the proper precautions are not taken.

Anti-fatigue mats are recommended for all employees whose work requires them to stand the entire workday. Mobile employees should invest in an inexpensive shoe insole that will absorb the shock and allow them to move from position to position without the hazard of tripping, slipping, and falling. In either case, the results will greatly improve if the proper footwear is being used and maintained, and the daily exercises are being practiced in the morning, at lunch, and after work. If all of these recommendations are followed, it is very likely that employers will decrease their pay-out in the medical care of the employee's feet, ankles, legs, knees, lower extremities, and backs.

Tips for the Well-Heeled Worker

Employees should maintain well-fitting, well-padded shoes. If the arch support of the shoes has decreased and the soles are disintegrating, then the foot is no longer being supported. This leads to a decrease in the shock absorption from the soles and to improper foot alignment, and may cause bone and joint problems.

Regularly replacing shoes is key to decreasing foot pain, especially in standing employees. Some tips from the American Podiatric Medical Association for choosing proper footwear are: the shoe must grip the heel tightly, the forefoot area must be wide and allow movement, the inner aspect of the shoe should be straight from heel to toe, and there should be fastening across the arch to decrease pronation. The fastening keeps the shoe tight against the foot and helps to prohibit the foot from turning inside and transmitting excessive body weight to the sole.

The ideal time to purchase shoes is at the end of a workday due to the swelling that can accumulate throughout the day. Shoes need to be tried on before purchase and must be walked in, because when a person is standing or walking, their toes and arch structure spread out. This changes the fitting of the shoes because of the widening of the forefoot.

Section 9.2

Improving Foot Protection

"Footwear Safety FactSheet," 2006. Reprinted with permission from the Texas Department of Insurance, Division of Workers' Compensation. This fact sheet was published with information from the Houston, TX, Parks and Recreation Department; Simon Fraser University; the Canadian Centre for Occupational Health and Safety; the American Standards Institute; and the Texas Department of Insurance, Division of Workers' Compensation (DWC), and is considered factual at development.

Protective footwear worn in the workplace is designed to protect the foot from physical hazards such as falling objects, stepping on sharp objects, heat and cold, wet and slippery surfaces, and exposure to corrosive chemicals. As a worker, you should know the risks in your workplace and when selecting footwear, consider the safety hazards in your work area. This will help you select the right protective footwear. Ask your supervisor what protective footwear and other personal protective equipment is required. Also, The American National Standards Institute (ANSI) Standard Z41-1999 "Personal Protection—Protective Footwear" should be consulted. There is also the ANSI Z41 "User Guide for Protective Footwear."

When purchasing new protective footwear, it's important to get the right fit and comfort so they will not cause calluses, ingrown toenails, or simply tired feet that are common among workers who spend most of their working time standing or do a lot of walking. Although these may not be considered as occupational injuries, they can have serious consequences for health and safety at the workplace. They can cause discomfort, pain, and fatigue. Fatigue can cause a worker an injury affecting the muscles and joints. Also, a worker who is tired and suffering pain is less alert and more likely to act unsafely, which can cause an accident.

Before wearing new shoes or boots on the job, wear them at home until you're sure they fit well. Keep them clean until it is decided they fit and you are keeping them, that way there should not be a problem exchanging them for a different size or style. Always check the store's return policy prior to purchasing footwear.

What should I know about safety footwear?

- If you are at risk for foot injury at your workplace, you should wear the appropriate protective footwear.

- If foot protection is required in your workplace, your employer should implement a complete foot safety protection program including: selection, fit testing, training, maintenance, and inspection of footwear.

- Safety footwear is designed to protect feet against a wide variety of injuries. Impact, compression, and puncture are the most common types of foot injury.

- Choose footwear according to the hazards in your workplace.

- Ensure that the footwear has the proper sole for the working conditions.

- Use metatarsal protection (top of the foot between the toes and ankle) where there is a potential for injury.

What built-in protection features come in safety footwear?

- High-cut shoes or boots provide ankle support and keep sparks, molten metals, and chemicals from getting into the footwear.

- Reinforced safety toe, reinforced toecap, or steel toecap footwear will absorb the blow if a heavy object falls on the foot.

- Reinforced metal soles protect feet from punctures.

- Steel midsoles protect the foot against penetration by sharp objects.

- Non-slip footwear prevents the wearer from slipping on certain surface type.

- Insulated footwear provides protection in cold temperatures.

Are there special shoes or boots for special working conditions?

- Metal-free footwear is recommended when working around electricity.

- Footwear with rubber or wooden soles is recommended for traction on wet floors.

- Treated footwear is recommended because it is resistant to chemicals and corrosives.

What should I know about the fit and care of safety footwear?

Fit

- Walk in new footwear to ensure fit and comfort.

- Shoes/boots should have ample toe room (toes should be about one-half inch from the front).

- Make allowances for socks or special arch supports when buying shoes/boots.

- Shoes/boots should fit snugly around the heel and ankle when laced.

- Lace up shoes/boots fully to ensure comfort.

Care

- Apply a protective coating to make footwear water-resistant.

- Inspect footwear regularly for damage.

- Repair or replace worn or defective footwear.

How should I care for my feet?

Feet are subject to a great variety of skin and toenail disorders. Workers can avoid many of them by following simple rules of foot care:

- Wash feet daily with soap, rinse thoroughly and dry, especially between the toes.

- Trim toenails straight across and not too short. Do not cut into the corners.

- Wear clean socks or stockings and change them daily.

Some feet sweat more than others and are more prone to athlete's foot. Again, following a few simple guidelines may help:

- Select shoes made of leather or canvas—not synthetic materials.

- Keep several pairs of shoes on hand and rotate shoes daily to allow them to air out.

- For some workers, non-colored wool or cotton socks may be recommended since dyes may cause or aggravate skin allergies.

- Use foot powder.

- See a doctor for persistent ingrown toenails, calluses, corns, fungal infection, and more serious conditions such as flat feet and arthritis.

Remember to practice safety; don't learn it by accident.

Section 9.3

Foot Comfort and Safety at Work

"OSH Answers: Foot Comfort and Safety at Work," http://www.ccohs.ca/oshanswers/prevention/ppe/foot_com.html. Canadian Centre for Occupational Health and Safety (CCOHS), 2001. Reproduced with permission of CCOHS, 2006.

Why is foot comfort important?

Foot troubles may be perceived as a trivial matter, especially at work. However, as the old saying goes, "When your feet hurt, you hurt all over."

There are two major categories of work-related foot injuries. The first category includes foot injuries from punctures, crushing, sprains, and lacerations. They account for 10 percent of all reported disabling injuries. The second group of injuries includes those resulting from slips, trips, and falls. They account for 15 percent of all reported disabling injuries. Slips and falls do not always result in a foot injury, but lack of attention to foot safety plays an important role in their occurrence.

These two categories of foot injuries, however, do not exhaust the whole range of foot problems at work. There are also other conditions such as calluses, ingrown toenails, or simply tired feet that are common among workers. Although these may not be considered as occupational injuries in the strictest sense, they can have serious consequences for health and safety at the workplace. They cause discomfort, pain, and fatigue. Fatigue sets up the worker for further injuries affecting the muscles and joints. Also, a worker who is tired and suffering pain is less alert and more likely to act unsafely. An accident of any kind may result.

What are some causes of foot problems?

Some foot problems are so common that they can occur in virtually any workplace and under any working conditions (see Table 9.1). There are no comprehensive statistics on these kinds of problems with feet. Surveys suggest that two out of every three workers suffer from some form of a foot problem.

How does the working position contribute to the foot problem?

Common foot problems occur both on and off the job. Still, there is no doubt that some work-related factors can lead to foot problems, especially jobs that require long periods of standing. Since the human foot is designed for mobility, maintaining an upright stance is extremely tiring. Standing for hours, day after day, not only tires the worker's feet but can also cause permanent damage. Continuous standing can cause the joints of bones of the feet to become misaligned (that is, cause flat feet) and can cause inflammation that can lead later to rheumatism and arthritis.

How does the flooring contribute to the foot problems?

The type of flooring used in the workplace has an important influence on comfort, especially on tender feet. Hard, unyielding floors like concrete are the least comfortable surfaces to work on. Working on a

Table 9.1. Causes of foot problems.

Foot Problems	Common Causes
Severely aching feet, blisters, calluses, corns, rheumatism, arthritis, malformations of toes, fallen arches (flat feet), bunions, sprains	Long periods of standing, hard flooring, and poorly fitted footwear: high heels, pointed shoes, lack of arch support, too loose or too tight footwear
Sweaty feet, fungal infections (athlete's foot)	Hot and humid environment, strenuous work, foot wear with synthetic (nonporous) uppers

hard floor has the impact of a hammer, pounding the heel at every step. Slippery floors are hazardous for slips and falls that can result in sprained ankles or broken foot bones.

How does the footwear contribute to the foot problems?

Footwear that fits poorly or is in need of repair also contributes heavily to foot discomfort. Pointed toes and high heels are particularly inappropriate for working footwear.

Prolonged standing, hard flooring, and inappropriate footwear are common working conditions. Are there jobs that are safe for feet? Statistics show there are not, really. Among teachers and workers in clerical occupations that belong to "safe" jobs, foot injuries account for from 15 percent to more than 20 percent of all disabling injuries. Not knowing about the need for foot protection in workplaces like schools or offices can play a role in the onset of foot problems.

Table 9.2. Examples of workplace foot injuries.

Injuries	Common Causes
Crushed or broken feet, amputations of toes or feet	Feet trapped between objects or caught in a crack, falls of heavy objects, moving vehicles (lift trucks, bulldozers, etc.), conveyor belts (feet drawn between belt and roller)
Punctures of the sole of the foot	Loose nails, sharp metal, or glass objects
Cuts or severed feet or toes, lacerations	Chain saws, rotary mowers, unguarded machinery
Burns	Molten metal splashes, chemical splashes, contact with fire, flammable, or explosive atmospheres
Electric shocks	Static electricity, contact with sources of electricity
Sprained or twisted ankles, fractured or broken bones because of slips, trips, or falls	Slippery floors, littered walkways, incorrect footwear, poor lighting

Additional hazards for foot injury exist in outdoor jobs such as logging, hydro linework, or fishing which involve freezing temperatures, or wetness in low temperature: frostbite and trench foot. [See sections on frostbite, trench foot, and chilblains in Chapter 30 for more information.]

How can foot injuries be prevented?

There is no workplace where a worker is immune to foot injury. However, the hazards differ according to the workplace and the types of tasks the worker does. The first step in developing a strategy to reduce foot problems is to identify the relevant hazards at the workplace. Such hazards should be assessed in each workplace, no matter how safe or how dangerous it may seem.

How can the job design improve foot safety?

Aching, flat, or tired feet are common among workers who spend most of their working time standing.

The most important goal of job design is to avoid fixed positions especially fixed standing positions. Good job design includes varied tasks requiring changes in body position and using different muscles. Job rotation, job enlargement, and teamwork are all ways to make work easier on the feet.

- Job rotation moves workers from one job to another. It distributes standing among a group of workers and shortens the time each individual spends standing. However, it must be a rotation where the worker does something completely different such as walking around or sitting at the next job.

- Job enlargement includes more and different tasks in a worker's duties. If it increases the variety of body positions and motions, the worker has less chance of developing foot problems.

- Teamwork gives the whole team more control and autonomy in planning and allocation of the work. Each team member carries a set of various operations to complete the whole product. Teamwork allows workers to alternate between tasks which, in turn, reduces the risk of overloading the feet.

- Rest breaks help to alleviate foot problems where redesigning jobs is impractical. Frequent short breaks are preferable to fewer long breaks.

How can the workplace design improve foot safety?

However, redesigning the job alone will not effectively reduce foot problems if it is not combined with the proper design of the workplace.

- For standing jobs, an adjustable work surface is the best choice. If the work surface is not adjustable, two solutions include installing a platform to raise the shorter worker or a pedestal to raise the object for a taller worker.

- Work station design should allow the worker room to change body position.

- A foot-rail or footrest enables the worker to shift weight from one leg to the other. This ability reduces the stress on the lower legs and feet.

- Where possible, a worker should be able to work sitting or standing at will. Even when work can only be done while standing, a seat should be provided for resting purposes.

How can one improve the foot safety in workplaces where foot injuries occur frequently?

Job and workplace designs also have the potential to increase foot safety in workplaces that are specifically hazardous. Here are some examples:

- Separating mobile equipment from pedestrian traffic and installing safety mirrors and warning signs can decrease the number of accidents that might result in cut or crushed feet or toes.

- Proper guarding of machines such as chain saws or rotary mowers can avoid cuts or severed feet or toes.

- Effective housekeeping reduces the number of accidents at workplaces. For example, loose nails, other sharp objects, and littered walkways are hazards for foot injury.

- Using color contrast and angular lighting to improve depth vision in complicated areas such as stairs, ramps, and passageways reduces the hazard of tripping and falling.

How can the kind of floor improve foot comfort?

Standing or working on a hard, unyielding floor can cause a lot of discomfort. Wood, cork, carpeting, or rubber—anything that provides some flexibility—is gentler on workers' feet. Where resilient floors are not practical, footwear with thick, insulating soles and shock-absorbing insoles can alleviate discomfort. Anti-fatigue matting can also be useful wherever workers have to stand or walk. They provide a cushioning which reduces foot fatigue. However, the use of matting requires caution. When installed improperly, it can lead to tripping and slipping accidents.

Special anti-slip flooring or matting can reduce slipping accidents. If installed properly, these mats are useful, but workers may find that their feet burn and feel sore. The non-slip properties of the flooring mat cause their shoes to grab suddenly on the flooring making their feet slide forward inside the shoes. Friction inside the shoes produces heat that creates soreness and, eventually, calluses. A non-slip resilient insole can reduce this discomfort.

What should I know about footwear?

Proper footwear is important, not only for foot comfort but also for one's general well-being. Improper footwear can cause or aggravate existing foot problems. Unfortunately, being fashionable sometimes takes precedence over choosing well-fitting, supportive safety footwear. However, many safety footwear manufacturers produce safety footwear that does look fashionable.

The best way to involve workers in programs to protect their feet is to provide:

- training and information on the health hazards of wearing improper shoes,
- the principles for selecting proper ones, and,
- the simple rules of general foot care.

What should I know when I buy footwear for work?

Good footwear should have the following qualities:

- The inner side of the shoe must be straight from the heel to the end of the big toe.
- The shoe must grip the heel firmly.
- The forepart must allow freedom of movement for the toes.
- The shoe must have a fastening across the instep to prevent the foot from slipping when walking.
- The shoe must have a low, wide-based heel; flat shoes are recommended.

111

People buying footwear for work should take the following advice:

- Do not expect that footwear which is too tight will stretch with wear.

- Have both feet measured when buying shoes. Feet normally differ in size.

- Buy shoes to fit the bigger foot.

- Buy shoes late in the afternoon when feet are likely to be swollen to their maximum size.

- Ask a doctor's advice if properly fitting shoes are not available.

- Consider using shock-absorbing insoles where the job requires walking or standing on hard floors.

When selecting footwear, one should remember that tight socks or stockings can cramp the toes as much as poorly-fitted shoes. Wrinkled socks, or socks that are too large or too small, can cause blisters. White woolen or cotton socks may be recommended since colored socks cause skin allergies in some people.

What type of footwear is appropriate for cold conditions?

Selection should be made to suit the specific working condition. Working outdoors in cold weather poses a special requirement on selecting the proper footwear. "Normal" protective footwear is not designed for cold weather. "Insulated" footwear gives little temperature protection in the sole for it has no extra insulation there. Loss of heat through steel toe caps (commonly blamed for increased heat loss) is insignificant.

Foot protection against cold weather can be resolved by the following:

- Insulating the legs by wearing warmers—"dancercize" type.

- Wearing insulating overshoes over work footwear.

- Wearing insulating muffs around the ankles and over the top of the footwear.

How should I care about feet?

Feet are subject to a great variety of skin and toenail disorders. Workers can avoid many of them by following simple rules of foot care:

- Wash feet daily with soap, rinse thoroughly and dry, especially between the toes.

- Trim toenails straight across and not too short. Do not cut into the corners.

- Wear clean socks or stockings and change them daily.

Some feet sweat more than others and are more prone to athlete's foot. Again, following a few simple guidelines may help:

- Select shoes made of leather or canvas—not synthetic materials.

- Keep several pairs of shoes on hand and rotate shoes daily to allow them to air out.

- For some workers, non-colored woolen or cotton socks may be recommended since dyes may cause or aggravate skin allergies.

- Use foot powder.

- If problems persist, see a doctor.

In cases of persisting ingrown toenails, calluses, corns, fungal infection, and more serious conditions such as flat feet and arthritis, see a doctor and follow the doctor's advice.

What exercises can I do at the workstation?

Standing still requires considerable muscular effort. Even so, it is not exercise—only a strain. It does not allow for the alternate contracting and relaxing of muscles of the feet and legs.

To keep feet healthy, it is necessary to compensate for working in a stationary position. One action that can be done frequently on the job is alternately to contract and relax the calf muscles, and flex and straighten ankles and knees. Another bit of advice is to walk whenever practical instead of riding. More information on exercise for feet can be obtained from a foot specialist or from a local fitness center.

Section 9.4

Preventing Injuries from Slips, Trips, and Falls

This section contains excerpts from "Preventing Injuries from Slips, Trips, and Falls," Circular 869, Copyright © 2006, The University of Florida Cooperative Extension—Institute of Food and Agriculture Sciences. All rights reserved. Reprinted with permission. Revised May 2006. Please visit the Institute of Food and Agriculture Sciences website at http://edis.ifas.ufl.edu/AS042 for the complete text and references.

The Problem

For 2003, the National Safety Council reported that falls resulted in over 7 million visits to emergency rooms—leading all other causes of ER visits. Over 16,000 Americans died as the result of a fall in 2003.

In the workplace, the Bureau of Labor Statistics reported 4.4 million injuries for 2003. About a third of these resulted in days away from work, and of these, over 250,000 were falls, accounting for almost 20 percent of disabling workplace injuries. Injuries due to falls in the workplace typically resulted in 7 to 14 days away from work. About 700 workers died from a workplace fall in 2003.

The average direct cost for one disabling workplace injury has been estimated at $34,000. Taking into account indirect costs would make this number much higher. Estimates for indirect costs of injuries range from two to five times the direct cost. In the case of a death on the job, the average cost has recently been estimated at $1.15 million. Add to these the personal and family costs and trauma, and it is evident that slips, trips, and falls should be avoided.

A thorough analysis of falls in Florida agriculture was conducted in 1991, based on an analysis of workers' compensation records. Falls accounted for nearly 25 percent of all serious disabling work injuries: 17 percent were elevated falls, 8 percent were same-level falls. Elevated falls accounted for 26 percent of the injuries in fruit and vegetable production occupations. Same-level falls accounted for 12 percent in both livestock and horticultural production occupations.

In addition, 32 percent of all elevated falls in Florida agriculture were from ladders, while 25 percent were from vehicles and other mobile equipment. Same-level falls were on walking or working surfaces in 76 percent of the incidents.

The back was the most frequently injured part of the body in falls: 37 percent of the injuries were from elevated falls, while 29 percent were from same-level falls. The joints—wrist, elbow and shoulder, or the ankle, knee and hip—accounted for 32 percent of elevated falls and 47 percent of same-level falls.

Most injuries are sprains and strains: 52 percent from elevated falls, 46 percent from same-level falls. Fractures are the result of 19 percent of elevated falls and 10 percent of same-level falls. Bruises and contusions account for most of the remaining injuries.

Types of Falls

Falls are of two basic types: elevated falls and same-level falls. Same-level falls are most frequent, but elevated falls are more severe.

- **Same-level falls:** high frequency—low severity
- **Elevated falls:** lower frequency—high severity

Same-level falls are generally slips or trips. Injury results when the individual hits a walking or working surface or strikes some other object during the fall. Over 60 percent of elevated falls are from less than 10 feet.

Examples of same-level falls are described below.

Slip and Fall

Slips are primarily caused by a slippery surface and compounded by wearing the wrong footwear. In normal walking, two types of slips occur. The first of these occurs as the heel of the forward foot contacts the walking surface. Then, the front foot slips forward, and the person falls backward.

The second type of fall occurs when the rear foot slips backward. The force to move forward is on the sole of the rear foot. As the rear heal is lifted and the force moves forward to the front of the sole, the foot slips back and the person falls.

The force that allows you to walk without slipping is commonly referred to as "traction." Common experience shows that dry concrete sidewalks have good traction, while icy surfaces or freshly waxed floors can have low traction. Technically, traction is measured as the "coefficient of friction." A higher coefficient of friction means more friction, and therefore more traction. The coefficient of friction depends on two things: the quality of both the walking surface and the soles of your shoes.

To prevent slips and falls, a high coefficient of friction (COF) between the shoe and walking surface is needed. On icy, wet, and oily surfaces, the COF can be as low as 0.10 with shoes that are not slip resistant. A COF of 0.40 to 0.50 or more is needed for excellent traction. To put these figures in perspective, a brushed concrete surface and a rubber heel will often show a COF greater than 1.0. Leather soles on a wet smooth surface, such as ceramic tile or ice, may have a COF as low as 0.10.

Providing dry walking and working surfaces and slip-resistant foot-wear is the answer to slips and their resultant falls and injuries. Obviously, high heels, with minimal heel-to-surface contact, taps on heels, and shoes with leather or other hard, smooth-surfaced soles lead to slips, falls, and injuries. Shoes with rubber-cleated, soft soles and heels provide a high COF and are recommended for most agricultural work.

In work areas where the walking and working surface is likely to be slippery, non-skid strips or floor coatings should be used. Since a COF of 0.40 to 0.50 is preferred for walking and working surfaces, we should strive for a surface which provides a minimum of 50 percent of this friction. If the working surface is very slippery, no footwear will provide a safe COF.

Trip and Fall

Trips occur when the front foot strikes an object and is suddenly stopped. The upper body is then thrown forward, and a fall occurs.

As little as a three-eighth inch rise in a walkway can cause a person to "stub" his toe resulting in a trip and fall. The same thing can happen going up a flight of stairs: only a slight difference in the height of subsequent steps and a person can trip and fall.

Step and Fall

Another type of working and walking surface fall is the "step and fall." This occurs when the front foot lands on a surface lower than expected, such as when unexpectedly stepping off a curb in the dark. In this type of fall, the person normally falls forward. A second type of step and fall occurs when one steps forward or down, and either the inside or outside of the foot lands on an object higher than the other side. The ankle turns, and one tends to fall forward and sideways.

Contributing Factors

Proper housekeeping in work and walking areas can contribute to safety and the prevention of falls. Not only is it important to maintain a safe working environment and walking surface, these areas must also be kept free of obstacles which can cause slips and trips. One method which promotes good housekeeping in work environments is the painting of yellow lines to identify working and walking areas. These areas should never be obstructed by objects of any kind.

Adequate lighting to ensure proper vision is also important in the prevention of slips and falls. Moving from light to dark areas, or vice versa, can cause temporary vision problems that might be just enough to cause a person to slip on an oil spill or trip over a misplaced object.

Carrying an oversized object can also obstruct one's vision and result in a slip or a trip. This is a particularly serious problem on stairs.

Behaviors that Lead to Falls

In addition to wearing the wrong footwear, there are specific behaviors which can lead to slips, trips, and falls. Walking too fast or running can cause major problems. In normal walking, the most force is exerted when the heel strikes the ground, but in fast walking or running, one lands harder on the heel of the front foot and pushes harder off the sole of the rear foot; thus, a greater COF is required to prevent slips and falls. Rapid changes in direction create a similar problem.

Other problems that can lead to slips, trips, and falls are: distractions; not watching where one is going; carrying materials which obstruct view; wearing sunglasses in low-light areas; and failure to use handrails. These and other behaviors, caused by lack of knowledge, impatience, or bad habits developed from past experiences, can lead to falls, injuries, or even death.

Learning How to Fall

Naturally, the goal is not to slip, trip, and fall; however, the possibility of a fall still exists. There are correct ways to fall, however, the following procedures are recommended:

- Tuck your chin in, turn your head, and throw an arm up. It is better to land on your arm than on your head.

- While falling, twist or roll your body to the side. It is better to land on your buttocks and side than on your back.

- Keep your wrists, elbows and knees bent. Do not try to break the fall with your hands or elbows. When falling, the objective is to have as many square inches of your body contact the surface as possible, thus, spreading out the impact of the fall.

More about Shoes and Boots

According to the National Safety Council (NSC), there are 110,000 injuries each year to the feet and toes of United States workers, representing 19 percent of all disabling work injuries.

The most important protection is to wear the proper footwear for your work and environment. In most agricultural occupations the shoes or boots should provide three major types of protection.

- The soles and heels should be slip-resistant.
- The toe of the shoe should resist crushing injuries.
- The shoe should support the ankle.

ANSI sets standards for shoes and boots. Never purchase work shoes that do not meet these standards. A typical ANSI rating could be I-75 C-25. This means the toe will withstand 75 foot-pounds of impact and 2,500 pounds of compression.

Chevron or cleat-designed soles are definitely the best for slippery situations because of the suction or squeezing action they provide. The softer soles are better for slippery indoor conditions; the harder, more rugged cleat-type sole is preferred for tough outdoor use.

Leather covering the foot and ankle portion of the foot is preferred in most work environments. However, when working in wet environments or around chemicals, oils, greases, or pesticides, boots made of polyvinyl chloride (PVC), a blend of PVC and polyurethane, or neoprene should be used. Rubber is satisfactory for wet conditions, but not with pesticides or petroleum products.

When purchasing work shoes or boots, it is best to purchase them from a reputable dealer who handles quality footwear. A dealer who is informed of your work and work environment will be able to provide the correct footwear for you. Quality footwear for work is expensive; but not nearly as expensive or painful as broken foot bones or other injuries from a slip, trip, or fall.

—by Carol J. Lehtola, Charles M. Brown, and William J. Becker

Chapter 10

Diagnostic and Therapeutic Injection of the Ankle and Foot

The ankle and foot are susceptible to multiple injuries and inflammatory conditions[6] that are amenable to diagnostic and therapeutic injection.[7] This chapter covers the anatomy, pathology, diagnosis, and injection technique at common sites for which these procedures are applicable. These areas include the plantar fascia, ankle joint, tarsal tunnel, interdigital space, and first metatarsophalangeal joint.

Plantar Fascia

The plantar fascia, a band of connective tissue deep to the fat layer of the base (plantar aspect) of the foot, spans from the medial plantar tuberosity of the calcaneus to the base of the digits. It helps support the medial longitudinal arch of the foot.

Indications and Diagnosis

The plantar fascia is frequently a site of chronic pain.[8,9] Patients typically complain of pain that starts with the first step on arising in the morning or after prolonged sitting. Pain onset is usually insidious but also may commence after a traumatic injury. Diagnosis is made by eliciting pain with palpation in the region of the origin of the plantar fascia. Pain may be worsened by passive dorsiflexion of the foot.

Overpronation, pes cavus, and restricted foot dorsiflexion are common with this condition, although foot pronation itself has not been demonstrated to be a predisposing factor.[10]

Timing and Other Considerations

In plantar fasciitis, corticosteroid injection is a treatment option, usually after other therapeutic modalities have failed. These therapies include active stretching, and use of nonsteroidal anti-inflammatory drugs (NSAIDs), cushioning heel cups, nighttime plantar fascia splints, and foot orthoses.[11-13] Corticosteroid injection effectively provides pain relief,[14] although it carries the risk of plantar fascia rupture[15] and fat pad atrophy.

Technique

Pharmaceuticals and equipment are listed in Table 10.1. The patient is placed in the lateral recumbent position with the affected side down. The physician identifies the medial aspect of the foot and palpates the soft tissue just distal to the calcaneus, locating the point of maximal tenderness or swelling.

Approach and Needle Entry

At the defined soft tissue area, a 25-gauge, 1.5-inch needle is inserted perpendicular to the skin. The needle should be inserted directly down past the midline of the width of the foot. The physician should not inject into the fat pad at the base of the foot.

The pharmaceutical material is injected slowly and evenly through the middle one-third of the width of the foot while the needle is being withdrawn. The physician should avoid injecting through the base of the foot, because this approach can result in the complications of pharmaceutical leakage and fat pad atrophy.

The patient should remain in the supine position for several minutes after the injection. The physician may put the injected region through passive range of motion. The patient should remain in the office for 30 minutes after the injection to be monitored for adverse reactions. In general, patients should avoid any strenuous activity involving the injected region for at least 48 hours. Patients should be cautioned that they may experience worsening symptoms during the first 24 to 48 hours. This is related to a possible steroid flair, which can be treated with ice and NSAIDs (such as ibuprofen, naproxen). A follow-up examination within three weeks should be arranged.

Table 10.1. Equipment and pharmaceuticals.

Site	Syringe	Needle	Anesthetic	Corticosteroid	Hydrocortisone equivalents per injection (mg)
Plantar fascia	5 mL	25 gauge, 1.5 inch	2 mL of 1% lidocaine (Xylocaine) or 0.25% or 0.5% bupivacaine (Marcaine)	1 mL of Celestone* or 1 mL of 40 mg per mL of methylprednisolone (Solumedrol)	150 / 200
Ankle joint	10 mL (30 to 60 mL if aspirating)	25 gauge, 1 to 1.5 inch (18 gauge, 1.5 inch if aspirating)†	3 to 5 mL of 1% lidocaine or 0.25% or 0.5% bupivacaine	1 mL of Celestone or 1 mL of Solumedrol	150 / 200
Tarsal tunnel	3 to 5 mL	25 gauge, 1 or 1.5 inch	1 to 2 mL of 1% lidocaine or 0.25% or 0.5% bupivacaine	0.5 mL of Celestone or 0.5 mL of Solumedrol	75 / 100
Interdigital space	3 to 5 mL	25 gauge, 1.5 inch	2 mL of 1% lidocaine or 0.25% or 0.5% bupivacaine	0.5 mL of Celestone or 0.5 mL of Solumedrol	75 / 100
First metatarsophalangeal joint	3 mL (10 mL if aspirating)	25 to 27 gauge, 1 or 1.5 inch†	1 mL of 1% lidocaine or 0.25% or 0.5% bupivacaine	0.25 to 0.5 mL of Celestone or 0.25 to 0.5 mL of Solumedrol	37.5 to 57.5 / 50 to 100

*—1 mL of Celestone is 3 mg each of betamethasone sodium phosphate and betamethasone acetate.
†—A hemostat is needed to immobilize the needle when injection follows aspiration.

Ankle Joint

The ankle joint is formed by the articulation of the talus with the tibia and fibula. The medial and lateral malleoli of the tibia and fibula stabilize the talus.

Indications and Diagnosis

Arthritis of the ankle joint may occur in athletes with a history of trauma to the area, and in older patients, and can be an indication for corticosteroid joint injection. Besides osteoarthritis, rheumatoid arthritis, and acute traumatic arthritides, other indications for joint injection include crystalloid deposition disease, mixed connective tissue disease, and synovitis.[16,17] Pain and disability are the usual presenting complaints, and examination can reveal pain with limitation of motion, tenderness, swelling, crepitus, and deformity. Gait disturbance, erythema, and warmth to palpation also may be present. Radiographs may be helpful to support the diagnosis.

Timing and Other Considerations

Aspiration of the joint must be performed if infection is suspected. Infection is an absolute contraindication to corticosteroid joint injection. Aspiration also can be useful for confirming certain arthropathies such as crystalloid deposition disease and Lyme arthritis.

Technique

Pharmaceuticals and equipment are listed in Table 10.1. The patient is placed in the supine position with the ankle relaxed. The physician identifies the space between the anterior border of the medial malleolus and the medial border of the tibialis anterior tendon and palpates this space for the articulation of the talus and tibia.

Approach and Needle Entry

As with any joint aspiration or injection procedure, sterile technique must be followed. The needle is inserted into the identified space and directed posterolaterally. Reduced resistance will be felt on entering the joint space, making aspiration and the free flow of pharmaceuticals possible. When aspiration precedes injection, the needle is held with a hemostat while the syringe is changed. Follow-up care is the same as that described for injection of the plantar fascia.

Tarsal Tunnel

The tarsal tunnel is formed by the medial malleolus and a fibrous ligament, the flexor retinaculum. The posterior tibial nerve passes through the tunnel and can be compressed by any condition that reduces the space of the tunnel. The medial plantar, lateral plantar, and calcaneal branches of the posterior tibial nerve innervate the base of the foot.

Indications and Diagnosis

Patients with arthritis of the tarsal tunnel may complain of a burning sensation, pain, and paresthesias over the distribution of the posterior tibial nerve and its branches that worsen with weight bearing.[18] Symptoms are often related to chronic conditions such as impingement syndromes and hyperpronation, or may be secondary to acute trauma.[19,20] Eliciting a positive Tinel sign by tapping over the tarsal tunnel typically causes discomfort in the medial one-third of the distal plantar foot, although the entire plantar foot surface may be affected.

Timing and Other Considerations

Injection is a modality that is performed after a treatment program that can include stretching, rest, and the use of shoe inserts or orthoses, and NSAIDs.[21]

Technique

Pharmaceuticals and equipment are listed in Table 10.1. The patient is placed in the lateral recumbent position with the affected foot down. Behind the medial malleolus, the point over the posterior tibial nerve where percussion elicits the symptoms is identified. Having the patient actively invert the foot against resistance will help the physician identify the posterior tibial tendon. The nerve lies posterior to the tendon.

Approach and Needle Entry

At approximately 2 cm proximal to the identified location, the needle is inserted at an angle of 30 degrees to the surface of the skin and directed distally. This injection is relatively superficial. The final needle depth will be determined by the amount of subcutaneous tissue. The physician should aspirate before injecting to ensure that the needle is not in an artery or a vein. The pharmaceutical agent is injected slowly. Follow-up care is the same as that previously described.

Interdigital Space

The interdigital spaces of the foot are sites for the occurrence of painful neuromas, a condition termed Morton neuroma. The second and third common digital branches of the medial plantar nerve are the most frequent sites for development of interdigital neuromas.

Indications and Diagnosis

Morton neuromas develop secondary to chronic trauma and repetitive stress, as occurs in persons wearing tight-fitting or high-heeled shoes.[22] Pain and paresthesias are usually insidious at onset and are located in the interdigital space of the affected nerve. In some cases, the interdigital space between the affected toes may be widened as a result of an associated ganglion or synovial cyst. Pain is elicited in the affected interdigital space when the metatarsal heads of the foot are squeezed together. Injection with one percent lidocaine (Xylocaine) can be helpful in confirming the diagnosis.

Timing and Other Considerations

Treatment for Morton neuroma can include the use of NSAIDs, metatarsal pads, orthoses, proper footwear, and injection. Injection may be considered as an early therapeutic option.[23] Surgery is a last resort.

Technique

Pharmaceuticals and equipment are listed in Table 10.1. The patient is placed in a supine position with the knee in a supported flexed position (that is, with a pillow beneath it) and the foot in a relaxed neutral position. The physician palpates the area of tenderness and fullness on the dorsum of the foot between the affected metatarsal heads.

Approach and Needle Entry

Injection is performed by inserting the needle on the dorsal foot surface in the distal to proximal direction, at an angle of 45 degrees, and down to the area of fullness between the metatarsal heads. Position is key, because plantar fat pad atrophy can occur if the fat pad is injected.[24] Follow-up care is the same as that previously described.

First Metatarsophalangeal Joint

The first metatarsophalangeal joint varies in size and shape, and it may be difficult to palpate in patients with conditions such as advanced degenerative arthritis.

Indications and Diagnosis

Diagnostic aspiration or therapeutic injection of the first metatarsophalangeal joint can be performed in the management of advanced osteoarthritis, rheumatoid arthritis, and other inflammatory arthritides such as gout, or for synovitis or an arthrosis such as "turf toe."[25-27] Turf toe, a painful ligamentous injury resulting from hyperextension of the first metatarsophalangeal joint, often occurs in football linemen. Diagnosis of the specific underlying condition entails eliciting supporting historic and physical findings and, possibly, diagnostic laboratory tests and imaging studies.

Timing and Other Considerations

Treatment is specific to the underlying condition. Injection may be considered as a diagnostic or therapeutic adjunct. Aside from diagnostic aspiration, therapeutic injection may be used early in the course of certain inflammatory arthritides, such as gout.

Technique

Pharmaceuticals and equipment are listed in Table 10.1. The patient is placed in a supine position with the knee in a supported flexed position (e.g., with a pillow beneath the knee), and the foot is firmly supported by the table. The physician palpates the joint line on the dorsum of the foot and passively flexes and extends the toe to locate the joint line.

Approach and Needle Entry

Distal traction may be applied to the great toe to open the joint space. The needle is inserted on the dorsomedial or dorsolateral surface. The needle should be angled 60 to 70 degrees to the plane of the foot and pointed distally to match the slope of the joint. The joint space is not deep below the skin surface. The physician should aspirate before injecting; the injectable agent should flow without major resistance when the needle is positioned properly in the joint space. Follow-up care is the same as that previously described.

—*by Alfred F. Tallia, MD, MPH,*
and Dennis A. Cardone, DO, CAQSM

References

1. Cardone, D.A., Tallia, A.F. Joint and soft tissue injection. *Am Fam Physician* 2002; 66:283-8.

2. Tallia, A.F., Cardone, D.A. Diagnostic and therapeutic injection of the shoulder region. *Am Fam Physician* 2003; 67:1271-8.

3. Cardone, D.A., Tallia, A.F. Diagnostic and therapeutic injection of the elbow region. *Am Fam Physician* 2002; 66:2097-100.

4. Tallia, A.F., Cardone, D.A. Diagnostic and therapeutic injection of the wrist and hand region. *Am Fam Physician* 2003; 67:745-50.

5. Cardone, D.A., Tallia, A.F. Diagnostic and therapeutic injection of the hip and knee region. *Am Fam Physician* 2003; 67:2147-52.

6. Omey, M.L., Micheli, L.J. Foot and ankle problems in the young athlete. *Med Sci Sports Exerc* 1999; 31(7 suppl):S470-86.

7. Kerlan, R.K., Glousman, R.E. Injections and techniques in athletic medicine. *Clin Sports Med* 1989; 8:541-60.

8. Barrett, S.J., O'Malley, R. Plantar fasciitis and other causes of heel pain. *Am Fam Physician* 1999; 59: 2200-6.

9. Silko, G.J., Cullen, P.T. Indoor racquet sports injuries. *Am Fam Physician* 1994; 50:374-80,383-4.

10. Cornwall, M.W., McPoil, T.G. Plantar fasciitis: etiology and treatment. *J Orthop Sports Phys Ther* 1999; 29:756-60.

11. Bedinghaus, J.M., Niedfeldt, M.W. Over-the-counter foot remedies. *Am Fam Physician* 2001; 64:791-6.

12. Young, C.C., Rutherford, D.S., Niedfeldt, M.W. Treatment of plantar fasciitis. *Am Fam Physician* 2001; 63:467-74,477-8.

13. Ryan, J. Use of posterior night splints in the treatment of plantar fasciitis. *Am Fam Physician* 1995; 52:891-8,901-2.

14. Furey, J.G. Plantar fasciitis. The painful heel syndrome. *J Bone Joint Surg* [Am] 1975; 57:672-3.

15. Beals, T.C., Pomeroy, G.C., Manoli, A. 2d. Posterior tendon insufficiency: diagnosis and treatment. *J Am Acad Orthop Surg* 1999; 7:112-8.

16. Padeh, S., Passwell, J.H. Intraarticular corticosteroid injection in the management of children with chronic arthritis. *Arthritis Rheum* 1998; 41:1210-4.

17. Khoury, N.J., el-Khoury, G.Y., Saltzman, C.L., Brandser, E.A. Intraarticular foot and ankle injections to identify source of pain before arthrodesis. *AJR Am J Roentgenol* 1996; 167:669-73.

18. Lau, J.T., Daniels, T.R. Tarsal tunnel syndrome: a review of the literature. *Foot Ankle Int* 1999; 20:201-9.

19. Oh, S.J., Meyer, R.D. Entrapment neuropathies of the tibial (posterior tibial) nerve. *Neurol Clin* 1999; 17: 593-615,vii.

20. Schwartzman, R.J., Maleki, J. Postinjury neuropathic pain syndromes. *Med Clin North Am* 1999; 83:597-626.

21. Malusky, L.P. Podiatric procedures. In Roberts, J.R., Hedges, J.R., eds. *Clinical procedures in emergency medicine.* 3d ed. Philadelphia: Saunders, 1998: 879-80.

22. Wu, K.K. Morton's interdigital neuroma: a clinical review of its etiology, treatment, and results. *J Foot Ankle Surg* 1996; 35:112-9.

23. Greenfield, J., Rea, J. Jr., Ilfeld, F.W. Morton's interdigital neuroma. Indications for treatment by local injections versus surgery. *Clin Orthop* 1984; 185: 142-4.

24. Basadonna, P.T., Rucco, V., Gasparini, D., Onorato, A. Plantar fat pad atrophy after corticosteroid injection for an interdigital neuroma: a case report. *Am J Phys Med Rehabil* 1999; 78:283-5.

25. Boxer, M.C. Osteoarthritis involving the metatarsophalangeal joints and management of metatarsophalangeal joint pain via injection therapy. *Clin Podiatr Med Surg* 1994; 11:125-32.

26.   Solan, M.C., Calder, J.D., Bendall, S.P. Manipulation and injection for hallux rigidus. Is it worthwhile? *J Bone Joint Surg* [Br] 2001; 83:706-8.

27.   Mizel, M.S., Michelson, J.D. Nonsurgical treatment of monarticular nontraumatic synovitis of the second metatarsophalangeal joint. *Foot Ankle Int* 1997; 18:424-6.

Chapter 11

Gait Analysis and Other Diagnostic Tests

A gait analysis test is completely noninvasive. The patient is usually evaluated using a team approach. The team examines the patient and determines the extent of the testing for each individual case. Markers are then placed on the patient at specific anatomical locations, and the subject walks down a walkway at a predetermined speed. An array of measuring devices is focused on the walkway and data is collected through a central computer. The main source of data is a computerized video analysis system that collects motion data, and a force plate that measures external forces on the lower extremity. The tests require about two hours. The data is then stored and processed through computerized reduction and analysis. Experts in biomechanics then review this data and a report is produced summarizing the data, relevant findings, and recommended treatment options.

Using the data gathered during a gait analysis session, a solid surface three-dimensional model of a patient's motion can be developed using available software. This model allows physicians and health care providers visualize the data in a format other than charts and graphs.

Pain in the lower extremities is often felt during movement only, and will frequently radiate from the actual site of the injury or dysfunction. Many tests available to physicians of the lower extremity are limited in their ability to discover the source of this discomfort and measure the success of treatment. Some of the options available are as follows:

"Gait Analysis Lab," © 2002 Rosalind Franklin University of Medicine and Science. Reprinted with permission.

- Physicians and therapists can manually evaluate patients for variations in the range of motions of a body segment.

- A radiograph can show structural defects.

- An MRI can show abnormal tissue structure.

- Electromyograms can show defects in the transmission of signals in the various neuromuscular groups.

- Isokinetic machines can measure relative strength of a muscle group.

Most of these tests are considered passive or static measurements in that little or no activity is initiated by the patient on the affected area and under the same conditions when the pain is occurring.

Gait analysis, on the other hand, provides the patient with an active or dynamic measurement. This is testing during movement, thereby allowing the dysfunction to occur in a near natural state while under controlled testing conditions.

By studying the motion of the lower extremities, combined with the forces acting on those extremities, gait experts are usually able to identify the source of the pain or dysfunction. Often treatment based on other diagnostic methods means treating symptoms of the dysfunction. This results in a lengthy trial and error period because identification of the source of the problem can not be made without continuous movement of the lower extremity. Gait analysis allows for such movement and exertion of the lower extremities; thus the source of the pain or dysfunction can usually be identified and treated.

Available Tests

Computerized Gait Analysis

Computerized video cameras capture the motion while force plates record the ground reactive forces. This data is then used to calculate the parameters of gait and other motions such as muscle forces, joint movements, power, work, and energy. The recorded data is then compared to standard parameters in similar patient populations from a database.

Electromyography

Surface electrodes record the electrical activity of muscles during standard movements. This test may be performed separately or synchronized with the computerized gait analysis.

Foot Pressure Analysis (F-Scan Pedobarograph)

In-shoe disposable sensors record the pressures under the foot during walking or running. Similar sensors in the walkway can show barefoot pressures with ambulation. These tests are helpful in the diabetic population to predict ulcers and can be used to test orthotic and bracing devices.

Force Platform Analysis

This provides data on the ground reactive forces as a patient walks or stands on the plates. It is usually used in conjunction with the computerized video analysis, but can also be used independently to provide data on center of gravity and relative stability of patients.

Laser Topographical Anatomy

Uses laser beams to map surface anatomy accurately and reliably. It is generally used for orthotic purposes, but it also has the potential of measuring wound volumes of ulcerations to document the healing of such wounds.

Stability or Instability in Stance

Using the force plates and pressure sensor, tests similar to the balance master system can be performed to measure postural stability in the geriatric population.

Three-Dimensional Computer Modeling

Using the data gathered during a gait analysis session, a solid surface three-dimensional model of a patient's motion can be developed using available software. This model allows physicians and health care providers to visualize the data in a format other than charts and graphs.

Chapter 12

Common Foot Surgeries

Chapter Contents

Section 12.1

Foot Surgery and Other Procedures

This section contains excerpts from "Taking Care of Your Feet" by Michelle Meadows, *FDA Consumer Magazine*, U.S. Food and Drug Administration, March-April 2006.

Types of Foot Surgery and Less-Invasive Procedures

Common types of foot surgery include surgery to correct bunions, surgery for fungal nails when medications don't work, and surgery to reduce arthritis pain. For people who have chronic ingrown toenails, a procedure called matrixectomy may be used to prevent recurring problems. Jane Andersen, DPM, a podiatrist in Chapel Hill, NC, says, "We numb the toe and remove the smallest amount of the nail on the side, usually about one-eighth of an inch, and then use a chemical to kill the root or remove the root of the nail surgically."

Sometimes, bunions can be treated without surgery, but when bunions limit or affect one's daily activities, bunion surgery may be appropriate. Pain is the big factor here. Joshua Kaye, DPM, a podiatrist in Los Angeles, says, "Bunion surgery may also be warranted if there is chronic inflammation and the person gets no relief from nonsteroidal antiinflammatory drugs and other conservative treatments."

Kaye says there are two main components to bunion problems. "One problem is the pain associated with shoe pressure against the bony enlargement," he says. "The second condition is a stiff toe joint that causes internal joint pain during movement of the big toe. Both or either of these problems can occur."

Advanced surgical techniques have improved outcomes for bunion surgery. The type of surgery needed depends on the patient's age, activity level, and degree of deformity. Kaye says he doesn't only remove the "bump of bone," which won't usually produce lasting results. "We realign the bone and use a surgical screw for stable bone alignment," he says. Recovery time usually takes about four weeks.

"The precision in which the bone is cut, shaped, and realigned is critical," Kaye says. Though consumers may see lasers publicized to treat bunions, lasers can't cut bone or correct bunions, he says. Lasers are not cleared by the U.S. Food and Drug Administration (FDA) for these indications.

According to the American College of Foot and Ankle Surgeons (ACFAS), there have also been advances in less invasive foot and ankle surgery. Newer surgical plates and screws let surgeons repair fractures with less trauma. Smaller incisions mean less bleeding and tissue damage.

In ankle arthroscopy, surgeons look at the ankle joint with a fiber optic camera system. This technique has been applied to knee surgery for several years, but now it's being used for bones and joints in the foot and ankle. This type of surgery can relieve inflammation from arthritis and ligament damage, with reduced recovery time as compared to open surgical procedures.

Before considering any surgery, people should always explore and discuss the nonsurgical options with their doctor, and the benefits and risks of surgery. It is also important to consider the doctor's experience and results with the procedure.

Cosmetic Foot Surgery

The American Orthopaedic Foot and Ankle Society (AOFAS) has released statements warning about trends in cosmetic surgery to improve the appearance of the foot. "Some women are getting surgeries to shorten toes and narrow their feet so they can fit into fashionable shoes," says Sharon Dreeben, MD, chairwoman of the AOFAS Public Education Committee and an orthopedic surgeon in La Jolla, CA.

"A woman recently called asking if I would inject collagen into her heel, and she will probably go doctor shopping to find someone who will do it," Dreeben says. "Some people want more padding to have cushion for high heels. But cosmetic foot surgery can result in chronic pain, infection, and nerve injury."

Dreeben has had to fix problems from cosmetic foot surgery that went wrong. "One woman had bunion surgery even though she hadn't been experiencing pain," she says. "She ended up with more problems, including nerve pain and difficulty walking."

The AOFAS defines cosmetic foot surgery as surgery that is aimed at only improving appearance. Dreeben says, "Foot surgery should only be used if the goal is to provide pain relief, improve function, or enhance quality of life during normal activities of daily living."

"I tell people: One difference between cosmetic surgery on the face and cosmetic surgery on the feet is that you don't walk around on your face. When you readjust one piece in the foot, it can affect everything."

Shock Wave Therapy

The most common cause of heel and arch pain is painful stretching or tearing of the plantar fascia, which runs along the bottom of the foot and supports the arch of the foot. Extracorporeal shock wave treatment is an outpatient procedure in which a medical device uses shock waves to relieve chronic heel pain. A dome filled with water is placed against the heel so shock waves pass through. The shock waves increase blood flow to trigger the healing process so that inflammation and pain subside.

FDA-approved devices for this procedure are the OssaTron, made by SANUWAVE Inc. of Marietta, GA; The Epos Ultra, made by Dornier MedTech, Kennesaw, GA; and the Orbasone Pain Relief System, made by Orthometrix Inc., White Plains, NY. People who have bleeding disorders, who are taking blood-thinning medication, or who are pregnant, should not undergo shock wave therapy. Complications can include mild neurological symptoms and tears in the tissue in the bottom of the foot.

Section 12.2

Forefoot Surgery

When Is Foot Surgery Necessary?

Many foot problems do not respond to "conservative" management. Your podiatric physician can determine when surgical intervention may be helpful. Often when pain or deformity persists, surgery may be appropriate to alleviate discomfort or to restore the function of your foot.

Bunions

A common deformity of the foot, a bunion is an enlargement of the bone and tissue around the joint of the big toe. Heredity frequently plays a role in the occurrence of bunions, as it does in other foot conditions. When symptomatic, the area may become red, swollen, and inflamed, making shoe gear and walking uncomfortable and difficult. If conservative care fails to reduce these symptoms, surgical intervention may be warranted. Your podiatric physician will determine the type of surgical procedure best suited for your deformity, based on a variety of information which may include x-rays and gait examination.

Hammer Toes

A hammer toe deformity is a contracture of the toe(s), frequently caused by an imbalance in the tendon or joints of the toes. Due to the "buckling" effect of the toe(s), hammer toes may become painful secondary to footwear irritation and pressure. Corn and callus formation may occur as a hammer toe becomes more rigid over time, making it difficult to wear shoes. Your podiatric physician may suggest correction of this deformity through a surgical procedure to realign the toe(s).

Neuroma

An irritation of a nerve may produce a neuroma, which is a benign enlargement of a nerve segment, commonly found between the third and fourth toes. Several factors may contribute to the formation of a neuroma.

Trauma, arthritis, high-heeled shoes, or an abnormal bone structure are just some of the conditions that may cause a neuroma. Symptoms such as burning or tingling in the ball of the foot or in the adjacent toes and even numbness are commonly seen with this condition. Other symptoms include swelling between the toes and pain in the ball of the foot when weight is placed on it.

Those suffering from the condition often find relief by stopping their walk, taking off their shoe, and rubbing the affected area. At times, the patient will describe the pain as similar to having a stone in his or her shoe.

Your podiatric physician will suggest a treatment plan. If conservative treatment does not relieve the symptoms, then your podiatric physician will decide, on the basis of your symptoms, whether surgical treatment is appropriate.

Bunionette (Tailor's Bunion)

A protuberance of bone at the outside of the foot behind the fifth (small) toe, the bunionette or "small bunion" is caused by a variety of conditions including heredity, faulty biomechanics (the way one walks), or trauma, to name a few. Pain is often associated with this deformity, making shoes very uncomfortable and at times even walking becomes difficult. If severe and conservative treatments fail to improve the symptoms of this condition, surgical repair may be suggested. Your podiatric physician will develop a surgical plan specific to the condition present.

Bone Spurs

A bone spur is an overgrowth of bone as a result of pressure, trauma, or reactive stress of a ligament or tendon. This growth can cause pain and even restrict motion of a joint, depending on its location and size. Spurs may also be located under the toenail plate, causing nail deformity and pain. Surgical treatment and procedure is based on the size, location, and symptoms of the bone spur. Your podiatric physician will determine the surgical method best suited for your condition.

Preoperative Testing and Care

As with anyone facing any surgical procedure, those undergoing foot and ankle surgery require specific tests or examinations before surgery to improve a successful surgical outcome. Prior to surgery, the podiatric physician will review your medical history and medical conditions. Specific diseases, illnesses, allergies, and current medications need to be evaluated. Other tests that help evaluate your health status may be ordered by the podiatric physician, such as blood studies, urinalysis, EKG, x-rays, a blood flow study (to better evaluate the circulatory status of the foot/legs), and a biomechanical examination. A consultation with another medical specialist may be advised by a podiatric physician, depending on your test results or a specific medical condition.

Postoperative Care

The type of foot surgery performed determines the length and kind of aftercare required to assure that your recovery from surgery is rapid and uneventful. The basics of all postoperative care involve to some degree each of the following: rest, ice, compression, and elevation. Bandages, splints, surgical shoes, casts, crutches, or canes may be necessary to improve and ensure a safe recovery after foot surgery. A satisfactory recovery can be hastened by carefully following instructions from your podiatric physician.

Your Feet Aren't Supposed to Hurt

Remember that foot pain is not normal. Healthy, pain-free feet are a key to your independence. At the first sign of pain, or any noticeable changes in your feet, seek professional podiatric medical care. Your feet must last a lifetime, and most Americans log an amazing 75,000 miles on their feet by the time they reach age 50. Regular foot care can make sure your feet are up to the task. With proper detection, intervention, and care, most foot and ankle problems can be lessened or prevented. Remember that the advice provided in this text should not be used as a substitute for a consultation or evaluation by a podiatric physician.

Section 12.3

Ankle Replacement Surgery (Ankle Arthroplasty)

"Ankle Replacement," © 2006 A.D.A.M., Inc. Reprinted with permission. Updated July 5, 2005, by A.D.A.M. editorial staff and Kevin B. Freedman, MD, MSCE.

Alternative names: Ankle arthroplasty—total; Total ankle arthroplasty

Definition: Ankle replacement involves replacing the damaged parts of the three bones that make up the ankle joint with artificial joint parts (prosthetic components) made of high-quality metal and plastic. The parts are typically held in place by bone cement. The artificial joints come in different sizes to fit the patient.

Description

The patient may receive general anesthesia (unconscious, no pain) or a spinal anesthetic (awake, but no feeling below the waist). Patients receiving spinal anesthesia also receive medicine to help them relax during the operation.

The surgeon makes an incision in the front of the ankle to expose the ankle joint. After gently pushing the tendons to the side, the surgeon disconnects the shin bone (tibia) and the smaller lower leg bone (fibula) from the main bone of the ankle (talus). The damaged surfaces of the bones are removed, and the artificial joint is attached. Screws are also commonly used to help support the artificial ankle. After putting the tendons back into place, the surgeon closes the wound with stitches. A brace may be used to keep the ankle from moving.

Indications

Ankle replacement surgery may be performed if the ankle joint has been severely damaged. Causes of damage include:

- osteoarthritis;
- rheumatoid arthritis;
- fracture;
- arthritis due to previous ankle surgery.

Risks

Risk for any type of surgery includes:

- bleeding;
- blood clot;
- infection.

Additional risks for ankle replacement surgery include:

- loosening of the artificial joint over time;
- nerve damage;
- blood vessel damage;
- bone break during surgery;
- ankle weakness, stiffness, instability;
- dislocation of the artificial joint;
- allergic reaction to the implant.

Expectations after Surgery

The patient will be in the hospital up to four days. Physical therapy to improve ankle motion may be prescribed a few days after the procedure. To avoid swelling, the foot may be raised higher than the heart while sleeping or resting.

Convalescence

Recovery can take two to three months. The patient should stay off their foot for several weeks, and use a walker or crutches. High-impact activities, such as step aerobics, should be avoided while recovering from ankle replacement surgery.

A successful ankle replacement will eliminate pain and allow the ankle to move up and down. In general, total ankle replacements last from 10 to 15 years, depending on the patient's activity level and overall health.

It is important to note that there are few, medium- to long-term studies yet on the newer total ankle replacement procedures. Early results are promising, but complication rates may be as high as 25 percent. Discuss the risks and benefits of this procedure with your health care provider.

References

Su, E.P., Kahn, B., Figgie, M.P. Total ankle replacement in patients with rheumatoid arthritis. *Clin Orthop Relat Res.* 2004 July; (424):32-8.

Knect, S.I., Estin, M., Callaghan, J.J., et al. The Agility total ankle arthroplasty. Seven- to sixteen-year follow-up. *J Bone Joint Surg Am.* 2004 June; 86-A(6):1161-71.

Hebert, M.B., Coetzee, J.C. *The Agility Total Ankle Replacement: A Prospective Outcome Study with Minimum Two Year Follow-Up.* Washington, DC. American Academy of Orthopaedic Surgeons' 2005 Annual Meeting. Podium Presentation. February 24, 2005. Paper No: 126.

Section 12.4

Diabetics Fare Worse after Ankle Fracture Surgery

From Duke University Medical Center News Office, August 15, 2005.
© 2005 Duke University Medical Center. Reprinted with permission.

In the largest analysis of its kind, Duke University Medical Center researchers have found that patients with diabetes who require surgery for ankle fractures have significantly higher rates of complications and higher hospital costs compared to non-diabetic patients.

Specifically, the researchers found that diabetics experienced one additional day of hospitalization (an average of 4.7 versus 3.6 days) with costs approximately 20 percent higher ($12,898 versus $10,794). Additionally, diabetics had higher mortality rates (0.26 percent versus 0.11 percent) and higher rates of postoperative complications (4.63 percent versus 3.27 percent).

Demonstrating this link between diabetes and worse outcomes is important, the researchers said, because ankle fractures are one of the most common injuries treated by orthopedic surgeons, and the study's findings provide guidance on how to improve the care for these patients and reduce health care expenditures.

The results of the Duke analysis were published August 15, 2005, in the *Journal of Bone and Joint Surgery*.

"While a number of smaller studies have indicated that diabetic patients tended to have worse outcomes after ankle surgery, this is the first large-scale analysis of a cross-section of patients across the U.S.," said Shanti Ganesh, MPH, lead author of the study and fourth-year medical student at Duke University School of Medicine.

"This analysis demonstrated that diabetic patients, no matter how severe the ankle fracture, were more likely to experience higher rates of postoperative complications, mortality, and non-routine discharge, with accompanying longer lengths of hospital stay and higher hospital charges," Ganesh said.

For their analysis, the Duke team consulted the Nationwide Inpatient Samples (NIS) database and identified 169,598 patients who underwent surgery for ankle fractures. The NIS, sponsored by the U.S. Agency for Healthcare Research and Quality, is a publicly available database of more than 8 million patients from more than 1,000 U.S. hospitals. The hospitals vary by region, size, location, teaching status, and ownership.

"The strength of this analysis is that it provides a nationally representative and real-world picture of what happens to ankle fracture patients in the U.S.," said Ricardo Pietrobon, MD, senior member of the research team and director of Duke's Center for Excellence in Surgical Outcomes (CESO), which supported the analysis. "We were unable to extrapolate from the data gathered from smaller, single-center studies what the situation was nationwide." Now we have specific data that allows us to quantify the added risks and costs of diabetes for these patients," Pietrobon continued. "This information is crucial in improving outcomes and quality of life for our patients undergoing surgery to repair ankle fractures."

Of the 169,598 ankle fracture patients, the Duke team identified 9,174 (5.71 percent) with diabetes. The diabetic patients tended to be more than 10 years older than the non-diabetic patients, and when they did suffer ankle fractures, they tended to be more severe than those suffered by non-diabetic patients.

Ganesh said that the results of the study indicate that physicians taking care of ankle fracture patients should appreciate the effect that diabetes can have on the treatment and recovery of their patients. Strategies could include close monitoring of glucose levels during and after surgery and the prophylactic use of medications to prevent the formation of deep venous thrombosis (DVT), which can occur in surgery patients who are bedridden for extended periods of time.

It is also widely appreciated that diabetic patients tend to have slower healing rates than non-diabetic patients, Ganesh continued. This can be important not only during hospitalization, but also after discharge, when patients typically begin rehabilitation activities, she added.

One interesting finding, which the researchers said was not a focus of the current study and confirms other findings, was that the percentage of patients with diabetes steadily increased over the 12-year period from 1988 to 2000.

The researchers estimate that of the 260,000 Americans who fracture their ankles every year, about 25 percent will require surgery to stabilize the ankle.

Other Duke members of the team, in addition to Ganesh and Pietrobon, were Deng Pan, Nina Lightdale, MD, and James Nunley, MD. William Cecilio, Catholic University of Parana, Brazil, was also a member of the team.

Section 12.5

Risks of Cosmetic Foot Surgery Outweigh Benefits

This section contains "Position Statement on Cosmetic Foot Surgery" © 2003 American Orthopaedic Foot and Ankle Society (AOFAS) and "Cosmetic Foot Surgery to Beautify Feet Has Serious Risks" © 2004 AOFAS. Both documents are reprinted with permission.

AOFAS Position Statement on Cosmetic Foot Surgery

Recent articles in women's magazines and other consumer publications have touted cosmetic foot surgery performed solely to change the appearance of the foot. Cosmetic foot surgery does not include surgery performed to provide pain relief, improve function, or enhance the quality of life during normal activities of daily living. The American Orthopaedic Foot and Ankle Society (AOFAS) warns consumers that the risks inherent in such surgery far outweigh the benefits. Cosmetic foot surgery should not be considered in any circumstances and the Society does not condone its practice.

All surgical procedures have inherent risks, including, but not limited to, wound problems, infection, nerve injury, recurrence of deformity, post-surgical pain, and scar formation. There are also risks associated with anesthesia. Post-surgical complications could lead to an inability to walk or wear shoes comfortably. In deciding when to proceed with surgery, a patient and surgeon must consider all the risks and benefits of a procedure. When the potential benefits outweigh the potential risks, then surgical intervention may be warranted. The most substantial benefit of surgery is the reduction or elimination of pain and the improvement of function, often through the correction of deformity. Cosmetic foot surgery fails to provide pain relief, improve function, or enhance the quality of life during normal activities of daily living.

Studies have shown that many of the most prevalent forefoot deformities including bunions, hammer toes, claw toes, corns, neuromas, and bunionettes are associated with the repetitive use of ill-fitting shoes. Such shoes include high heels and those that are too narrow, too small, or with a toe box shape that causes the front of the foot to be deformed to fit into the shoe. If deformities are corrected and a person resumes use of ill-fitting shoes, the deformity likely will recur.

In light of the risks associated with surgical procedures and the increased risk of recurrent deformity with the repetitive use of ill-fitting shoes, the AOFAS recommends that surgery not be performed simply to improve the appearance of the foot. Surgery should never be performed in the absence of pain, functional limitation, or reduced quality of life.

Cosmetic Foot Surgery to Beautify Feet Has Serious Risks

An alarming trend in women's health and fashion has been the advocacy of cosmetic surgery to improve the appearance of women's feet or to accommodate their feet to high fashion shoes. Among the surgeries being touted by some are shortening of the toes, narrowing of the feet, injecting the fat pad with collagen or other substances, and other procedures performed solely to change the appearance of the feet, rather than provide pain relief or improve foot function.

The American Orthopaedic Foot and Ankle Society (AOFAS) warns consumers that the risks inherent in such surgery can far outweigh the benefits. The AOFAS advisory notes that foot surgery should not be performed in the absence of pain or functional limitation.

"The public needs to be aware of the risks associated with these procedures," counseled AOFAS President Glenn B. Pfeffer, MD, San Francisco, CA. "Women need to know what they are getting into." He noted that the trend towards the practice of cosmetic surgery raises serious concern when one considers the risks of surgery on painless feet. "Complications can include infection, nerve injury, prolonged swelling of a toe, and even chronic pain with walking," Pfeffer said.

The AOFAS decided to take a public stance on cosmetic foot surgery after recent consumer magazine articles ran stories on women who had surgery so that their feet would look "prettier" and fit better into their shoes. Since ill-fitting shoes are the cause of most forefoot deformities, the obvious choice would be to wear better fitting shoes.

"I think it's reprehensible for a physician to correct someone's feet so they can get into Jimmy Choo shoes," said Sharon Dreeben, MD, La Jolla, CA, chair of the AOFAS Public Education Committee. "To perform surgery with significant risk in order to put the foot back into the very device that caused the problem is inappropriate," said Dr. Dreeben. "Continuing to wear ill-fitting shoes will likely lead to a reoccurrence of the foot deformity, pain, or new forefoot problems. At worst, cosmetic surgery may result in a woman being unable to wear any shoes, let alone fashionable shoes."

Dr. Dreeben added that fashionable shoes can be widened or otherwise modified or the wearer can choose to wear shorter heels. "Changing the shoe to fit the foot is a perfectly acceptable practice," she said. "What the Society discourages is changing the foot to fit the shoe."

The American Orthopaedic Foot and Ankle Society is the leading organization of orthopaedic foot and ankle specialists. Its members are the orthopaedic surgeons who specialize in foot care.

Chapter 13

Orthoses (Limb Braces)

Chapter Contents

Section 13.1

Orthotics Demystified

"What Is an AFO? Orthotics Demystified" is reprinted with permission from the Eleanor and Lou Gehrig MDA/ALS Newsletter, Volume 13, Number 4, Winter 2001. © 2001 Eleanor and Lou Gehrig MDA/ALS Research Center of Columbia University Medical Center.

The field of medicine is filled with jargon, abbreviations, and acronyms. The field of orthotics (or limb braces) is no different. Unfortunately the terms are often used without explanation and are familiar only to those who regularly use them. What follows is an attempt to demystify orthotics and the practitioners who recommend and make them.

About ten years ago, the word *orthosis* began to be used in place of the traditional word *brace*. Orthosis comes from the Greek *ortho*, meaning "straight." (One function of an orthosis or brace may be to keep a limb straight.) An orthosis is the same thing as an orthotic device. There are four main types of orthotic devices (or orthoses). Two of these four types may be used by people who have weakness due to amyotrophic lateral sclerosis (ALS): orthoses that stabilize and support a joint, and thereby prevent movement and orthoses that assist movement or help to compensate for loss of movement.

Orthoses are named for the joints they encompass. A short leg brace (below the knee) is known as an AFO (ankle-foot orthosis) because it deals with weakness in the foot and ankle. A KAFO controls the knee, ankle, and foot, and extends above the knee.

Orthoses are made of metal, plastic, or a combination of these two materials. Metal orthoses do not touch the skin and attach to the outside of a shoe. However, metal orthoses are heavier than plastic ones and are therefore not often used for people with ALS who have limb weakness. Plastic orthoses come into direct contact with the skin and fit inside a shoe. Care must be taken if there is swelling in the foot or ankle: the close contact with skin can cause pressure and discomfort. People with diabetes and those who have problems with circulation or sensation must also use plastic orthoses with caution in order to avoid skin irritation and pressure.

The type of orthosis most commonly used by people with ALS is an AFO. One type of AFO is a posterior leaf orthosis (PLO), also called a posterior leaf spring (PLS) by some orthotics professionals. The PLO or PLS is the lightest in weight of the AFOs and is used mainly when a person has "footdrop." A footdrop occurs when there is weakness in the muscles in the front of the lower leg that lift up the toes and foot when one takes a step. A PLO or PLS holds the foot at a right angle to the leg and prevents the foot from dragging. If a person also has weakness in the other muscles around the ankle (e.g., the muscles that turn the foot in or out, or allow one to push down with the foot), he or she may need an AFO that is more solid than a PLO/PLS. In this case, more plastic is used to hold the ankle in place and therefore prevent the ankle from being twisted or sprained.

Orthoses are prescribed by a physician and fabricated by an orthotist. Orthotists are the professionals who know the latest styles and materials that are used to make orthoses. He or she is responsible for measuring the client for the orthosis and ensuring its proper fit once it is made. The physical therapist is the clinician responsible for teaching the person with ALS how to walk using the orthosis. Both the therapist and orthotist should instruct the user in the following areas:

- checking the skin for pressure areas

- how to apply and remove the orthosis easily

- the best type of shoe to use with an orthosis (sorry, no high heels)

- a wearing schedule (i.e., how often to wear the orthosis on the first day, the second day, etc.)

If a person has weakness in the foot and ankle and is having difficulty walking, a physician may prescribe an orthosis. Alternatively, the medical doctor may prescribe a physical therapist to evaluate the person for an orthosis. The physical therapist can provide input and make recommendations to the medical doctor and orthotist based on orthoses that have been found to be most beneficial. The ideal situation is when the orthotist and therapist work together with a person with ALS to determine which type of orthosis will best suit his or her individual needs. Usually, outpatient departments of hospitals, rehabilitation centers, and some skilled nursing facilities will have both therapists and orthotists on staff.

Section 13.2

Ankle Foot Orthosis (AFO)

AFO stands for ankle foot orthosis. This kind of brace is usually made of plastic. Orthoses are named for the parts of the body they control. An orthosis provides correction, support, or protection to a part of the body.

How do I get used to my new orthosis?

A new orthosis must be broken in slowly. When first wearing your new orthosis, start a little at a time.

- Begin with two hours on and one hour off.

- During the next two or three days, gradually increase the time the orthosis is used until it is being worn for the amount of time that your orthotist or therapist prescribed.

How do I wear my orthosis?

- Always wear a sock or stocking under the orthosis. It helps to reduce friction and decreases irritation of your skin from sweat.

- The sock you wear should be taller than the orthosis. You may even choose to wear a knee-high sock for more comfort.

- Cotton socks allow air to circulate better and absorb sweat. For more comfort, use talcum powder and change your sock after sweating.

- Inspect your socks to ensure they are wrinkle free.

- Be sure that the straps on your orthosis are snug and your heel is completely back in the orthosis to ensure a proper fit.

- Shoes worn with your orthosis should have good support and the correct heel height for which your orthosis was designed.

Ask your orthotist or therapist which shoes are best for your orthosis.

- Do not wear your orthosis barefooted or with slippers, sandals, loafers, or any shoe without a back.

How do I care for my orthosis?

Since your orthosis will be worn for long periods of time, it may become very dirty. The following tips will help you keep it clean:

- Clean your orthosis frequently inside and out with a damp cloth. Let it dry fully before you put it back on.

- Use a towel or let your orthosis dry at room temperature. Do not place your orthosis in front of a heater. Do not use a hair dryer for drying, or leave it in the sun or a hot car.

- A solution of one tablespoon of unscented bleach in a gallon of water can be used to clean your orthosis.

- Velcro can be kept clean with soap and water and can be kept free of lint and hair with a wire brush, toothbrush, or fine-toothed comb.

- Metal joints should be lubricated occasionally with silicon spray or a light oil such as WD40® or 3-in-1 Oil®.

How do I care for my skin?

- Any part of the body covered by the orthosis should be washed daily with warm water and mild soap.

- Be sure to clean the bottoms of your feet and between your toes to eliminate bacteria and dirt collection.

- Your body should be completely dry before wearing your orthosis.

- Remember to keep socks clean, dry and wrinkle-free. Inspect skin daily.

Why do I need to examine my skin?

- It should become a habit to inspect your skin daily. People with decreased sense of touch are not as likely to notice that their skin is irritated. Irritation is especially common in bony areas such as the shin or sides of the feet. Even minor irritations should be treated.

- An orthosis should provide steady pressure, not sharp pain. Inspect your skin daily for bruises, calluses, or blisters.

- A new orthosis may cause redness, but this should disappear within 15 minutes once the orthotic is removed.

- Swelling may occur after prolonged standing or during hot, humid weather. If this occurs, you should remove the orthosis, sit or lie down, and elevate your leg above your heart until the swelling subsides.

Safety is important!

For your safety, it is important to quickly inspect the orthosis every day.

- Check rivets and screws for tightness.
- Check plastic and metal uprights for cracks.
- Check straps and buckles for proper fit.
- With daytime foot and leg orthoses, shoes should be worn at all times because the footplate is slippery and can cause a trip on uneven surfaces.

Part Two

Common Foot Conditions

Chapter 14

Understanding and Treating Athlete's Foot

Athlete's Foot

Although the words *ringworm*, *jock itch*, and *athlete's foot* may sound funny, if you have one of these skin infections, you're probably not laughing. The good news is that tinea, the name for this category of common skin infections, is usually easy to treat. Read on to learn some fast facts about foot fungus.

The Basics on Tineal Infections

Tinea (pronounced: tih-nee-uh) is the medical name for a group of related fungal skin infections that affect the skin, nails, or scalp, including athlete's foot, jock itch, and ringworm (despite its name, ringworm isn't a worm at all). These infections are caused by several types of mold-like fungi called dermatophytes (pronounced: der-mah-tuh-fites) that live on the dead tissues of your skin, hair, and nails.

This chapter begins with "Athlete's Foot." This information was provided by TeensHealth, one of the largest resources online for medically reviewed health information written for parents, kids, and teens. For more articles like this one, visit www.TeensHealth.org, or www.KidsHealth.org. © 2004 The Nemours Center for Children's Health Media, a division of The Nemours Foundation. Reviewed by Patrice Hyde, MD, March 2004. "Over-the-Counter Remedies for Athlete's Foot," © 2001 Medical College of Wisconsin, is reprinted with permission of Medical College of Wisconsin HealthLink, www.healthlink.mcw.edu. Article created and reviewed by Joan M. Bedinghaus, MD, and Mark W. Niedfeldt, MD, October 30, 2001.

What Is Athlete's Foot?

The medical name for athlete's foot is tinea pedis. Usually athlete's foot affects the soles of the feet and the areas between the toes, and it may also spread to the toenails. Athlete's foot can also spread to the palms of your hands, groin, or underarms if you touch your feet and then touch another area of your body. Athlete's foot doesn't just aggravate athletes; anyone whose feet tend to be damp or sweaty can get this infection. The fungi that cause athlete's foot thrive in warm, moist environments.

The signs and symptoms of athlete's foot include itching, burning, redness, and stinging on the soles of the feet. The skin may flake, peel, blister, or crack.

How Can I Prevent Getting Athlete's Foot?

Athlete's foot is contagious. It's often spread in damp areas, such as public showers or pool areas. To prevent getting athlete's foot, dry your feet—and the spaces between your toes—thoroughly after showering or swimming. Use a clean towel. (Avoid sharing towels because doing so can spread the infection.) If you use public showers, like those in the locker room, wearing waterproof shoes or flip-flops is a good way to protect your feet.

To keep your feet as dry as possible, try not to wear the same shoes or sneakers all the time, and don't wear socks that make your feet sweat or trap moisture. Cotton or wool socks are a good bet. You can also find socks made of special "moisture wicking" fabrics in many sports stores—these are designed to keep feet dry. If possible, choose sneakers that are well ventilated—some sneakers contain small ventilation holes that help to keep your feet dry.

How Is Athlete's Foot Treated?

A doctor can often diagnose athlete's foot simply by examining the affected area. Your doctor may also take a small scraping of the skin on your foot. This sample is then examined under a microscope or sent to a laboratory for culture to see if the fungi that cause athlete's foot are present.

If you have athlete's foot, over-the-counter antifungal creams and sprays may solve the problem. Most mild cases of athlete's foot usually clear up within two weeks, but it is common for athlete's foot to recur (come back), so some people use medicated powders and sprays to prevent this from happening.

If an athlete's foot infection is more serious, it can take longer than a couple of weeks to get better. In these cases, it's a good idea to see your doctor, who may prescribe a stronger antifungal cream, spray, or pill.

Over-the-Counter Remedies for Athlete's Foot

Athlete's foot is a fungal infection of the skin of the foot, usually between the toes. Heat and dampness are key factors. Characterized by cracking and peeling of the skin, athlete's foot generally responds well to over-the-counter medications.

Lamisil-AT is as effective as any prescription athlete's foot cream, and is usually effective with one week of treatment. Other athlete's foot creams that are effective include Desenex (undecylenic acid), Lotrimin (clotrimazole), Monistat-Derm (miconazole), and Tinactin (tolnaftate), all of which require four weeks of treatment.

While a tube of Lamisil-AT costs considerably more than the other antifungal agents, one tube is generally enough. The other antibiotics may require additional tubes and be more expensive in the long term.

Tea tree oil is also marketed as a treatment for athlete's foot. One study found it to be as effective as tolnaftate in reducing symptoms of the condition, but no more effective than a placebo in curing it. Washing and drying feet twice a day may also help treat and prevent athlete's foot.

If the athlete's foot infection appears on the entire sole of the foot or on top of the foot, it requires systemic antifungal therapy. In other words, a lotion or spray will not work. A doctor must prescribe an oral antifungal medication instead.

Chapter 15

Foot Odor

Smelly feet can be not only embarrassing but uncomfortable as well. But once you understand the problem, you'll be able to take steps to reduce the odor.

Causes of Foot Odor

Feet smell for two reasons: you wear shoes and your feet sweat. The interaction between your perspiration and the bacteria that thrive in your shoes and socks generates the odor. So any attempt to reduce foot odor has to address both your sweating and your footwear. The feet and hands contain more sweat glands than any other part of the body (about 3,000 glands per square inch) and provide a ready supply of perspiration. You're probably familiar with the phenomenon of sweaty palms, but sweat on your hands doesn't produce the same strong odor as sweaty feet. That's because your hands are usually exposed to the air and the sweat has a chance to evaporate.

Feet, however, are trapped inside shoes, where temperatures can easily reach 102° F. The perspiration moisture combines with the dark warmth to create a fertile breeding ground for the bacteria that normally live on our skin. The bacteria produce isovaleric acid, the substance associated with foot odor. The more moisture there is, the more

Reproduced with permission from "Smelly (Malodorous) Feet," in Johnson TR, (ed): *Your Orthopaedic Connection*. Rosemont, IL, American Academy of Orthopaedic Surgeons. Available at http://orthoinfo.aaos.org. Co-developed by the American Orthopaedic Foot and Ankle Society. Published May 2002.

bacteria proliferate, and the greater the odor. Smelly feet can also be caused by an inherited condition called hyperhidrosis, or excessive sweating, which primarily affects males. Stress, some medications, fluid intake, and hormonal changes also can increase the amount of perspiration your body produces.

Preventing Foot Odor

Fortunately, smelly feet generally can be controlled with a few preventive measures. The American Orthopaedic Foot and Ankle Society recommends that you do the following:

- Practice good foot hygiene to keep bacteria levels at a minimum.
  - Bathe your feet daily in lukewarm water, using a mild soap. Dry thoroughly.
  - Change your socks and shoes at least once a day.
  - Dust your feet frequently with a nonmedicated baby powder or foot powder. Applying antibacterial ointment also may help.
  - Check for fungal infections between your toes and on the bottoms of your feet. If you spot redness or dry, patchy skin, get treatment right away.
- Wear thick, soft socks to help draw moisture away from the feet. Cotton and other absorbent materials are best.
- Avoid wearing nylon socks or plastic shoes. Instead, wear shoes made of leather, canvas, mesh, or other materials that let your feet breathe.
- Don't wear the same pair of shoes two days in a row. If you frequently wear athletic shoes, alternate pairs so that the shoes can dry out. Give your shoes at least 24 hours to air out between wearings; if the odor doesn't go away, discard the shoes.
- Always wear socks with closed shoes.

These preventive measures also can help prevent athlete's foot, which can flourish in the same environment as sweaty feet. However, athlete's foot won't respond to an antibacterial agent because it's caused by a fungus infection. Use an antifungal powder and good foot hygiene to treat athlete's foot.

Treating Foot Odor

Persistent foot odor can indicate a low-grade infection or a severe case of hereditary sweating. In these cases, your doctor may prescribe a special ointment. You apply it to the feet at bedtime and then wrap your feet with an impermeable covering such as kitchen plastic wrap.

Soaking your feet in strong black tea for 30 minutes a day for a week can help. The tannic acid in the tea kills the bacteria and closes the pores, keeping your feet dry longer. Use two tea bags per pint of water. Boil for 15 minutes, then add two quarts of cool water. Soak your feet in the cool solution. Alternately, you can soak your feet in a solution of one part vinegar and two parts water.

A form of electrolysis called iontophoresis also can reduce excessive sweating of the feet, but requires special equipment and training to administer. In the most severe cases of hyperhidrosis, a surgeon can cut the nerve that controls sweating. Recent advances in technology have made this surgery much safer, but you may notice compensatory sweating in other areas of the body afterwards.

Chapter 16

Plantar Warts

Warts are one of several soft tissue conditions of the foot that can be quite painful. They are caused by a virus, which generally invades the skin through small or invisible cuts and abrasions. They can appear anywhere on the skin, but technically only those on the sole are properly called plantar warts.

Children, especially teenagers, tend to be more susceptible to warts than adults; some people seem to be immune.

Identification Problems

Most warts are harmless, even though they may be painful. They are often mistaken for corns or calluses—which are layers of dead skin that build up to protect an area which is being continuously irritated. The wart, however, is a viral infection.

It is also possible for a variety of more serious lesions to appear on the foot, including malignant lesions such as carcinomas and melanomas. Although rare, these conditions can sometimes be misidentified as a wart. It is wise to consult a podiatric physician when any suspicious growth or eruption is detected on the skin of the foot in order to ensure a correct diagnosis.

Plantar warts tend to be hard and flat, with a rough surface and well-defined boundaries; warts are generally raised and fleshier when

---

"Warts" is reprinted with permission from the American Podiatric Medical Association, http://www.apma.org. © 2005. All rights reserved.

163

they appear on the top of the foot or on the toes. Plantar warts are often gray or brown (but the color may vary), with a center that appears as one or more pinpoints of black. It is important to note that warts can be very resistant to treatment and have a tendency to reoccur.

Source of the Virus

The plantar wart is often contracted by walking barefoot on dirty surfaces or littered ground where the virus is lurking. The causative virus thrives in warm, moist environments, making infection a common occurrence in communal bathing facilities.

If left untreated, warts can grow to an inch or more in circumference and can spread into clusters of several warts; these are often called mosaic warts. Like any other infectious lesion, plantar warts are spread by touching, scratching, or even by contact with skin shed from another wart. The wart may also bleed, another route for spreading.

Occasionally, warts can spontaneously disappear after a short time, and, just as frequently, they can recur in the same location.

When plantar warts develop on the weight-bearing areas of the foot—the ball of the foot, or the heel, for example—they can be the source of sharp, burning pain. Pain occurs when weight is brought to bear directly on the wart, although pressure on the side of a wart can create equally intense pain.

Tips for Prevention

- Avoid walking barefoot, except on sandy beaches.
- Change shoes and socks daily.
- Keep feet clean and dry.
- Check children's feet periodically.
- Avoid direct contact with warts—from other persons or from other parts of the body.
- Do not ignore growths on, or changes in, your skin.
- Visit your podiatric physician as part of your annual health checkup.

Self Treatment

Self treatment is generally not advisable. Over-the-counter preparations contain acids or chemicals that destroy skin cells, and it takes an expert to destroy abnormal skin cells (warts) without also destroying surrounding healthy tissue. Self treatment with such medications especially should be avoided by people with diabetes and those with cardiovascular or circulatory disorders. Never use them in the presence of an active infection.

Professional Treatment

It is possible that your podiatric physician will prescribe and supervise your use of a wart-removal preparation. More likely, however, removal of warts by a simple surgical procedure, performed under local anesthetic, may be indicated.

Lasers have become a common and effective treatment. A procedure known as CO_2 laser cautery is performed under local anesthesia either in your podiatrist's office surgical setting or an outpatient surgery facility. The laser reduces post-treatment scarring and is a safe form for eliminating wart lesions.

Tips for Individuals with Warts

- Avoid self treatment with over-the-counter preparations.

- Seek professional podiatric evaluation and assistance with the treatment of your warts.

- Diabetics and other patients with circulatory, immunological, or neurological problems should be especially careful with the treatment of their warts.

- Warts may spread and are catching. Make sure you have your warts evaluated to protect yourself and those close to you.

Chapter 17

Heel Pain

Chapter Contents

Section 17.1

Common Causes of Heel Pain

Heel Pain Has Many Causes

In our pursuit of healthy bodies, pain can be an enemy. In some instances, however, it is of biological benefit. Pain that occurs right after an injury or early in an illness may play a protective role, often warning us about the damage we've suffered.

When we sprain an ankle, for example, the pain warns us that the ligament and soft tissues may be frayed and bruised, and that further activity may cause additional injury.

Pain, such as may occur in our heels, also alerts us to seek medical attention. This alert is of utmost importance because of the many afflictions that contribute to heel pain.

Heel Pain

Heel pain is generally the result of faulty biomechanics (walking gait abnormalities) that place too much stress on the heel bone and the soft tissues that attach to it. The stress may also result from injury, or a bruise incurred while walking, running, or jumping on hard surfaces; wearing poorly constructed footwear; or being overweight.

The heel bone is the largest of the 26 bones in the human foot, which also has 33 joints and a network of more than 100 tendons, muscles, and ligaments. Like all bones, it is subject to outside influences that can affect its integrity and its ability to keep us on our feet. Heel pain, sometimes disabling, can occur in the front, back, or bottom of the heel.

Heel Spurs

A common cause of heel pain is the heel spur, a bony growth on the underside of the heel bone. The spur, visible by x-ray, appears as a protrusion that can extend forward as much as half an inch. When there is no indication of bone enlargement, the condition is sometimes referred to as "heel spur syndrome."

Heel spurs result from strain on the muscles and ligaments of the foot, by stretching of the long band of tissue that connects the heel and the ball of the foot, and by repeated tearing away of the lining or membrane that covers the heel bone. These conditions may result from biomechanical imbalance, running or jogging, improperly fitted or excessively worn shoes, or obesity.

Plantar Fasciitis

Both heel pain and heel spurs are frequently associated with an inflammation of the band of fibrous connective tissue (fascia) running along the bottom (plantar surface) of the foot, from the heel to the ball of the foot. The inflammation is called plantar fasciitis. It is common among athletes who run and jump a lot, and it can be quite painful.

The condition occurs when the plantar fascia is strained over time beyond its normal extension, causing the soft tissue fibers of the fascia to tear or stretch at points along its length; this leads to inflammation, pain, and possibly the growth of a bone spur where it attaches to the heel bone.

The inflammation may be aggravated by shoes that lack appropriate support, especially in the arch area, and by the chronic irritation that sometimes accompanies an athletic lifestyle.

Resting provides only temporary relief. When you resume walking, particularly after a night's sleep, you may experience a sudden elongation of the fascia band, which stretches and pulls on the heel. As you walk, the heel pain may lessen or even disappear, but that may be just a false sense of relief. The pain often returns after prolonged rest or extensive walking.

Excessive Pronation

Heel pain sometimes results from excessive pronation. Pronation is the normal flexible motion and flattening of the arch of the foot that allows it to adapt to ground surfaces and absorb shock in the normal walking pattern.

As you walk, the heel contacts the ground first; the weight shifts first to the outside of the foot, then moves toward the big toe. The arch rises, the foot generally rolls upward and outward, becoming rigid and stable in order to lift the body and move it forward. Excessive pronation—

excessive inward motion—can create an abnormal amount of stretching and pulling on the ligaments and tendons attaching to the bottom back of the heel bone. Excessive pronation may also contribute to injury to the hip, knee, and lower back.

Disease and Heel Pain

Some general health conditions can also bring about heel pain.

- Rheumatoid arthritis and other forms of arthritis, including gout, which usually manifests itself in the big toe joint, can cause heel discomfort in some cases.

- Heel pain may also be the result of an inflamed bursa (bursitis), a small, irritated sac of fluid; a neuroma (a nerve growth); or other soft-tissue growth. Such heel pain may be associated with a heel spur or may mimic the pain of a heel spur.

- Haglund deformity ("pump bump") is a bone enlargement at the back of the heel bone, in the area where the Achilles tendon attaches to the bone. This sometimes painful deformity generally is the result of bursitis caused by pressure against the shoe and can be aggravated by the height or stitching of a heel counter of a particular shoe.

- Pain at the back of the heel is associated with inflammation of the Achilles tendon as it runs behind the ankle and inserts on the back surface of the heel bone. The inflammation is called Achilles tendonitis. It is common among people who run and walk a lot and have tight tendons. The condition occurs when the tendon is strained over time, causing the fibers to tear or stretch along its length, or at its insertion on to the heel bone. This leads to inflammation, pain, and the possible growth of a bone spur on the back of the heel bone. The inflammation is aggravated by the chronic irritation that sometimes accompanies an active lifestyle and certain activities that strain an already tight tendon.

- Bone bruises are common heel injuries. A bone bruise or contusion is an inflammation of the tissues that cover the heel bone. A bone bruise is a sharply painful injury caused by the direct impact of a hard object or surface on the foot.

Stress fractures of the heel bone also can occur, although infrequently.

Children's Heel Pain

Heel pain can also occur in children, most commonly between ages 8 and 13, as they become increasingly active in sports activity in and out of school. This physical activity, particularly jumping, inflames the growth centers of the heels; the more active the child, the more likely the condition will occur. When the bones mature, the problems disappear and are not likely to recur. If heel pain occurs in this age group, podiatric care is necessary to protect the growing bone and to provide pain relief. Other good news is that heel spurs do not often develop in children.

Prevention

A variety of steps can be taken to avoid heel pain and accompanying afflictions:

- Wear shoes that fit well—front, back, and sides—and have shock-absorbent soles, rigid shanks, and supportive heel counters.

- Wear the proper shoes for each activity.

- Do not wear shoes with excessive wear on heels or soles.

- Prepare properly before exercising. Warm up and do stretching exercises before and after running.

- Pace yourself when you participate in athletic activities.

- Don't underestimate your body's need for rest and good nutrition.

- If obese, lose weight.

Podiatric Medical Care

If pain and other symptoms of inflammation—redness, swelling, heat—persist, you should limit normal daily activities and contact a doctor of podiatric medicine.

The podiatric physician will examine the area and may perform diagnostic x-rays to rule out problems of the bone.

Early treatment might involve oral or injectable antiinflammatory medication, exercise and shoe recommendations, taping or strapping, or use of shoe inserts or orthotic devices. Taping or strapping supports the foot, placing stressed muscles and tendons in a physiologically restful state. Physical therapy may be used in conjunction with such treatments.

171

A functional orthotic device may be prescribed for correcting biomechanical imbalance, controlling excessive pronation, and supporting of the ligaments and tendons attaching to the heel bone. It will effectively treat the majority of heel and arch pain without the need for surgery.

Only a relatively few cases of heel pain require more advanced treatments or surgery. If surgery is necessary, it may involve the release of the plantar fascia, removal of a spur, removal of a bursa, or removal of a neuroma or other soft-tissue growth.

Heel Pain Tips

- If you have experienced painful heels try wearing your shoes around your house in the evening. Don't wear slippers or socks or go barefoot. You may also try gentle calf stretches for 20 to 30 seconds on each leg. This is best done barefoot, leaning forward towards a wall with one foot forward and one foot back.

- If the pain persists longer than one month, you should visit a podiatrist for evaluation and treatment. Your feet should not hurt, and professional podiatric care may be required to help relieve your discomfort.

- If you have not exercised in a long time, consult your podiatric physician before starting a new exercise program.

- Begin an exercise program slowly. Don't go too far or too fast.

- Purchase and maintain good shoes and replace them regularly.

- Stretch each foot and Achilles tendon before and after exercise.

- Avoid uneven walking surfaces or stepping on rocks as much as possible.

- Avoid going barefoot on hard surfaces.

- Vary the incline on a treadmill during exercise. Nobody walks uphill all the time.

- If it hurts, stop. Don't try to "work through the pain."

Your podiatric physician/surgeon has been trained specifically and extensively in the diagnosis and treatment of all manner of foot conditions. This training encompasses all of the intricately related systems and structures of the foot and lower leg including neurological, circulatory, skin, and the musculoskeletal system, which includes bones, joints, ligaments, tendons, muscles, and nerves.

Section 17.2

Plantar Fasciitis

What's the problem?

Plantar fasciitis/heel pain syndrome is an inflammation of a thick band of tissue at the bottom of the foot called the plantar fascia. The inflammation of the plantar fascia, at its origin at the heel bone (calcaneus), causes the classic symptoms of pain at the bottom and/or side of the heel facing the opposite foot, often the most painful upon arising in the morning or when standing after sitting for prolonged periods. We call this post-static pain—pain after rest. This is because the plantar fascia is tight after rest, and the stretching inflames the painful area even more, therefore increasing the discomfort. The pain can exist with or without a "heel spur." It is the feeling of most physicians that treat this condition often that the pain is caused by the stretching and inflammation of the plantar fascia, and not by the bone spur. The spur is a result of pulling of the plantar fascia at the heel bone, resulting in proliferation of bone, often referred to as a "heel spur."

How does it feel?

The classic symptoms are pain and a feeling of stiffness in the bottom and/or side of the heel. This pain is often a sharp pain that is described as a feeling of stepping on a stone or nail. The pain often reduces after a few steps, though it may still persist. This pain can also occur when walking after sitting for a prolonged time, such as sifting at work, driving a car, etc.

Let's do a test!

A thorough examination by a doctor of the clinical signs and symptoms will usually result in a clear diagnosis. X-rays will usually be taken to determine if any abnormality is present in the heel bone (calcaneus).

On occasion, fractures, bone cysts, or foreign objects (pieces of metal, splinters, broken needles, glass) can be discovered as the cause of heel pain. If the presentation is not clear, other diagnostic tests may be utilized. Bone scans are often used if a bone cyst or abnormality in the bone is suspected or if a fracture is suspected. An MRI may be performed if a small "stress" type fracture is suspected. Additionally, an MRI is useful in determining the status of the surrounding tissue and can determine if there is a tear of the fascia or any other soft tissue and bone abnormalities. A CT scan is useful when suspecting a fracture of the heel bone and the extent of the fracture. Additionally, blood tests can be utilized to rule out arthritic or infectious disorders.

How did this happen?

Plantar fasciitis heel pain syndrome can occur via a myriad of causes. Risk factors such as weight gain, foot type (flat feet, high arched feet), a high level of activity, sports, overuse, improper shoe gear, improper support of the feet, trauma, tightness of muscles, and daily activities can trigger the classic symptoms. Often, there is no single cause, but a culmination of several risk factors. It is imperative to address all of these factors to treat this condition successfully.

What can I do for it?

Switching shoe gear to a well supportive running shoe can be effective. Reducing your level of activity helps. When you are off your feet, the injury is healing, it's getting better. When you are standing with inadequate foot support, it is getting injured. An orthotic or arch support can support your foot well enough to virtually eliminate the injury that is occurring while standing and walking.

What will my doctor do for it?

Your podiatrist will perform a thorough examination and history of your condition. He/she will explain the cause of the problem and offer you various treatment options. X-rays will usually be taken to assess the status of the heel bone (calcaneus) and to check for other findings such as arthritis, foreign objects, fractures, etc. There are numerous treatment options, and the treatment protocol will vary according to the severity of the patient's symptoms.

Treatment options can include oral antiinflammatory medications, heel cushions, heel cups, physical therapy, stretching exercises, taping/strapping of the foot, over-the-counter inserts, custom orthoses, injections, soft tissue wraps, weight loss, change of shoes, casting, night splints, and surgery. Each option has advantages and disadvantages, and must be tailored to the needs and unique characteristics of each patient.

Conservative care is successful 85 percent of the time, and surgical treatment is usually performed 5-10 percent of the time. The surgical techniques differ according to the surgeon's preference. The surgery is usually performed as an outpatient and can be performed "traditionally," with removal of the spur and surgical release of the ligament, or via newer techniques utilizing endoscopic equipment. This newer technique utilizes two very small incisions and surgically releases a portion of the plantar fascia, and the "spur" is left undisturbed. The technique utilized should be discussed with the patient and will depend on x-ray and clinical findings.

Extracorporeal shock wave therapy (ESWT) is a newer method that utilizes sound waves/shock waves to help alleviate the pain associated with plantar fasciitis. This method has been used in Europe for many years and has been used in the United States for the past two to three years. ESWT is presently an FDA approved modality for plantar fasciitis. Although there are only a limited number of doctors performing this procedure, it is becoming more widely available. As a general rule, ESWT is an excellent alternative to surgery for those patients that haven't responded to approximately six months of conservative therapy with no relief of symptoms.

Can I prevent it from happening again?

Controlling body weight, wearing supportive shoes, and having additional support in your shoes can decrease the chance of recurrence. Additionally, stretching the Achilles tendon and hamstrings and maintaining flexibility are extremely important in preventing recurrence of the problem. Most importantly, pain and discomfort are your body's signals that a problem exists. Prompt attention and treatment can often result in significant relief with the avoidance of complications.

Chapter 18

Arch-Related Problems

The foot is made up of a complex interaction of bones, ligaments, and muscles. These structures help the foot alternate between being a mobile, flexible adaptor and a stable, rigid lever. The foot is broken down into two functional parts, the forefoot and the rearfoot. Overall, the foot functions in three primary ways:

1. It provides a stable platform of support.

2. It attenuates impact upon loading.

3. It assists in efficient forward propulsion of the body.

When we walk there is a load placed on the foot and the leg. The human foot has a definite, although varying, capacity to accept weight before injury results. The amount of weight tolerated before injury occurs varies with the time course of loading and the individual's ability to dissipate the loading force. By modifications of footwear, it is possible to change the load delivered to the body at foot strike and thus decrease injury. Shoewear and orthotics may play an important role in maintaining normal foot function.

The prescription of inserts or orthotics, as well as shoewear or modification of shoewear has three important functions:

1. The first is to provide protection to the foot and ankle.

2. The second is to help prevent injury by decreasing the stress on the leg. This is thought to occur through improved impact absorption or attempting to improve the alignment of the leg through compensation for malalignment.

3. The third possible function is enhancement of performance.

In order for proper function, the foot variation must be identified. People tend to have either a flat foot (pes planus) or a high arch foot (pes cavus). Regardless of the variation, the shoe must fit the foot and not vice versa.

Flat feet are generally excessively mobile and the foot has a tendency to move too much. In this case, the ligaments and muscle associated with this area tend to be stressed more than normal. This person tends to have a wide forefoot and a narrow heel which makes it difficult in shoe fitting. Breakdown is most often seen on the inside of the sole which leaves the foot in an unsupported position. Shoewear should conform to the foot which will give it the support it needs to function properly.

The individual with a cavus or high arch foot will generally have less motion within the joints of the foot and require more room on the top portion of the foot. This foot tends to wear out the outside of the outsole as well as flatten out the outside of the midsole. This foot is often associated with a tight Achilles tendon which results in excessive wear in the forward part of the sole under the ball of the foot.

When choosing a shoe for this foot type, a relatively high heel to relieve stress on the Achilles tendon and a midsole with good shock-absorption to dissipate the forces upon ground contact should be considered. The front of the shoe should be flexible under the ball of the foot. Together this will decrease the chance of injury related to this type of rigid and nonadapting foot.

Orthotics are another important adjunct that can be used in order for normal foot function to occur. Orthotics function to keep the foot in a neutral position and decrease or eliminate abnormal compensatory motions and unnecessary stresses. There are three types of orthotics: soft, semirigid, and rigid.

A soft orthotic's function is to provide cushion, improve shock absorption, decrease shear force, and redistribute pressure. This type of orthotic is indicated for a rigid foot. It provides little support which is not needed in this particular instance. The most important aspect is to cushion the rigid foot and decrease the force so that injury is prevented.

The next is a semirigid orthotic. This orthotic functions to control or balance the malaligned foot as well as provide some flexibility and shock absorption. It has increased compliance and is the most common orthotic prescribed. Those individuals with flat feet are the beneficiaries of this type of orthotic.

Finally, the rigid orthotic serves to control gross unwanted motion. It is not accommodating and offers no shock absorption or cushioning. This type of orthotic is indicated for the neurologic patient that has poor control of their feet.

The effect proper footwear and orthotic type have on particular foot variations has already been discussed. With flat feet, exercises may also be prescribed as a way to increase the arch. This increase in the arch height would increase its stability and function more optimally. Some exercises are as follows:

1. The individual stands on a towel and, with their toes, grabs it.

2. The individual stands holding a Thera-Band® [an elastic resistance exercise product], turned 90 degrees from the band. Then, rotates 90 degrees while standing on one foot. The muscles in the stance leg are being strengthened with this exercise.

3. While standing on one leg, the individual concentrates on increasing and decreasing the arch of the foot.

In the flat foot, the problem may be corrected with shoe modification, orthotic prescription, or muscle strengthening. These have all been shown to decrease stress and, hence, injury to the foot and leg. Flat fleet are more commonly seen than high arch feet. Persons with high arch feet often have tight heel cords. Therefore, stretching of the calf muscles is important. This can be done as described below.

1. Stand facing a wall with your arms straight and palms touching the wall.

2. Put one foot in front of the other with the leg being stretched behind.

3. Slowly lean forward keeping the heel of the back leg on the ground. Stop and hold the position when a stretch is felt. Hold the stretch for 30 seconds and repeat five times.

Exercises are not all that helpful in reversing the condition of a rigid foot. Shoe and orthotic management are the keys to dealing with this type of rigid foot. In cases where individuals lack the knowledge of shoewear modification, orthotic type, and exercises warranted, they should consult a professional who will guide them with the proper education that is needed.

Chapter 19

Neuromas

Chapter Contents

Section 19.1

What Is a Neuroma?

A neuroma is a painful condition, also referred to as a "pinched nerve"
or a nerve tumor. It is a benign growth of nerve tissue frequently found
between the third and fourth toes that brings on pain, a burning sensation, tingling, or numbness between the toes and in the ball of the
foot.

The principal symptom associated with a neuroma is pain between
the toes while walking. Those suffering from the condition often find
relief by stopping their walk, taking off their shoe, and rubbing the
affected area. At times, the patient will describe the pain as similar
to having a stone in his or her shoe. The vast majority of people who
develop neuromas are women.

Symptoms

- pain in the forefoot and between the toes
- tingling and numbness in the ball of the foot
- swelling between the toes
- pain in the ball of the foot when weight is placed on it

How You Get a Neuroma

Although the exact cause for this condition is unclear, a number
of factors can contribute to the formation of a neuroma.

- **Biomechanical deformities,** such as a high-arched foot or a
  flat foot, can lead to the formation of a neuroma. These foot types
  bring on instability around the toe joints, leading to the development of the condition.

- **Trauma** can cause damage to the nerve, resulting in inflammation or swelling of the nerve.

182

- **Improper footwear** that causes the toes to be squeezed together is problematic. Avoid high-heeled shoes higher than two inches. Shoes at this height can increase pressure on the forefoot area.

- **Repeated stress,** common to many occupations, can create or aggravate a neuroma.

What You Can Do for Relief

- Wear shoes with plenty of room for the toes to move, low heels, and laces or buckles that allow for width adjustment.

- Wear shoes with thick, shock-absorbent soles and proper insoles that are designed to keep excessive pressure off of the foot.

- High heels should be avoided whenever possible because they place undue strain on the forefoot and can contribute to a number of foot problems.

- Resting the foot and massaging the affected area can temporarily alleviate neuroma pain. Use an ice pack to help to dull the pain and improve comfort.

- For simple, undeveloped neuromas, a pair of thick-soled shoes with a wide toe box is often adequate treatment to relieve symptoms, allowing the condition to diminish on its own. For more severe conditions, however, podiatric medical treatment or surgery may be necessary to remove the tumor.

- Use over-the-counter shoe pads. These pads can relieve pressure around the affected area.

Treatment by Your Podiatric Physician

Treatment options vary with the severity of each neuroma, and identifying the neuroma early in its development is important to avoid surgical correction. Podiatric medical care should be sought at the first sign of pain or discomfort; if left untreated, neuromas tend to get worse.

The primary goal of most early treatment regimens is to relieve pressure on areas where a neuroma develops. Your podiatric physician will examine and likely x-ray the affected area and suggest a treatment plan that best suits your individual case.

- **Padding and taping:** Special padding at the ball of the foot may change the abnormal foot function and relieve the symptoms caused by the neuroma.

- **Medication:** Antiinflammatory drugs and cortisone injections can be prescribed to ease acute pain and inflammation caused by the neuroma.

- **Orthotic devices:** Custom shoe inserts made by your podiatrist may be useful in controlling foot function. An orthotic device may reduce symptoms and prevent the worsening of the condition.

- **Surgical options:** When early treatments fail and the neuroma progresses past the threshold for such options, podiatric surgery may become necessary. The procedure, which removes the inflamed and enlarged nerve, can usually be conducted on an outpatient basis, with a recovery time that is often just a few weeks. Your podiatric physician will thoroughly describe the surgical procedures to be used and the results you can expect. Any pain following surgery is easily managed with medications prescribed by your podiatrist.

Your Feet Aren't Supposed to Hurt

Remember that foot pain is not normal, and any disruption in foot function limits your freedom and mobility. It is important to schedule an appointment with your podiatrist at the first sign of pain or discomfort in your feet, and follow proper maintenance guidelines to ensure their proper health for the rest of your life. The advice in this section should not be used as a substitute for a consultation or evaluation by a podiatric physician.

Neuroma Tips

- Wear shoes with plenty of room for the toes to move, low heels, and laces or buckles that allow for width adjustment.

- Wear shoes with thick, shock-absorbent soles and proper insoles that are designed to keep excessive pressure off of the foot.

- High heels should be avoided whenever possible because they place undue strain on the forefoot and can contribute to a number of foot problems.

- Resting the foot and massaging the affected area can temporarily alleviate neuroma pain. Use an ice pack to help to dull the pain and improve comfort.

- For simple, undeveloped neuromas, a pair of thick-soled shoes with a wide toe box is often adequate treatment to relieve symptoms, allowing the condition to diminish on its own. For more severe conditions, however, podiatric medical treatment or surgery may be necessary to remove the tumor.

- Use over-the-counter shoe pads. These pads can relieve pressure around the affected area.

Section 19.2

Morton Neuroma

Text in this section was written by David A. Cooke, MD, Diplomate, American Board of Internal Medicine. © 2007 Omnigraphics, Inc.

Morton neuroma is a common, painful foot condition caused by compression of nerve tissue between bones in the foot. It typically causes burning pain or numbness in one or two toes.

Causes

The cause of this condition is a neuroma, a benign nerve tumor. These tumors are composed of disorganized nerve fibers and scar tissue, often forming a small ball-like mass. The exact cause of these neuromas is not known, but they are believed to occur after repeated injury to a given nerve. Improper footwear, such as high-heeled shoes or shoes that are excessively narrow in the toe, may contribute by pressing the foot bones together and pinching the nerves that run between them. It is most commonly seen in women between 35–60 years of age, possibly for this reason.

Morton neuromas most commonly occur in the forward part of the foot, between the third and fourth metatarsal bones. However, it can occur between other toes. If the neuroma is very small, it may not cause any symptoms. However, as the neuroma becomes larger, it becomes easily pinched between the metatarsal bones. This pinching and irritation leads to the symptoms of the condition.

Symptoms

Symptoms of Morton neuroma are usually sharp or burning pain on the sole of the foot, which radiates towards the tips of one or two toes. The pain is usually worse with standing or walking. Standing on tiptoes often triggers symptoms, as it increases pressure on the neuroma. Runners, ballet dancers, and women who frequently wear high heels are most commonly affected.

Diagnosis

Primary care physicians can usually diagnose Morton neuromas, although podiatrists and orthopedists frequently see the problem as well. The history of localized pain is usually suggestive. In most cases, compression of the web space between the two toes, or pressing the metatarsal bones together, will reproduce the pain. MRI can be useful if the diagnosis is in question, but is not usually necessary.

Treatment

Treatment of Morton neuroma usually consists of modifying footwear. Avoiding high heels or narrow-toed shoes improves matters significantly. Padding the shoe in the area of the neuroma may be helpful. Often, specially designed shoes or custom orthotics are used to reduce pressure on the affected area of the foot.

When these measures fail, other treatments are available. Injections of corticosteroids near the neuroma may reduce swelling and inflammation, which improves pain. Anesthetic agents may also be injected into the neuroma, helping to reduce painful sensation from the area.

For persistent cases, surgery is the major option. Surgical release of the metatarsal ligament reduces pressure from the adjacent bones on the neuroma. Alternatively, the neuroma can be surgically removed, in a procedure called interdigital neurectomy. This procedure effectively relieves pain in most cases, but because part of the nerve is removed, the adjacent toes are usually permanently numb afterwards.

Preventative Measures

The best way to avoid development of Morton neuromas is to ensure that you wear properly fitting footwear, and to try to avoid foot injuries.

Chapter 20

Metatarsalgia (Pain in the Ball of the Foot)

Note: Metatarsalgia is not an injury; it's actually a symptom or a group of symptoms. These may include pain in the ball of the foot, with or without bruising, and inflammation. Metatarsalgia can have a number of causes and, as a result, a number of treatments.

What to look for: Localized pain in the ball of the foot, on the bottom of the foot, in the area of the sole of the foot just before the toes. Metatarsalgia, the scientific name for this problem, is a painful but common occurrence. It is often localized in the metatarsal heads (the areas just before the second, third, and fourth toes), or it may be more isolated, in the area near the big toe. One of the hallmarks of this disorder is pain in the ball of the foot during weight-bearing activities (running, walking, standing, etc.). Sharp or shooting pains in the toes also may be present, and pain in the toes and/or ball of the foot may increase when the toes are flexed. Accompanying symptoms may include tingling or numbness in the toes. It is common to experience acute, recurrent, or chronic pain as a result of this problem. Some patients describe the feeling as being like "walking over pebbles," and others, whose pain is localized in one area, may wonder if they actually have a stone bruise.

"Metatarsalgia," © 2005 The American College of Foot and Ankle Orthopedics and Medicine (ACFAOM); reprinted with permission. For additional information from ACFAOM, visit http://www.acfaom.org.

Other notes: There is no one specific cause of metatarsalgia. The podiatric community has narrowed it down to a handful of factors, all of which have a common denominator: a forced change of the dynamics of the foot. In plain English, that means the foot is not moving as it should, and as a result, one or more of the metatarsal heads has become painful, often because of inflammation. More specific information on the causes of metatarsalgia appears below.

What it means to you: If you've noticed pain in your forefoot, which gets worse during walking, running, or standing, and/or pain in your toes, particularly when flexing them, you have some of the classic symptoms of metatarsalgia. Another hallmark is increased pain when going barefoot, particularly when standing or walking on a hard surface like tile, concrete, marble, or asphalt, as opposed to carpet or grass. You may notice that over time, you begin to adjust your stride to avoid putting pressure on the ball of the foot.

The good news is that while painful and annoying, metatarsalgia is generally treatable with conservative measures, particularly once the origin of the problem is identified.

What causes it?

Metatarsalgia develops when something changes or threatens the normal mechanics (working action) of the foot. Ultimately, this creates excessive pressure in the ball of the foot, and that leads to metatarsalgia. Some of the causes of metatarsalgia include the following:

- **Being overweight:** Nobody likes to talk about it, but the plain truth is that the more weight is brought to bear on the foot, the greater the pressure is on the forefoot when taking a step. As men and women age, the fat pad in the foot tends to thin out, creating less cushioning and making them more susceptible to pain in the ball of the foot. Keeping body weight within a healthy range can decrease your chance of having metatarsalgia; if a case already exists, losing weight can lessen its severity. In many cases, weight loss alone can eliminate the symptoms entirely.

- **Wearing shoes that do not fit properly:** Shoes with a narrow, tight toe box, or shoes that cause a great deal of pressure to be put on the ball of the foot (high heels, for example) are often the cause of metatarsalgia. Because such footwear inhibits the walking process and forces the wearer to alter his or her step to adjust to the shoe, the mechanics of the foot are compromised.

- **A bunion or arthritis** in the big toe can weaken the big toe, and cause extra stress on the ball of the foot. This also can occur after surgery on the big toe, such as a bunionectomy, when the patient does not allow the foot to rest long enough before resuming normal activity; postoperative pain will often cause the patient to modify his or her stride, causing problems to the forefoot. (Note: A bunionectomy will not cause metatarsalgia; a too-short recuperative period, however, will).

- **Stress fractures** of the metatarsal, or toe, bones often cause pain and force an individual to change their stride, thus bringing more pressure to the ball of the foot and stressing that area as well. (This is not uncommon among athletes such as runners, although they are not by any means the only ones who get stress fractures.)

- **Certain foot shapes** contribute to metatarsalgia, according to podiatric physicians. A high-arched foot, or a foot with an extra-long metatarsal bone, can cause pressure on the forefoot region and contribute to pain and inflammation there.

- **Claw toes or hammertoes** can press the metatarsals toward the ground and cause stress on the ball of the foot.

- **Arthritis, gout, or other inflammatory joint disorders** can produce pain in the ball of the foot.

- **What else?** Sometimes, a combination of the factors listed above will lead to metatarsalgia, and sometimes, the condition will appear with no apparent cause, to the frustration of patient and physician, since often a recurrence of the problem can be avoided by pinpointing the reason it developed in the first place.

What cures it?

Some of the best treatments come from being proactive. Keep body weight at a healthy level, and stick to shoes that fit properly, particularly in the toe area. Avoid high heels whenever possible. A regular checkup with a podiatric physician who can assess other risk factors, such foot shape, also will allow you to take preventive measures.

If you have pain in the ball of your foot already, don't panic. Treatment is generally conservative. However, it is imperative to have any foot problem checked by a podiatric physician. This healthcare professional can help you determine whether or not the problem is, in fact, metatarsalgia, since there are other problems which have similar symptoms but require different treatment.

Once your podiatric professional has diagnosed metatarsalgia, he or she will make recommendations based upon the severity of your condition. In many cases, he or she will want to know what factors in your daily routine may have contributed to the condition. Make sure you tell him or her whether your job requires a lot of standing or walking, what type of shoes you wear, what kind of exercise you do, and so forth. Let him or her know if you go barefoot often, and if you do, what surface your feet come into contact with as a result. Note: If you have diabetes, it is essential that you let your doctor know.

Assuming you have a routine case of metatarsalgia, with no complicating factors, such as diabetes, your podiatric physician generally will probably recommend one or more of the following measures, based upon your particular case of metatarsalgia:

- **Rest:** Elevate your feet after periods of standing and walking. This will take pressure off the ball of the foot, and allow it to recover. Using an ice pack at the site of the pain for 20 minutes on, 20 minutes off, may provide additional relief.

- **Wearing appropriate footwear:** Your podiatric physician will let you know whether you should change the type of shoes you wear.

- **Keeping body weight in a healthy range:** Your general practitioner can help you determine whether you are overweight, and if so, can provide you with information on better dietary habits.

- **Exercising:** The podiatric physician may recommend a regimen of exercises for your feet and/or ankles to build strength and flexibility

- **Non-steroidal anti-inflammatory medications or simple painkillers:** Your podiatric physician can decide whether medication will help reduce your symptoms. Whether medication is necessary depends upon the patient, and upon the progression of the case. In cases of more severe inflammation and pain, the doctor may decide to utilize injectable steroids, which can treat the pain at its source.

- **Orthoses or other shoe inserts:** If the podiatric physician feels the case warrants it, he or she may prescribe orthotic inserts, which can help align your foot inside your shoe. He or she may recommend an insert that can be purchased in a drugstore or shoe store instead. In some cases, a pad that allows some cushioning under the ball of the foot will be the doctor's choice.

- **What else?** Occasionally, if other factors are complicating the problem, such as hammertoes or a trapped or pinched nerve in the foot, the podiatric physician will recommend corrective surgery. However, it is important to note that the vast majority of patients are helped by the steps outlined above.

Who is most susceptible?

Metatarsalgia isn't confined to one particular gender or age group, although it is women who wear high heels, and those types of shoes contribute significantly to the problem. However, athletes of either gender (this includes those "weekend warrior" types) who run, walk, play tennis, etc., in worn-out, too-tight, or improper shoes can develop the problem, as can anyone who for, whatever reason, wears shoes that cause the forefoot to receive too much pressure. Remember that a lack of shoe cushioning also can play a role, so make sure athletic shoes, work shoes, and others are replaced according to the recommendation of your podiatric physician. (Note, too, that athletic shoes are activity-specific; in other words, tennis shoes are for tennis, not running, and so forth.)

As previously mentioned, overweight individuals may find themselves more prone to pain in the ball of the foot; of course, having that pain in and of itself does not signify overweight. (Consult with a doctor to ascertain that you are within a healthy weight range, and ask for a sensible, medically supervised dietary plan if you are not.)

How can they be prevented?

Controlling your weight and wearing proper footwear are important, as is letting yourself recover from injuries to your feet. If you find you have forefoot pain, back off on the exercise and try some rest, ice, and so forth. And of course, have regular podiatric checkups to assess your risk factors. Don't forget to see your podiatric physician at the first sign of foot pain or discomfort, and get a diagnosis and treatment plan before the problem has a chance to worsen.

Do these symptoms always mean metatarsalgia?

No—there are several problems with similar symptoms. Your podiatric professional knows how to diagnose and treat them, although treatment can vary, according to the specific problem. Using home remedies and waiting for the problem to go away on its own is not a good idea. After all, if your feet hurt, nothing else matters.

191

Who can help me?

The American College of Foot and Ankle Orthopedics and Medicine (ACFAOM) stands ready to help you find a podiatric physician in your area. Simply click on their foot-help-finder link online at http://www. acfaom.org/directory.shtml to find the professional who can help you find the most effective treatment.

Chapter 21

Muscle Cramps and Contractions

Chapter Contents

Section 21.1

Leg Cramps and Foot Pain

A muscle cramp or "charley horse" is a strong, painful contraction or tightening of a muscle that comes on suddenly and lasts from a few seconds to several minutes. It often occurs in the calf and foot while you are lying in bed or while you are exercising. It is important to note whether the cramps occurs while you are resting or while you are exercising as the cause of each are different. After the hard, tense cramp disappears, soreness in the muscle may last for hours. Muscle cramps may be brought on by a number of conditions:

Parkinson Disease (PD)

In PD the most common cause of muscle cramps, called dystonia, is a relative lack of dopamine stimulation in the brain. Such cramps usually occur at night, when you are resting, when your drug levels of levodopa, dopamine agonists (Mirapex, Requip) are low or "off." Such cramps, which usually occur in one or both legs, are called "off dystonia." "Off dystonia" responds to additional dopamine stimulating drugs: a dopamine agonist such as Mirapex or Requip, levodopa, or a combination of levodopa and Comtan.

Less often the legs cramps occur while the drugs are working or "on." This is called "on dystonia." "On dystonia" is usually but not always associated with dyskinesia. Some people may have both "off" and "on" dystonia at different times during the day. The leg cramps of "off" and "on" dystonia are usually more severe on the side of the worse PD. The cramps can occur on the side of the worse PD, the cramps can occur in both legs, in the calves, and/or the feet. The cramps can also involve the arms, the trunk, and, rarely, the back. The cramps of "on" or "off" dystonia usually, but not always, occur when the arm or leg is resting.

194

Other Nervous System Diseases

Leg and arm cramps may occur in multiple sclerosis, amyotrophic lateral sclerosis (ALS), spinal stenosis, peripheral nerve disease, muscular dystrophy, muscle injury, poliomyelitis, or post polio syndrome. The cramps in these disorders, unlike in PD, usually but not always occur during activity and are relieved by rest.

Activity

A muscle that is tired, a muscle that is improperly stretched, or one that is held in an awkward position may develop a cramp. Leg and foot cramps may occur if you wear high heels, if you jog, if you kick while swimming. Leg and foot cramps may occur if you crouch, or squat. Arm and finger cramps may occur if you type, write extensively, or play piano.

Claudication (Leg Cramps) from Peripheral Vascular Disease

Leg cramps may be caused by decreased blood flow to the legs. Although there is no actual muscle contraction, symptoms may include cramping pain in one or both calves that occurs with activity and is relieved by rest. Such cramps often begin after walking a specific distance. The cramping, called claudication, is caused by hardening and narrowing of the arteries (atherosclerosis) that supply blood to the legs, or arms, or other parts of the body. If the arteries to the heart are narrowed such pain is called angina pectoris. The arteries in the legs are more often affected than the arteries to the arms. As an artery to the leg is narrowed by atherosclerosis, the leg muscles do not get enough blood, especially during when they are active, such as walking, when more blood is required. When the muscle is in a resting state, the blood supply may be adequate.

The main symptom of peripheral vascular disease in the leg is a tight or squeezing pain in the calf, foot, thigh, or buttock that occurs during exercise. As the condition worsens, leg pain may occur after only minimal activity or even when at rest.

In addition to the pain of claudication, other symptoms of peripheral vascular disease include: numb, tingling, or cold skin on the feet or legs; loss of hair on the feet or legs; irregular toenail growth. In addition the feet may turn pale or dusky when they are lowered and improve when they are elevated.

195

Claudication from Spinal Stenosis

Claudication, cramps when walking, may NOT be caused by disease of the arteries to the legs, but by pressure on the nerves to the legs from spinal stenosis. This is called neurogenic claudication. It may be difficult to separate the two types of claudication. As a rule if claudication, cramps when walking, occurs and the pulses in the legs are good, the claudication is probably related to spinal stenosis.

Fluid, Electrolyte, or Mineral Imbalance

If you exercise during hot weather a loss of sodium, potassium, and fluid may occur resulting in cramps called "exercise" or "heat" cramps. Similarly dehydration caused by vomiting, diarrhea, or increased sweating may also result in a loss of sodium, potassium, and fluid and may cause cramps.

Medical Conditions

Hyperthyroidism (an over active thyroid), hypothyroidism (an under active thyroid), increased blood calcium, decreased blood calcium, decreased blood magnesium (from starvation or dehydration), diabetes, hypoglycemia, liver disease with cirrhosis (scarring of the liver), and kidney disease with or without dialysis (resulting in fluid and electrolyte imbalance) may all result in leg cramps.

Toxins

Toxins including tetanus (lockjaw), a bacterial infection that can be caused from a dirty wound and the venom from a black widow spider bite may result in cramps.

Drugs

Drugs, other than drugs for PD, that can cause muscle cramps include: water pills (diuretics), antipsychotic medications, such as chlorpromazine (Thorazine) or haloperidol (Haldol), estrogens, alcohol, drugs called calcium channel blockers that are used to treat high blood pressure, lithium. Muscle cramps may also occur when you suddenly stop taking some drugs such as steroids or opiates.

Section 21.2

Foot Spasms

"Hand or Foot Spasms," © 2006 A.D.A.M., Inc.
Reprinted with permission. Updated August 16, 2004, by
Joseph V. Campellone, MD.

Alternative names: Foot spasms; Carpopedal spasm; Spasms of the hands or feet

Definition: Spasms are contractions of the hands, thumbs, feet, or toes that are sometimes seen with muscle cramps, twitching, and convulsions (tetany). They can be severe and painful.

Considerations

Spasms of the hands or feet may be an important early sign of tetany, a potentially life-threatening condition. Tetany is a manifestation of an abnormality in calcium level, which can be linked to the following:

- lack of vitamin D
- lessened function of the parathyroid glands (hypoparathyroidism)
- alkalosis in the body
- ingestion of alkaline salts

These spasms are usually accompanied by the following symptoms:

- numbness, tingling, or a "pins-and-needles" feeling
- muscle weakness
- fatigue
- cramping
- twitching
- uncontrolled, purposeless, rapid motions

197

Common Causes

- muscle cramps, usually caused by sports or occupational muscle injury
- Parkinson disease and other neuromuscular conditions
- hypocalcemia
  - Causes diffuse, recurrent, or severe muscle cramping.
  - Severe hypocalcemia can produce convulsions.
- hyperventilation—calcium becomes temporarily unavailable to the body during hyperventilation
- damage to a single nerve or nerve group (mononeuropathy) or multiple nerves (polyneuropathy)
- multiple sclerosis
- various medications

Home Care

If vitamin D deficiency is the cause, supplemental vitamin D should be taken under the doctor's direction. Calcium supplements may also help.

Call Your Health Care Provider

If you notice recurrent spasms of your hands or feet, call your health care provider.

What to Expect at Your Health Care Provider's Office

Your provider will obtain your medical history and will perform a physical examination. Laboratory testing of blood and urine may also be done.

Medical history questions documenting hand or foot spasms in detail may include the following:

- Do the spasms appear to be involuntary or purposeless?
- Are they prolonged?
- At what age did the spasms first appear?
- Does the presence of spasms seem variable over weeks to months?

- Do spasms occur repeatedly (recurrent)?
- Do several spasms occur in a row (repetitive)?
- Are the spasms slow or rapid?
- Can the spasms be voluntarily suppressed?
- How long have you had spasms?
- Is it worse when you exercise?
- How much calcium-containing food do you eat (such as milk products)?
- What have you done to try to treat the spasms? How effective was it?
- What other symptoms are also present?
  - Do you have numbness or a "pins-and-needles" feeling?
  - Do you have muscle weakness?
  - Do you have fatigue?
  - Do you have muscle cramps elsewhere?
  - Do you have seizures?

Diagnostic tests may include the following:

- calcium levels (serum calcium)
- hormone levels
- renal function tests
- vitamin D levels (25-OH vitamin D)

Chapter 22

Toenail Problems

Chapter Contents

Section 22.1

Keeping Your Nails Healthy

"Nail Update: Keeping Your Nails Healthy," July 21, 2005, reprinted with permission from the American Academy of Dermatology. All rights reserved.

Healthy nails are an important part of overall health. When nails are in good physical shape, they are not only aesthetically pleasing, but they make it easier to perform everyday tasks. However, not many of us put a lot of thought into our nails, either finger or toe, until there appears to be something wrong.

Speaking at Academy '05, the American Academy of Dermatology's summer scientific session in Chicago, dermatologist Richard K. Scher, MD, professor of clinical dermatology, Columbia University, New York, NY, discussed common nail problems and how to keep them healthy.

"The nails can be windows to a patient's overall health, and while the nail itself is dead tissue, the areas under the cuticle and beneath the nail are alive," stated Dr. Scher. "These areas are particularly vulnerable to infection and damage, which is why it is important to see a dermatologist with any nail changes, so that the problem can be diagnosed and treated."

Cosmetics

Keeping the nails healthy and neat looking has become an important grooming ritual for both men and women as the number of consumers that frequent nail salons and use nail cosmetics at home has increased.

"Nail cosmetics and salon services are generally quite safe, but there are potential problem areas associated with the use of nail cosmetics and salon services: infection, allergic reactions, and mechanical damage to the nail," said Dr. Scher. "While these are fairly rare occurrences, they can be serious and consumers should take some simple measures to guard against these potential health concerns."

Contracting an infection is the most serious health risk related to nail cosmetics, particularly from manicure and pedicure tools and implements that have not been properly sterilized. Viral, bacterial, and fungal infections may be transmitted to unsuspecting consumers from improperly sterilized implements.

Most nail salons take sanitation very seriously and follow strict sanitation and disinfection guidelines, but consumers should not be afraid to ask how implements are cleaned. "Look at the salon with cleanliness in mind and ask yourself these questions: Are the stations clean? Does the nail technician wash her hands between clients? Are there dirty implements lying around? If the salon does not appear clean, then move on," recommended Dr. Scher, who also recommended that consumers bring their own tools and implements to be used at the salon in order to protect against infection.

Allergic reactions occur when a nail cosmetic ingredient sensitizes the skin which may result in itching, redness, blisters, and pain every time the ingredient is used. Some of the more common ingredients that can create an allergic reaction are the acrylic materials found in a wide variety of nail products. Another potential allergen is tosylamide formaldehyde resin, an ingredient found in some nail polishes. If consumers experience itching or burning of the skin following a nail salon service or the application of nail cosmetics at home, Dr. Scher recommends removing the product as soon as possible and visiting a dermatologist to determine which ingredient is responsible for the allergic reaction.

Fungus

Fungal infections, known as onychomycosis or tinea unguium, make up approximately 50 percent of all nail disorders and since the infection occurs under the nail plate or in the nail bed, it can be difficult to treat. Fungal infections often cause the end of the nail to separate from the nail bed, the skin on which the nail rests. Fungus—colored white, green, yellow, or black—may build up under the nail plate and discolor the nail bed. Toenails are more susceptible to fungal infections because they are confined in a warm, moist, weight-bearing environment. Candida or yeast infections are common in fingernails especially if the hands are always in water, as they are in professions such as fishermen, dishwashers, or those who work at aquariums or aquatic theme parks.

Fungal infections are contagious and organisms can sometimes spread from one person to another especially where the air is often moist and people's feet are bare. This can happen both at home and in public places like shower stalls, bathrooms, or locker rooms or they can be passed around by sharing a nail file or emery board. In fact, a recent study noted an increase in athlete's foot, a fungal infection that can grow and multiply on human skin, at boarding schools where students share the same living spaces.

"One way to reduce the risk of contracting toenail fungus is to always wear shower slippers in public showers, locker rooms, and around swimming pools," recommended Dr. Scher.

The Psoriatic Nail

Approximately 50 percent of patients with psoriasis, a disease of the immune system which causes skin lesions that range from patches of mild scaling to extensive thick, red, scaling plaques, have psoriatic changes in their finger and toenails.

"Nail changes in psoriasis fall into general categories that may occur singly or all together," stated Dr. Scher. "These changes can include a deeply pitted nail plate, yellow or yellow-pink discoloration of the nail, white areas under the nail plate, or a nail plate that flakes off in yellow patches."

In some cases, the nail is entirely lost due to psoriatic involvement of the nail matrix, where the nail and cuticle meet, and nail bed. Psoriasis of the fingernails also can resemble other conditions such as chronic infection or inflammation of the nail bed or nail fold, the hard skin overlapping the base and sides of the nails. Psoriasis of the toenails can resemble a chronic fungal infection.

Psoriatic nails can be treated by the dermatologist as part of the overall treatment of the disease and dermatologists are beginning to study the use of biologic treatments. "Therapies for the psoriatic nail have been limited because topical treatments do not penetrate down into the nail fold where the psoriasis is actually disfiguring the nail plate," said Dr. Scher. "The introduction of biologic therapies to control skin psoriasis also may be beneficial for patients with psoriatic nails since these treatments work with the body's immune system to prevent the body from triggering a psoriasis flare."

Nail Malignancies

Subungal, or under the nail, melanoma appears as a brown to black-colored streak underneath the nail, which is often mistaken for a bruise or the nail streaks that frequently occur in people with dark skin. Subungal melanoma accounts for approximately 2 percent of melanomas in Caucasians, and 30 to 40 percent of melanomas in patients with skin of color. Subungal melanoma occurs with equal frequency in males and females, appears most often in people over 50 years of age, but can develop at any age, and is seen most often under the nail of the thumb or the big toe.

"Subungal melanoma should be suspected whenever a nail streak appears without known injury to the nail, the nail discoloration does not gradually disappear as would a bruise or the size of the nail streak increases over time," said Dr. Scher. "It's important to see a dermatologist immediately if any changes are noticed on the nail since treatment for this condition should begin as soon as possible."

"Overall, it's important when caring for the nails at home or having a service in a salon, to make sure that the nails are being treated gently and safely," said Dr. Scher. "Paying careful attention to the nails can help ensure that any infections or diseases are identified early and that treatment is begun as soon as possible."

Section 22.2

Nail Ailments

Barometers of Health

Toenails often serve as barometers of our health; they are diagnostic tools providing the initial signal of the presence or onset of systemic diseases. For example, the pitting of nails and increased nail thickness can be manifestations of psoriasis. Concavity—nails that are rounded inward instead of outward—can foretell iron deficiency anemia. Some nail problems can be conservatively treated with topical or oral medications while others require partial or total removal of the nail. Any discoloration or infection on or about the nail should be evaluated by a podiatric physician.

Nail Ailments

Ingrown Toenails

Ingrown nails, the most common nail impairment, are nails whose corners or sides dig painfully into the soft tissue of nail grooves, often leading to irritation, redness, and swelling. Usually, toenails grow straight out. Sometimes, however, one or both corners or sides curve and grow into the flesh. The big toe is usually the victim of this condition but other toes can also become affected.

Ingrown toenails may be caused by the following:

- improperly trimmed nails (Trim them straight across, not longer than the tip of the toes. Do not round off corners. Use toenail clippers.)

- heredity

- shoe pressure; crowding of toes

- repeated trauma to the feet from normal activities

If you suspect an infection due to an ingrown toenail, immerse the foot in a warm salt water soak, or a basin of soapy water, then apply an antiseptic and bandage the area.

People with diabetes, peripheral vascular disease, or other circulatory disorders must avoid any form of self treatment and seek podiatric medical care as soon as possible.

Other "do-it-yourself" treatments, including any attempt to remove any part of an infected nail or the use of over-the-counter medications, should be avoided. Nail problems should be evaluated and treated by your podiatrist, who can diagnose the ailment, and then prescribe medication or another appropriate treatment.

A podiatrist will resect the ingrown portion of the nail and may prescribe a topical or oral medication to treat the infection. If ingrown nails are a chronic problem, your podiatrist can perform a procedure to permanently prevent ingrown nails. The corner of the nail that ingrows, along with the matrix or root of that piece of nail, are removed by use of a chemical, a laser, or by other methods.

Fungal Nails

Fungal infection of the nail, or onychomycosis, is often ignored because the infection can be present for years without causing any pain. The disease is characterized by a progressive change in a toenail's quality and color, which is often ugly and embarrassing.

In reality, the condition is an infection underneath the surface of the nail caused by fungi. When the tiny organisms take hold, the nail often becomes darker in color and foul smelling. Debris may collect beneath the nail plate, white marks frequently appear on the nail plate, and the infection is capable of spreading to other toenails, the skin, or even the fingernails. If ignored, the infection can spread and possibly impair one's ability to work or even walk. This happens because the resulting thicker nails are difficult to trim and make walking painful when wearing shoes. Onychomycosis can also be accompanied by a secondary bacterial or yeast infection in or about the nail plate.

Because it is difficult to avoid contact with microscopic organisms like fungi, the toenails are especially vulnerable around damp areas where people are likely to be walking barefoot, such as swimming pools, locker rooms, and showers, for example. Injury to the nail bed may make it more susceptible to all types of infection, including fungal infection. Those who suffer from chronic diseases, such as diabetes, circulatory problems, or immune-deficiency conditions, are especially prone to fungal nails. Other contributing factors may be a history of athlete's foot and excessive perspiration.

Prevention

- Proper hygiene and regular inspection of the feet and toes are the first lines of defense against fungal nails.

- Clean and dry feet resist disease.

- Washing the feet with soap and water, remembering to dry thoroughly, is the best way to prevent an infection.

- Shower shoes should be worn when possible in public areas.

- Shoes, socks, or hosiery should be changed more than once daily.

- Toenails should be clipped straight across so that the nail does not extend beyond the tip of the toe.

- Wear shoes that fit well and are made of materials that breathe.

- Avoid wearing excessively tight hosiery, which promote moisture.

- Socks made of synthetic fiber tend to "wick" away moisture faster than cotton or wool socks.

- Disinfect instruments used to cut nails.

- Disinfect home pedicure tools.

- Don't apply polish to nails suspected of infection—those that are red, discolored, or swollen, for example.

Treatment of Fungal Nails

Treatments may vary, depending on the nature and severity of the infection. A daily routine of cleansing over a period of many months may temporarily suppress mild infections. White markings that appear on the surface of the nail can be filed off, followed by the application of an over-the-counter liquid antifungal agent. However, even the best over-the-counter treatments may not prevent a fungal infection from coming back.

A podiatric physician can detect a fungal infection early, culture the nail, determine the cause, and form a suitable treatment plan, which may include prescribing topical or oral medication, and debridement (removal of diseased nail matter and debris) of an infected nail.

Newer oral antifungals, approved by the Food and Drug Administration, may be the most effective treatment. They offer a shorter treatment regimen of approximately three months and improved effectiveness. Podiatrists may also prescribe a topical treatment for onychomycosis, which can be an effective treatment modality for fungal nails.

In some cases, surgical treatment may be required. Temporary removal of the infected nail can be performed to permit direct application of a topical antifungal. Permanent removal of a chronically painful nail that has not responded to any other treatment permits the fungal infection to be cured and prevents the return of a deformed nail.

Trying to solve the infection without the qualified help of a podiatric physician can lead to more problems. With new technical advances in combination with simple preventive measures, the treatment of this lightly regarded health problem can often be successful.

Nail Care Tips

- Proper hygiene and regular inspection of the feet and toes are the first lines of defense against fungal nails.

- Clean and dry feet resist disease.

- Washing the feet with soap and water, remembering to dry thoroughly, is the best way to prevent an infection.

- Shower shoes should be worn when possible in public areas.

- Shoes, socks, or hosiery should be changed more than once daily.

- Toenails should be clipped straight across so that the nail does not extend beyond the tip of the toe.

- Wear shoes that fit well and are made of materials that breathe.

- Avoid wearing excessively tight hosiery, which promote moisture.

- Socks made of synthetic fiber tend to "wick" away moisture faster than cotton or wool socks.

- Disinfect instruments used to cut nails.

- Disinfect home pedicure tools.

- Don't apply polish to nails suspected of infection—those that are red, discolored, or swollen, for example.

Your podiatric physician/surgeon has been trained specifically and extensively in the diagnosis and treatment of all manner of foot conditions. This training encompasses all of the intricately related systems and structures of the foot and lower leg including neurological, circulatory, skin, and the musculoskeletal system, which includes bones, joints, ligaments, tendons, muscles, and nerves.

Section 22.3

Fungal Infections

Fungal infection of the nails is known as "onychomycosis." It is increasingly common with increased age. It rarely affects children.

Responsible Organisms

Onychomycosis can be due to the following:

- dermatophytes such as *Trichophyton rubrum* (*T rubrum*) and *Trichophyton interdigitale* (*T interdigitale*) (The infection is also known as tinea unguium.)
- yeasts such as *Candida albicans*
- molds, especially *Scopulariopsis brevicaulis* and *Fusarium species*

Clinical Features

Tinea unguium may affect one or more toenails and/or fingernails and most often involves the great toenail or the little toenail. It can present in one or several different patterns:

- lateral onychomycosis (A white or yellow opaque streak appears at one side of the nail.)
- subungual hyperkeratosis (Scaling occurs under the nail.)
- distal onycholysis (The end of the nail lifts up. The free edge often crumbles.)
- superficial white onychomycosis (Flaky white patches and pits appear on the top of the nail plate.)

210

- proximal onychomycosis (Yellow spots appear in the half-moon (lunula).)

- complete destruction of the nail

Tinea unguium often results from untreated tinea pedis (feet) or tinea manuum (hand). It may follow an injury to the nail.

Candida infection of the nail plate generally results from parony-chia and starts near the nail fold (the cuticle). The nail fold is swollen and red, lifted off the nail plate. White, yellow, green, or black marks appear on the nearby nail and spread. The nail may lift off its bed and is tender if you press on it.

Mold infections are usually indistinguishable from tinea unguium.

Onychomycosis must be distinguished from other nail disorders such as the following:

- bacterial infection, especially *Pseudomonas aeruginosa*, which turns the nail black or green

- psoriasis

- eczema or dermatitis

- lichen planus

- viral warts

- onychogryposis (nail thickening and scaling under the nail), common in the elderly

Nail Clippings

Clippings should be taken from crumbling tissue at the end of the infected nail. The discolored surface of the nails can be scraped off. The debris can be scooped out from under the nail.

Previous treatment can reduce the chance of growing the fungus successfully in culture; so it is best to take the clippings before any treatment is commenced:

- to confirm the diagnosis—antifungal treatment will not be successful if there is another explanation for the nail condition.

- to identify the responsible organism. Molds and yeasts may require different treatment from dermatophyte fungi.

Treatment may be required for a prolonged period and is expensive. Partially treated infection may be impossible to prove for many months as antifungal drugs can be detected even a year later.

Treatment

Fingernail infections are usually cured more quickly and effectively than toenail infections.

Mild infections affecting less than 80 percent of one or two nails may respond to topical antifungal medications but cure usually requires an oral antifungal medication for several months. Combined topical and oral treatment is probably the most effective regime.

Section 22.4

Mycotic Nails

"Mycotic Nails," reprinted with permission from the Cleveland Clinic Department of Orthopaedic Surgery, © 2006 The Cleveland Clinic Foundation, 9500 Euclid Avenue, Cleveland, OH 44195, www.clevelandclinic.org. Additional information is available from Cleveland Clinic toll-free 800-223-2273 or at www.clevelandclinic.org.

Mycotic nails are nails that are infected with a fungus. The nail may be discolored, yellowish-brown, or opaque, thick, brittle, and separated from the nail bed. In some cases the nail actually may be crumbly.

What causes the pain?

Mycotic infections of nails are caused by a fungal organism that is found in the atmosphere. This organism thrives in the dark, moist, warm environment of shoes, which promotes fungal growth. Prior injury to the nail may predispose the nail to developing a fungal infection. Also, a fungus can be passed from one person to another by sharing shoes or other personal items. Chronic athlete's foot can result in toenail infection, as can shoes that are moist, tight, and prevent air circulation.

Preventing mycotic nails is difficult. The fungal organisms that cause these infections are ubiquitous and difficult to control. You should maintain good hygiene by alternating shoes, changing hosiery on a daily basis, and treating injuries to the nails or toes promptly. Wearing properly fitted shoes and avoiding tight, constrictive shoes may also be helpful in preventing injury to the nail and nail plate which may predispose the nails to mycotic infections. Appropriate regular care to the toenails may also be helpful in avoiding fungal infections.

What are the benefits of treatment?

Mycotic nail infections are difficult to treat. If patients notice an infected nail they should not try to remove that part of the nail, since this can cause the infection to spread. Two standard forms of treatment are available:

- Antifungal creams, lotions, and gels can be applied to the affected area. They are used for mild fungal infections and to prevent the spreading of athlete's foot. Treatment can last several weeks and maintaining a fungus-free nail requires long-term use.

- Antifungal pills (oral medication) can cure an infection but have dangerous side effects, such as damage to the liver. Thus, they are only used when the infection is severe or difficult to treat. The pills are taking once or twice per day for a couple of weeks to several months.

Treatment for fungal infections in the nails may also include periodic removal of the damaged portion of the nail and thinning out of the thickened nails to prevent pain to the patient.

What are the risks of treatment? Is the treatment safe?

Even after treatment, fungal nail infections can recur.

What clinical trials and orthopaedic research are being conducted at the Cleveland Clinic Foot and Ankle Center?

Researchers at Cleveland Clinic are involved in ongoing studies that investigate new drugs and treatment approaches for managing disease. Participants in these clinical trials can play a more active role in their own health care, gain access to new research treatments before they are widely available, and help others by contributing to medical research. There are currently more than 1,700 active clinical studies underway.

Are there other resources that I can go to for more information?

Patients can go to the following resources for more information:

Cleveland Clinic Health Information Center [http://www .clevelandclinic.org, 800-223-2273]

American Academy of Orthopaedic Surgeons [See Chapter 48 for contact information.]

Why should I seek a second opinion regarding treatment?

As modern medical care grows more complex, patients can feel overwhelmed. The opportunity to consult a recognized authority about a particular diagnosis and treatment can bring peace of mind at an emotionally difficult time. A second opinion may be beneficial when:

- you are uncertain about having surgery.
- you still have questions or concerns about your current treatment.
- a controversial or experimental treatment is recommended.
- you have multiple medical problems.
- you have choices to make about treatment.

A convenient way to obtain a second opinion is e-Cleveland Clinic, a contemporary adaptation of the Cleveland Clinic's 80-year tradition as a nationally designated referral center. An easy-to-use, secure, from-home, second opinion service, e-Cleveland Clinic utilizes sophisticated internet technology to make the skills of some of its specialists available to patients and their physicians, anytime, anywhere. With e-Cleveland Clinic's personalized access, no patient need ever to feel unsure or uninformed when faced with what could potentially be one of the most important decisions of their life. To learn more about e-Cleveland Clinic, go to www.eclevelandclinic.org on the internet.

Part Three

Foot and Ankle Injuries

Chapter 23

Blisters, Calluses, and Corns

Did you ever get a blister from a new pair of shoes? Or maybe last fall you raked a lot of leaves and developed a callus on your hand? Or maybe you're a dancer and have noticed painful little bumps called corns on your toes?

Blisters, calluses, and corns can be uncomfortable, but they're also pretty common and easy to prevent. All three happen because of friction—which means that two surfaces rub against each other. In the case of these skin problems, one of the surfaces is your tender skin!

What's a Blister?

A blister is an area of raised skin with a watery liquid inside. Blisters form on hands and feet from rubbing and pressure, but they form a lot more quickly than calluses. You can get blisters on your feet the same day you wear uncomfortable or poor-fitting shoes. You can get blisters on your hands if you forget to wear protective gloves when you're using a hammer, a shovel, or even when you're riding your bike.

Areas on your body that form blisters and continue to be rubbed every day (like your feet because of the same pair of uncomfortable shoes you always wear to school) may go on to form calluses.

This information was provided by TeensHealth, one of the largest resources online for medically reviewed health information written for parents, kids, and teens. For more articles like this one, visit www.TeensHealth.org, or www.Kids Health.org. © 2004 The Nemours Center for Children's Health Media, a division of The Nemours Foundation. Reviewed by Patrice Hyde, MD, September 2004.

What's a Callus?

A callus is an area of thick skin. Calluses form at points where there is a lot of repeated pressure for a long period of time—such as the hours spent raking leaves. The skin hardens from the pressure over time and eventually thickens, forming a hard tough grayish or yellowish surface that may feel bumpy.

Calluses can be a form of protection for the hands. Gymnasts who perform on uneven parallel bars and other apparatus often get calluses on their hands, which take a lot of abuse. Guitar players also get calluses—on their fingers—from manipulating the strings. Once formed, calluses may make it easier for the person to swing around the bars or play the guitar.

Calluses on the feet, however, can be painful because you have to step on them all the time. They usually form on the ball of the foot. (The ball is the roundish part on the bottom of your foot, just behind your big toe.) Some calluses also form on the outside of the big or little toe or the heel. Tight shoes and high heels often cause calluses because they put a lot of pressure on your feet at points that aren't used to all of that stress.

What's a Corn?

Like calluses, corns are also areas of hard, thick skin. They're usually made up of a soft yellow ring of skin around a hard, gray center. They often form on the tops of the toes or in between toes. Like calluses, corns come from pressure or repeated rubbing of the toes. Corns usually develop after wearing shoes that are tight around the toe area.

How to Prevent Blisters, Calluses, and Corns

The best way to deal with blisters, calluses, and corns is to avoid getting them altogether. So how do you do that?

To avoid getting blisters and calluses on your hands, wear the right kind of gloves or protective gear. For instance, you might use work gloves during yard work or palm protectors called "grips" for gymnastics.

To keep your feet callus free, choose your shoes wisely. Try to shop for shoes in the afternoon—that's when your feet are their largest. Why? Because they get a little swollen from you walking on them all day! And be sure to try on both shoes and walk around a little bit before buying them. Even if they look really cool, don't get them if they don't feel right. Often, a different size or width can make a big differ-ence.

And even if you love a certain pair of shoes in your closet, don't wear them all the time. Mix it up by wearing a variety of shoes. That way, your feet will get a break and won't always be rubbed in the same places.

Caring for Blisters, Calluses, and Corns

If any skin problem gets red, inflamed, or looks infected, your mom or dad will want to check with your doctor. But more often blisters, calluses, and corns can be cared for at home.

- Blisters usually just need time to heal on their own. Keep a blis-ter clean and dry and cover it with a bandage until it goes away. While it heals, try to avoid putting pressure on the area or rub-bing it.

- You can help a callus go away faster by soaking it in warm, soapy water for 10 minutes, then rubbing it with a pumice (say: puh-mus) stone. The stone has a rough surface and can be used to rub off the dead skin. Be sure to ask your parent for help us-ing one. Shoe pads that go inside your shoes also can help relieve the pressure, so foot calluses can heal. Pumice stones and foot pads are sold in pharmacies.

- Corns take a little bit longer to go away. To help them heal, you can buy special doughnut-shaped pads that let the corn fit right into the hole in the middle to relieve pain and pressure. There are also pads that contain salicylic (say: sah-luh-sih-lik) acid, which takes off the dead skin to help get rid of the corn. If the corn sticks around for a while and keeps hurting, you may need to see a podia-trist (say: puh-dye-uh-trist), which is the fancy name for a foot doctor.

Chapter 24

Sprains and Strains

This chapter contains general information about sprains and strains, which are both very common injuries. Individual sections describe what sprains and strains are, where they usually occur, what their signs and symptoms are, how they are treated, and how they can be prevented. If you have further questions, you may wish to discuss them with your health care provider.

What is the difference between a sprain and a strain?

A sprain is a stretch and/or tear of a ligament (a band of fibrous tissue that connects two or more bones at a joint). One or more ligaments can be injured at the same time. The severity of the injury will depend on the extent of injury (whether a tear is partial or complete) and the number of ligaments involved.

A strain is an injury to either a muscle or a tendon (fibrous cords of tissue that connect muscle to bone). Depending on the severity of the injury, a strain may be a simple overstretch of the muscle or tendon, or it can result from a partial or complete tear.

What causes a sprain?

A sprain can result from a fall, a sudden twist, or a blow to the body that forces a joint out of its normal position and stretches or tears

"Questions and Answers about Sprains and Strains," National Institute of Arthritis and Musculoskeletal and Skin Diseases, U.S. Department of Health and Human Services, National Institutes of Health, May 2004.

the ligament supporting that joint. Typically, sprains occur when people fall and land on an outstretched arm, slide into a baseball base, land on the side of their foot, or twist a knee with the foot planted firmly on the ground.

Where do sprains usually occur?

Although sprains can occur in both the upper and lower parts of the body, the most common site is the ankle. More than 25,000 individuals sprain an ankle each day in the United States.

The ankle joint is supported by several lateral (outside) ligaments and medial (inside) ligaments (see Figure 24.1). Most ankle sprains happen when the foot turns inward as a person runs, turns, falls, or lands on the ankle after a jump. This type of sprain is called an inversion injury. The knee is another common site for a sprain. A blow to the knee or a fall is often the cause; sudden twisting can also result in a sprain.

Sprains frequently occur at the wrist, typically when people fall and land on an outstretched hand. A sprain to the thumb is common

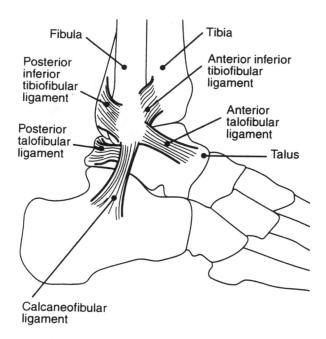

Figure 24.1. Lateral view of the ankle.

in skiing and other sports. This injury often occurs when a ligament near the base of the thumb (the ulnar collateral ligament of the metacarpophalangeal joint) is torn.

What are the signs and symptoms of a sprain?

The usual signs and symptoms include pain, swelling, bruising, instability, and loss of the ability to move and use the joint (called functional ability). However, these signs and symptoms can vary in intensity, depending on the severity of the sprain. Sometimes people feel a pop or tear when the injury happens.

Doctors closely observe an injured site and ask questions to obtain information to diagnose the severity of a sprain. In general, a grade I or mild sprain is caused by overstretching or slight tearing of the ligaments with no joint instability. A person with a mild sprain usually experiences minimal pain, swelling, and little or no loss of functional ability. Bruising is absent or slight, and the person is usually able to put weight on the affected joint.

When should you see a doctor for a sprain?

- You have severe pain and cannot put any weight on the injured joint.

- The injured area looks crooked or has lumps and bumps (other than swelling) that you do not see on the uninjured joint.

- You cannot move the injured joint.

- You cannot walk more than four steps without significant pain.

- Your limb buckles or gives way when you try to use the joint.

- You have numbness in any part of the injured area.

- You see redness or red streaks spreading out from the injury.

- You injure an area that has been injured several times before.

- You have pain, swelling, or redness over a bony part of your foot.

- You are in doubt about the seriousness of the injury or how to care for it.

A grade II or moderate sprain is caused by further, but still incomplete, tearing of the ligament and is characterized by bruising, moderate pain, and swelling. A person with a moderate sprain usually has more difficulty putting weight on the affected joint and experiences some loss of function. An x-ray may be needed to help the health care provider determine if a fracture is causing the pain and swelling. Magnetic resonance imaging is occasionally used to help differentiate between a significant partial injury and a complete tear in a ligament, or can be recommended to rule out other injuries.

People who sustain a grade III or severe sprain completely tear or rupture a ligament. Pain, swelling, and bruising are usually severe, and the patient is unable to put weight on the joint. An x-ray is usually taken to rule out a broken bone. When diagnosing any sprain, the provider will ask the patient to explain how the injury happened. He or she will examine the affected area and check its stability and its ability to move and bear weight.

What causes a strain?

A strain is caused by twisting or pulling a muscle or tendon. Strains can be acute or chronic. An acute strain is associated with a recent trauma or injury; it also can occur after improperly lifting heavy objects or overstressing the muscles. Chronic strains are usually the result of overuse: prolonged, repetitive movement of the muscles and tendons.

Where do strains usually occur?

Two common sites for a strain are the back and the hamstring muscle (located in the back of the thigh). Contact sports such as soccer, football, hockey, boxing, and wrestling put people at risk for strains. Gymnastics, tennis, rowing, golf, and other sports that require extensive gripping can increase the risk of hand and forearm strains. Elbow strains sometimes occur in people who participate in racquet sports, throwing, and contact sports.

What are the signs and symptoms of a strain?

Typically, people with a strain experience pain, limited motion, muscle spasms, and possibly muscle weakness. They can also have localized swelling, cramping, or inflammation and, with a minor or moderate strain, usually some loss of muscle function. Patients typically have pain in the injured area and general weakness of the muscle when they attempt to move it. Severe strains that partially or completely tear the muscle or tendon are often very painful and disabling.

How are sprains and strains treated?

Reduce Swelling and Pain

Treatments for sprains and strains are similar and can be thought of as having two stages. The goal during the first stage is to reduce swelling and pain. At this stage, health care providers usually advise patients to follow a formula of rest, ice, compression, and elevation (RICE) for the first 24 to 48 hours after the injury (see "RICE Therapy"). The provider may also recommend an over-the-counter or prescription nonsteroidal anti-inflammatory drug, such as aspirin or ibuprofen, to help decrease pain and inflammation.

For people with a moderate or severe sprain, particularly of the ankle, a hard cast may be applied. This often occurs after the initial swelling has subsided. Severe sprains and strains may require surgery to repair the torn ligaments, muscle, or tendons. Surgery is usually performed by an orthopaedic surgeon.

It is important that moderate and severe sprains and strains be evaluated by a health care provider to allow prompt, appropriate treatment to begin. The following section lists some signs that should alert people to consult their provider. However, a person who has any concerns about the seriousness of a sprain or strain should always contact a provider for advice.

RICE Therapy

- *Rest:* Reduce regular exercise or activities of daily living as needed. Your health care provider may advise you to put no weight on an injured area for 48 hours. If you cannot put weight on an ankle or knee, crutches may help. If you use a cane or one crutch for an ankle injury, use it on the uninjured side to help you lean away and relieve weight on the injured ankle.

- *Ice:* Apply an ice pack to the injured area for 20 minutes at a time, four to eight times a day. A cold pack, ice bag, or plastic bag filled with crushed ice and wrapped in a towel can be used. To avoid cold injury and frostbite, do not apply the ice for more than 20 minutes.

- *Compression:* Compression of an injured ankle, knee, or wrist may help reduce swelling. Examples of compression bandages are elastic wraps, special boots, air casts, and splints. Ask your provider for advice on which one to use, and how tight to safely apply the bandage.

* *Elevation:* If possible, keep the injured ankle, knee, elbow, or wrist elevated on a pillow, above the level of the heart, to help decrease swelling.

Begin Rehabilitation

The second stage of treating a sprain or strain is rehabilitation, whose overall goal is to improve the condition of the injured area and restore its function. The health care provider will prescribe an exercise program designed to prevent stiffness, improve range of motion, and restore the joint's normal flexibility and strength. Some patients may need physical therapy during this stage. When the acute pain and swelling have diminished, the provider will instruct the patient to do a series of exercises several times a day. These are very important because they help reduce swelling, prevent stiffness, and restore normal, pain-free range of motion. The provider can recommend many different types of exercises, depending on the injury. A patient with an injured knee or foot will work on weight-bearing and balancing exercises. The duration of the program depends on the extent of the injury, but the regimen commonly lasts for several weeks.

Another goal of rehabilitation is to increase strength and regain flexibility. Depending on the patient's rate of recovery, this process begins about the second week after the injury. The provider will instruct the patient to do a series of exercises designed to meet these goals. During this phase of rehabilitation, patients progress to more demanding exercises as pain decreases and function improves.

The final goal is the return to full daily activities, including sports when appropriate. Patients must work closely with their health care provider or physical therapist to determine their readiness to return to full activity. Sometimes people are tempted to resume full activity or play sports despite pain or muscle soreness. Returning to full activity before regaining normal range of motion, flexibility, and strength increases the chance of reinjury and may lead to a chronic problem.

The amount of rehabilitation and the time needed for full recovery after a sprain or strain depend on the severity of the injury and individual rates of healing. For example, a mild ankle sprain may require up to three to six weeks of rehabilitation; a moderate sprain could require two to three months. With a severe sprain, it can take up to eight to twelve months to return to full activities. Extra care should be taken to avoid reinjury.

Can sprains and strains be prevented?

There are many things people can do to help lower their risk of sprains and strains:

- Avoid exercising or playing sports when tired or in pain.
- Maintain a healthy, well-balanced diet to keep muscles strong.
- Maintain a healthy weight.
- Practice safety measures to help prevent falls (for example, keep stairways, walkways, yards, and driveways free of clutter; anchor scatter rugs; and salt or sand icy patches in the winter).
- Wear shoes that fit properly.
- Replace athletic shoes as soon as the tread wears out or the heel wears down on one side.
- Do stretching exercises daily.
- Be in proper physical condition to play a sport.
- Warm up and stretch before participating in any sports or exercise.
- Wear protective equipment when playing.
- Run on even surfaces.

Chapter 25

Foot Fractures Frequently Misdiagnosed as Ankle Sprains

Ankle injuries are commonly evaluated by primary care and emergency physicians. Most of these injuries do not pose a diagnostic dilemma and can be managed nonsurgically without a prolonged or costly work-up. However, the clinical presentation of some subtle fractures can be similar to that of routine ankle sprains, and they are commonly misdiagnosed as such. Many of these injuries, if left without a definitive diagnosis, result in long-term disability.

This chapter features subtle fractures to facilitate timely diagnosis and treatment of these less-common injuries. These fractures should be considered in the differential diagnosis of any acute ankle sprain, as well as any suspected sprain that does not improve with routine treatment.

Overall, optimal results are achieved with early diagnosis and treatment of these fractures. When treatment is delayed, patients tend to have a more complex clinical course.

Talar Dome Injuries

The dome of the talus articulates with the tibia and fibula, and has a key role in ankle motion and in supporting the axial load during weight-bearing.[1-4] Fractures of the talar dome are generally the result of inversion injuries of the ankle. They are located medially or laterally with equal frequency and occasionally through both.[3-5] Lateral talar dome fractures are almost always associated with trauma, while medial talar dome lesions can be traumatic or atraumatic in origin.

Although the etiology in atraumatic lesions is unclear, osteochondral fragments can separate from the surrounding cartilage surface and dissect into the joint space. As these osteochondral fragments (often referred to as osteochondritis dissecans lesions) become loose in the joint, they can cause pain, locking, crepitance, and swelling.[1,4,5]

Diagnosis

Clinical diagnosis of talar dome fractures can be highly challenging because there are no pathognomonic signs or symptoms.[5] The patient may have sustained a fall or a twisting injury to the ankle and may generally ambulate with an antalgic gait. In the acute setting, the symptoms of a talar dome fracture are similar to and often occur with an ankle sprain.[3,5]

In lateral talar dome lesions, tenderness is generally found anterior to the lateral malleoli, along the anterior lateral border of the talus.[3,6] In medial talar dome lesions, tenderness is usually located posterior to the medial malleolus, along the posterior medial border of the talar dome.[3,6] Chronic talar dome lesions—traumatic and atraumatic osteochondritis dissecans lesions—may have a clinical presentation similar to that of arthritis. Typical findings include crepitance, stiffness, and recurrent swelling with activity.[5]

Diagnosis of talar dome lesions can often be made with standard anteroposterior (AP), lateral, and mortise ankle radiographs. However, repeated radiographs may be necessary because initial films may appear normal. Secondary changes in the subchondral bone (visible on plain radiographs) caused by a compression fracture of the articular osteochondral surface may take weeks to appear.[2,4] In addition, small chondral fragments are radiolucent and not evident on standard radiographs.

Generally, the AP ankle view is best for visualizing deep, cup-shaped medial lesions,[1,4] although the lesions are often appreciated on the mortise view as well. Lateral lesions are best visualized on a mortise view and are generally thin and wafer-shaped.[1,4] If suggested by the clinical scenario, fractures not visualized with plain radiographs may require magnetic resonance imaging (MRI) or computed tomography (CT).[6] The fracture classification developed by Berndt and Harty is widely used to stage talar dome lesions.[5]

Treatment

An orthopedic surgeon should be consulted for treatment of talar dome lesions because of the high functional demands of the talar dome and the potential for complications. Stage I, II, and III medial lesions can usually be treated nonsurgically with six weeks in a nonweight-bearing cast.[1,3,5] Adequate reduction and immobilization are crucial for fracture healing and to avoid avascular necrosis of the fracture fragment.[5]

Patients with stage III lateral lesions, stage IV lesions, and persistent symptoms are generally treated surgically. Treatment options for fragment excision range from arthroscopy with or without subchondral bone drilling to open reduction internal fixation.[4,5]

Lateral Process Fractures

The lateral talar process is an osseous protuberance that articulates superolaterally with the fibula, helping to stabilize the ankle mortise, and inferomedially with the calcaneus, forming the lateral portion of the subtalar joint.[7] Lateral process fractures are the second most common talar fracture. From 33 to 41 percent of these fractures are missed on initial presentation.[8-11] Traditionally, the causative injuries are falls, motor vehicle crashes, or direct trauma. Some recent reports [7-9,12] implicate snowboarding accidents in these fractures.

Diagnosis

The patient usually has a history of a rapid inversion and dorsiflexion injury.[7-9] Fractures of the lateral process range from avulsion fractures of the capsular ligaments to intra-articular injuries involving the ankle and subtalar joints.[9]

Physical examination findings are similar to those in lateral ankle ligamentous injuries. Pain with plantar flexion, dorsiflexion, and subtalar joint movement is generally present.[7] Although the normal anatomy of the ankle may be obscured by soft tissue swelling, a helpful diagnostic indicator is point tenderness over the lateral process. The lateral process can be palpated anteriorly and inferiorly to the tip of the lateral malleolus.[8,11]

Fractures can usually be visualized on a standard ankle series.[9] A posterior subtalar effusion seen on the lateral view is highly suggestive of an occult lateral process fracture.[13] A CT scan can clearly show this injury and may be required to confirm a suspected fracture.[11]

Treatment

A nonweight-bearing, short leg cast can be used if anatomic position with less than 2 mm displacement can be maintained.[7,11] A nonweight-bearing cast should be maintained for four to six weeks, followed by two weeks in a walking cast and initiation of rehabilitation exercises.[7] For large and displaced fragments, the treatment of choice is usually surgical reduction and fixation.[7,8]

Posterior Process Fractures

The posterior process of the talus is composed of two tubercles, the lateral and medial. The lateral tubercle is the larger of the two and serves as the attachment of the posterior talocalcaneal and posterior talofibular ligaments.[9,14,15] The medial tubercle serves as the attachment for the posterior third of the deltoid ligament.[9,14,15] The undersurface of both tubercles forms the posterior fourth of the subtalar joint.[9,14]

An accessory bone known as the os trigonum is relatively common, posterior to the lateral tubercle.[6,15] The os trigonum can be a source of pathology, and a normal os trigonum may be confused with a fracture of the lateral tubercle.[2,9,14]

Again, these fractures have been commonly misdiagnosed as ankle sprains.[2,9,15,16] In one case series,[15] 17 of 20 patients with fractures were misdiagnosed with ankle sprains. Posterior process fractures can occur at either or both tubercles.[14-18] Lateral and medial tubercle fractures are discussed separately.

Fractures of the Posterior Process: Lateral Tubercle

Fractures of the lateral tubercle can be caused by hyperplantar flexion or inversion.[1,2,15] Hyperplantar flexion injuries tend to cause compression fractures, while inversion injuries tend to produce avulsion fractures.[1,2,15] Both of these injuries have been described after falls and have been associated with football and rugby kicking injuries, which place the ankle in a forced plantar flexed position.[19] If present, an os trigonum can be injured by the same mechanisms described above.[2,19]

Diagnosis: Clinically, patients with a fracture of the lateral tubercle present with pain and swelling in the posterolateral area of the ankle. The pain is often exacerbated by activities requiring plantar flexion.[15] Physical examination findings in lateral tubercle fractures of the posterior process are highly consistent for tenderness to deep palpation anterior to the Achilles tendon over the posterior talus. The pain is often reproduced with plantar flexion and occasionally accentuated with dorsiflexion of the great toe. This is caused by compression of the fracture fragment as the flexor hallucis longus tendon passes between the medial and lateral tubercle.[15]

Careful physical examination and correlation with radiographic findings may be necessary to differentiate a fracture of the lateral tubercle, a fracture of a fused os trigonum, a tear in the fibrous attachment of the os trigonum to the lateral tubercle, or a normal os trigonum.[2,6,19]

A lateral radiograph of the foot usually best visualizes the lateral tubercle and, if present, the os trigonum.[6,9] When evaluating the fracture line, a rough, irregular cortical surface suggests the presence of an acute fracture. In acute injuries, this rough irregular surface may help distinguish a fracture from a normal os trigonum, which generally has a smooth, rounded cortical surface.[15] In chronic cases, these differences may be less distinct, making the distinction between a fracture and a normal os trigonum difficult. When the diagnosis is unclear and clinical suspicion is present, an MRI or CT will clearly demonstrate this fracture.[16]

Treatment: Nondisplaced or minimally displaced fractures can be treated with a nonweight-bearing, short leg cast for four to six weeks.[9,15] After this period of immobilization, weight-bearing is allowed as tolerated. If symptoms persist, an additional four to six weeks of immobilization would be recommended.[6] If the fracture site continues to be symptomatic after six months, fragment excision is usually curative.[6,9] Larger and more displaced fractures may require open reduction internal fixation.[6,16]

Fractures of the Posterior Process: Medial Tubercle

Medial tubercle fractures are relatively rare.[17,18] They were first described by Cedell,[18] who presented four cases of medial tubercle fractures that had originally been treated as ankle sprains.

Diagnosis: Generally, medial tubercle fractures are secondary to dorsiflexion, pronation-type injuries, because the medial tubercle is avulsed by the deltoid ligament.[17,18]

On clinical assessment, there may be only slight pain with ambulation and range-of-motion testing.[6,18] Patients with medial tubercle fractures typically have swelling and pain posterior to the medial malleolus and anterior to the Achilles tendon.[17,18,20]

Visualization of the medial tubercle fracture on plain radiograph may be challenging, but the fracture can generally be seen on an oblique projection with the foot and ankle externally rotated 40 degrees and the beam centered 1 cm posterior and inferior to the medial malleolus.[16,17] However, CT or MRI may be necessary if the diagnosis is unclear.[16,17]

Treatment: Medial tubercle fractures are treated in a manner similar to that for lateral tubercle fractures.[17,18,20]

Fracture of the Anterior Process of the Calcaneus

The anterior process of the calcaneus is a saddle-shaped bony protuberance that articulates with the cuboid. It is attached to the cuboid by an interosseous ligament and to the cuboid and navicular bones by the strong bifurcate ligament.[21,22] Fractures of the anterior process account for approximately 15 percent of all calcaneal fractures and are commonly misdiagnosed as ankle sprains.[6,21,23,24]

Anterior process fractures result from avulsion or compression. Inversion plantar flexion can cause avulsion fractures of the anterior process. This injury tends to be extra-articular and accounts for most of the anterior process fractures that are initially diagnosed as ankle sprains.[21-23]

Anterior process fractures secondary to compression generally occur when the foot is forcefully dorsiflexed and the anterior process is pressed against the cuboid.[22] Because of the energy involved with this mechanism, anterior process fractures secondary to compression are often intra-articular and are commonly associated with other fractures.[7,23]

Diagnosis

Patients with anterior process fractures generally have a history of a previous inversion injury or involvement in a motor vehicle crash.[21] Clinically, patients generally show signs and symptoms similar to those of a lateral ankle sprain.[21,23] The pain may be minimal with standing but increases substantially with ambulation.[21,23] An important diagnostic feature is point tenderness over the calcaneocuboid joint that is localized approximately 1 cm inferior and 3 to 4 cm anterior to the lateral malleolus, just distal to the anterior talofibular ligament insertion.[21,23,24] Careful assessment of the point of maximal tenderness may help differentiate this fracture from a lateral ligament sprain.[21,23]

Although this fracture can be difficult to assess on routine radiographs of the foot and ankle, a careful inspection of the lateral view of the calcaneus often reveals this subtle fracture.[21,24] As the clinical scenario dictates, a CT scan or MRI may be necessary.[9,21,23] In addition, an accessory ossicle (calcaneus secondarium) may be located near the anterior process and could be misinterpreted as a fracture.[21,24]

Treatment

For small, nondisplaced fractures, early immobilization in a non-weight-bearing, short leg cast or compressive dressing for four to six weeks followed by range-of-motion exercises and a gradual return to weight-bearing has been successful.[21,23]

Although fracture healing may appear radiographically to be complete, approximately 25 percent of patients require more than a year before becoming asymptomatic.[21] Following nonsurgical management, most patients report satisfactory results and a return to preinjury activity levels.[21,23,24] Symptomatic nonunions or large, displaced fractures may require surgical intervention.[21,24]

Final Comment

The fractures discussed here can be serious injuries and cause prolonged disability. In general, extra-articular fractures of the talus and calcaneus can be managed with nonsurgical treatment. However, intra-articular fractures require special attention to ensure that the articular surface is restored to anatomic congruity and that the correct mechanical alignment is maintained. This step optimizes the chance for a full recovery and decreases the incidence of post-traumatic arthritis and associated morbidities.

Appropriate radiographs are essential to the diagnosis of these fractures but, in the work-up of an ankle injury, radiographs are not always required. The Ottawa ankle rules offer the physician clinical guidance as to which injuries require radiographs. Prospective studies have validated the effectiveness of these guidelines and shown the rules to be 100 percent sensitive for clinically significant fractures.[25,26]

Although fractures of the talus were very rarely encountered in the Ottawa ankle trials, the fractures discussed in this chapter would likely be identified using the Ottawa ankle rules, because of the inability of the patient to bear weight after the injury and during the examination.

Nevertheless, some patients with these fractures are able to ambulate and, because patients with these fractures generally do not present with tenderness along the posterior border of the lateral or medial malleolus, radiographic evaluation may not be indicated under the Ottawa guidelines. However, as with all guidelines, clinical judgment and experience may be grounds for radiographic analysis in unique cases. Furthermore, in the case of a suspected ankle sprain that does not improve as expected or is accompanied by tenderness over a potential fracture site, radiographic analysis at a follow-up evaluation may be indicated. The fracture may then be diagnosed and treated soon enough after the injury to avoid an adverse prognosis.

—by Daniel B. Judd, MD and David H. Kim, MD

References

1. Higgins, T.F., Baumgaertner, M.R. Diagnosis and treatment of fractures of the talus: a comprehensive review of the literature. *Foot Ankle Int* 1999; 20:595-605.

2. Keene, J.S., Lange, R.H. Diagnostic dilemmas in foot and ankle injuries. *JAMA* 1986; 256:247-51.

3. Nash, W.C., Baker, C.L. Jr. Transchondral talar dome fractures: not just a sprained ankle. *South Med J* 1984; 77:560-4.

4. Canale, S.T., Belding, R.H. Osteochondral lesions of the talus. *J Bone Joint Surg [Am]* 1980; 62:97-102.

5. Berndt, A.L., Harty, M. Transchondral fractures (osteochondritis dissecans) of the talus. *J Bone Joint Surg [Am]* 1959; 41:988-1020.

6. DeLee, J.C. Fractures and dislocations of the foot. In: Mann, R.A., Coughlin, M.J., eds. *Surgery of the foot and ankle.* 6th ed. St. Louis: Mosby, 1993:1465-1703.

7. Hawkins, L.G. Fracture of the lateral process of the talus. *J Bone Joint Surg* 1965; 47:1170-5.

8. Mukherjee, S.K., Pringle, R.M., Baxter, A.D. Fracture of the lateral process of the talus. A report of thirteen cases. *J Bone Joint Surg [Br]* 1974; 56:263-73.

9. Heckman, J.D. Fractures and dislocations of the foot. In: Rockwood, C.A., Green, D.P. *Rockwood and Green's fractures in adults*. 4th ed. Philadelphia: Lippincott-Raven, 1996:2313-16.

10. Heckman, J.D., McLean, M.R. Fractures of the lateral process of the talus. *Clin Orthop* 1985;199:108-13.

11. Tucker, D.J., Feder, J.M., Boylan, J.P. Fractures of the lateral process of the talus: two case reports and a comprehensive literature review. *Foot Ankle Int* 1988; 19:641-6.

12. Kirkpatrick, D.P., Hunter, R.E., Janes, P.C., Mastrangelo, J., Nicholas, R.A. The snowboarder's foot and ankle. *Am J Sports Med* 1998; 26:271-7.

13. Cimmino, C.V. Fracture of the lateral process of the talus. *Am J Roentgenol* 1963; 90:1277-80.

14. Nasser, S., Manoli, A. 2d. Fracture of the entire posterior process of the talus: a case report. *Foot Ankle* 1990; 10:235-8.

15. Paulos, L.E., Johnson, C.L., Noyes, F.R. Posterior compartment fractures of the ankle. A commonly missed athletic injury. *Am J Sports Med* 1983; 11:439-43.

16. Kim, D.H., Hrutkay, J.M., Samson, M.M. Fracture of the medial tubercle of the posterior process of the talus: a case report and literature review. *Foot Ankle Int* 1996; 17:186-8.

17. Nadim, Y., Tosic, A., Ebraheim, N. Open reduction and internal fixation of fracture of the posterior process of the talus: a case report and review of the literature. *Foot Ankle Int* 1999; 20:50-2.

18. Cedell, C.A. Rupture of the posterior talotibial ligament with the avulsion of a bone fragment from the talus. *Acta Orthop Scand* 1974; 45:454-61.

19. McDougall, A. The os trigonum. *J Bone Joint Surg [Br]* 1955; 37:257-65.

20. Stefko, R.M., Lauerman, W.C., Heckman, J.D. Tarsal tunnel syndrome caused by an unrecognized fracture of the posterior process of the talus (Cedell fracture). A case report. *J Bone Joint Surg [Am]* 1994; 76:116-8.

21. Degan, T.J., Morrey, B.F., Braun, D.P. Surgical excision for anterior-process fractures of the calcaneus. *J Bone Joint Surg [Am]* 1982; 64:519-24.

22. Jahss, M.H., Kay, B.S. An anatomic study of the anterior superior process of the os calcis and its clinical application. *Foot Ankle* 1983; 3:268-81.

23. Bradford, C.H., Larsen, I. Sprain-fractures of the anterior lip of the os calcis. *N Engl J Med* 1951; 244:970-2.

24. Hodge, J.C. Anterior process fracture or calcaneus secundarius: a case report. *J Emerg Med* 1999; 17:305-9.

25. Rubin, A., Sallis, R. Evaluation and diagnosis of ankle injuries. *Am Fam Physician* 1996; 54:1609-18.

26. Stiell, I.G., Greenberg, G.H., McKnight, R.D., Nair, R.C., McDowell, I., Reardon, M., et al. Decision rules for the use of radiography in acute ankle injuries. Refinement and prospective validation. *JAMA* 1993; 269:1127-32.

Chapter 26

Growth Plate Injuries

Chapter Contents

Section 26.1

Questions and Answers about Growth Plate Injuries

National Institute of Arthritis and Musculoskeletal and Skin Diseases Information Clearing House, National Institutes of Health, NIH Publication No. 02-5028, October 2001.

This section contains general information about growth plate injuries. It describes what the growth plate is, how injuries occur, and how they are treated. At the end of this book is a list of additional resources. If you have further questions after reading this section, you may wish to discuss them with your doctor.

What is the growth plate?

The growth plate, also known as the epiphyseal plate or physis, is the area of growing tissue near the end of the long bones in children and adolescents. Each long bone has at least two growth plates: one at each end. The growth plate determines the future length and shape of the mature bone. When growth is complete—sometime during adolescence—the growth plates close and are replaced by solid bone.

Who gets growth plate injuries?

These injuries occur in children and adolescents. The growth plate is the weakest area of the growing skeleton, weaker than the nearby ligaments and tendons that connect bones to other bones and muscles. In a growing child, a serious injury to a joint is more likely to damage a growth plate than the ligaments that stabilize the joint. An injury that would cause a sprain in an adult can be associated with a growth plate injury in a child.

Injuries to the growth plate are fractures. They comprise 15 percent of all childhood fractures. They occur twice as often in boys as in girls, with the greatest incidence among 14- to 16-year-old boys and 11- to 13-year-old girls. Older girls experience these fractures less often because their bodies mature at an earlier age than boys. As a result, their bones finish growing sooner, and their growth plates are replaced by stronger, solid bone.

Approximately half of all growth plate injuries occur in the lower end of the outer bone of the forearm (radius) at the wrist. These injuries also occur frequently in the lower bones of the leg (tibia and fibula). They can also occur in the upper leg bone (femur) or in the ankle, foot, or hip bone.

What causes growth plate injuries?

While growth plate injuries are caused by an acute event, such as a fall or a blow to a limb, chronic injuries can also result from overuse. For example, a gymnast who practices for hours on the uneven bars, a long-distance runner, or a baseball pitcher perfecting his curve ball can all have growth plate injuries.

In one large study of growth plate injuries in children, the majority resulted from a fall, usually while running or playing on furniture or playground equipment. Competitive sports, such as football, basketball, softball, track and field, and gymnastics, accounted for one-third of all injuries. Recreational activities, such as biking, sledding, skiing, and skateboarding, accounted for one-fifth of all growth plate fractures, while car, motorcycle, and all-terrain-vehicle accidents accounted for only a small percentage of fractures involving the growth plate.

Whether an injury is acute or due to overuse, a child who has pain that persists or affects athletic performance or the ability to move or put pressure on a limb should be examined by a doctor. A child should never be allowed or expected to "work through the pain."

Children who participate in athletic activity often experience some discomfort as they practice new movements. Some aches and pains can be expected, but a child's complaints always deserve careful attention. Some injuries, if left untreated, can cause permanent damage and interfere with proper growth of the involved limb.

Although many growth plate injuries are caused by accidents that occur during play or athletic activity, growth plates are also susceptible to other disorders, such as bone infection, that can alter their normal growth and development.

Additional Reasons for Growth Plate Injuries

- Child abuse can be a cause of skeletal injuries, especially in very young children, who still have years of bone growth remaining. One study reported that half of all fractures due to child abuse were found in children younger than age one, whereas only 2 percent of accidental fractures occurred in this age group.

- Injury from extreme cold (for example, frostbite) can also damage the growth plate in children and result in short, stubby fingers or premature degenerative arthritis.

- Radiation, which is used to treat certain cancers in children, can damage the growth plate. Moreover, a recent study has suggested that chemotherapy given for childhood cancers may also negatively affect bone growth. The same is true of the prolonged use of steroids for rheumatoid arthritis.

- Children with certain neurological disorders that result in sensory deficit or muscular imbalance are prone to growth plate fractures, especially at the ankle and knee. Similar types of injury are seen in children who are born with insensitivity to pain.

- The growth plates are the site of many inherited disorders that affect the musculoskeletal system. Scientists are just beginning to understand the genes and gene mutations involved in skeletal formation, growth, and development. This new information is raising hopes for improving treatment of children who are born with poorly formed or improperly functioning growth plates.

How are growth plate fractures diagnosed?

After learning how the injury occurred and examining the child, the doctor will use x-rays to determine the type of fracture and decide on a treatment plan. Because growth plates have not yet hardened into solid bone, they don't show on x-rays. Instead, they appear as gaps between the shaft of a long bone, called the metaphysis, and the end of the bone, called the epiphysis. Because injuries to the growth plate may be hard to see on x-ray, an x-ray of the noninjured side of the body may be taken so the two sides can be compared. Magnetic resonance imaging (MRI), which is another way of looking at bone, provides useful information on the appearance of the growth plate. In some cases, other diagnostic tests, such as computed tomography (CT) or ultrasound, will be used.

Since the 1960s, the Salter-Harris classification, which divides most growth plate fractures into five categories based on the type of damage, has been the standard. The categories are as follows:

Type I: The epiphysis is completely separated from the end of the bone or the metaphysis, through the deep layer of the growth plate.

The growth plate remains attached to the epiphysis. The doctor has to put the fracture back into place if it is significantly displaced. Type I injuries generally require a cast to keep the fracture in place as it heals. Unless there is damage to the blood supply to the growth plate, the likelihood that the bone will grow normally is excellent.

Type II: This is the most common type of growth plate fracture. The epiphysis, together with the growth plate, is separated from the metaphysis. Like type I fractures, type II fractures typically have to be put back into place and immobilized.

Type III: This fracture occurs only rarely, usually at the lower end of the tibia, one of the long bones of the lower leg. It happens when a fracture runs completely through the epiphysis and separates part of the epiphysis and growth plate from the metaphysis. Surgery is sometimes necessary to restore the joint surface to normal. The outlook or prognosis for growth is good if the blood supply to the separated portion of the epiphysis is still intact and if the fracture is not displaced.

Type IV: This fracture runs through the epiphysis, across the growth plate, and into the metaphysis. Surgery is needed to restore the joint surface to normal and to perfectly align the growth plate. Unless perfect alignment is achieved and maintained during healing, prognosis for growth is poor. This injury occurs most commonly at the end of the humerus (the upper arm bone) near the elbow.

Type V: This uncommon injury occurs when the end of the bone is crushed and the growth plate is compressed. It is most likely to occur at the knee or ankle. Prognosis is poor, since premature stunting of growth is almost inevitable.

Type VI: A newer classification, called the Peterson classification, adds a type VI fracture, in which a portion of the epiphysis, growth plate, and metaphysis is missing. This usually occurs with an open wound or compound fracture, often involving lawnmowers, farm machinery, snowmobiles, or gunshot wounds. All type VI fractures require surgery, and most will require later reconstructive or corrective surgery. Bone growth is almost always stunted.

What kind of doctor treats growth plate injuries?

For all but the simplest injuries, the doctor may recommend that the injury be treated by an orthopaedic surgeon (a doctor who specializes in bone and joint problems in children and adults). Some problems may require the services of a pediatric orthopaedic surgeon, who specializes in injuries and musculoskeletal disorders in children.

How are growth plate injuries treated?

As indicated in previously, treatment depends on the type of fracture. Treatment, which should be started as soon as possible after injury, generally involves a mix of the following:

Immobilization: The affected limb is often put in a cast or splint, and the child is told to limit any activity that puts pressure on the injured area.

Manipulation or surgery: If the fracture is displaced, the doctor will have to put the bones or joints back in their correct positions, either by using his or her hands (called manipulation) or by performing surgery (open reduction and internal fixation). After the procedure, the bone will be set in place so it can heal without moving. This is usually done with a cast that encloses the injured growth plate and the joints on both sides of it. The cast is left in place until the injury heals, which can take anywhere from a few weeks to two or more months for serious injuries. The need for manipulation or surgery depends on the location and extent of the injury, its effect on nearby nerves and blood vessels, and the child's age.

Strengthening and range-of-motion exercises: These treatments may also be recommended after the fracture is healed.

Long-term follow-up: Long-term follow-up is usually necessary to monitor the child's recuperation and growth. Evaluation includes x-rays of matching limbs at three- to six-month intervals for at least two years. Some fractures require periodic evaluations until the child's bones have finished growing. Sometimes a growth arrest line may appear as a marker of the injury. Continued bone growth away from that line may mean that there will not be a long-term problem, and the doctor may decide to stop following the patient.

What is the prognosis for growth in the involved limb of a child with a growth plate injury?

About 85 percent of growth plate fractures heal without any lasting effect. Whether an arrest of growth occurs depends on the following factors, in descending order of importance:

- **Severity of the injury:** If the injury causes the blood supply to the epiphysis to be cut off, growth can be stunted. If the growth plate is shifted, shattered, or crushed, a bony bridge is more likely to form and the risk of growth retardation is higher. An open injury in which the skin is broken carries the risk of infection, which could destroy the growth plate.

- **Age of the child:** In a younger child, the bones have a great deal of growing to do; therefore, growth arrest can be more serious, and closer surveillance is needed. It is also true, however, that younger bones have a greater ability to remodel.

- **Which growth plate is injured:** Some growth plates, such as those in the region of the knee, are more responsible for extensive bone growth than others.

- **Type of growth plate fracture:** The five fracture types are described in the section, "How are growth plate fractures diagnosed?" Types IV and V are the most serious.

Treatment depends on the above factors and also bears on the prognosis.

The most frequent complication of a growth plate fracture is premature arrest of bone growth. The affected bone grows less than it would have without the injury, and the resulting limb could be shorter than the opposite, uninjured limb. If only part of the growth plate is injured, growth may be lopsided and the limb may become crooked.

Growth plate injuries at the knee are at greatest risk of complications. Nerve and blood vessel damage occurs most frequently there. Injuries to the knee have a much higher incidence of premature growth arrest and crooked growth.

What are researchers trying to learn about growth plate injuries?

Researchers continue to develop methods to optimize the diagnosis and treatment of growth plate injuries and to improve patient outcomes. Examples of such work include the following:

- removal of a growth-blocking "bridge" or bar of bone that can form across a growth plate following a fracture (After the bridge is removed, fat, cartilage, or other materials are inserted in its place to prevent the bridge from forming again.)

245

- the investigation of drugs that protect the growth plate during radiation treatment

- development of methods to regenerate musculoskeletal tissue by using principles of tissue engineering

To improve the early diagnosis of growth plate injuries, the National Institute of Arthritis and Musculoskeletal and Skin Diseases (NIAMS) is supporting a study to evaluate the use of MRI to visualize young bones and enable prompt, appropriate treatment. In May 1997, the NIAMS, together with the National Institute of Child Health and Human Development (NICHD), the American Academy of Orthopaedic Surgeons (AAOS), and the Orthopaedic Research and Education Foundation, supported a conference on skeletal growth and development. The resulting publication, "Skeletal Growth and Development: Clinical Issues and Basic Science Advances," can be obtained from the AAOS at the address listed in Chapter 48—A Directory of Foot and Ankle Health Resources near the end of this book. In March 2000, the NIAMS supported the First International Conference on Growth Plate.

The NIAMS is working with the NICHD, the National Institute of Dental and Craniofacial Research, and the National Institute of Diabetes and Digestive and Kidney Diseases, to support a research initiative in the area of skeletal growth and development. The purpose of the initiative is to:

- stimulate research to identify and understand the action of the genes that regulate skeletal development;

- evaluate factors that affect growth plate function;

- develop animal models to study disturbances in skeletal growth and development;

- find new ways to correct musculoskeletal deformities.

Section 26.2

Sever Disease:
Injury to the Heel Growth Plate

What is Sever disease?

Sever disease occurs in children when the growing part of the heel is injured. This growing part is called the growth plate. The foot is one of the first body parts to grow to full size. This usually occurs in early puberty. During this time, bones often grow faster than muscles and tendons. As a result, muscles and tendons become tight. The heel area is less flexible. During weight-bearing activity (activity performed while standing), the tight heel tendons may put too much pressure at the back of the heel (where the Achilles tendon attaches). This can injure the heel.

When is my child most at risk for Sever disease?

Your child is most at risk for this condition when he or she is in the early part of the growth spurt in early puberty. Sever disease is most common in physically active girls 8 to 10 years old and in physically active boys 10 to 12 years old. Soccer players and gymnasts often get Sever disease, but children who do any running or jumping activity may be affected. Sever disease rarely occurs in older teenagers because the back of the heel has finished growing by the age of 15.

How do I know if my child's heel pain is caused by Sever disease?

In Sever disease, heel pain can be in one or both heels. It usually starts after a child begins a new sports season or a new sport. Your child may walk with a limp. The pain may increase when he or she stands on tiptoe. Your child's heel may hurt if you squeeze both sides

247

toward the very back. This is called the squeeze test. Your doctor may also find that your child's heel tendons have become tight.

How is Sever disease treated?

First, your child should cut down or stop any activity that causes heel pain. Apply ice to the injured heel for 25 minutes three times a day. If your child has a high arch, flat feet, or bowed legs, your doctor may recommend orthotics, arch supports, or heel cups. Your child should never go barefoot.

If your child has severe heel pain, medicines such as acetaminophen (one brand name: Tylenol) or ibuprofen (some brand names: Advil, Motrin, Nuprin) may help.

Will stretching exercises help?

Yes. It is important that your child performs exercises to stretch the hamstring and calf muscles, and the tendons on the back of the leg. The child should do these stretches five times each, two or three times a day. Each stretch should be held for 20 seconds.

Your child also needs to do exercises to strengthen the muscles on the front of the shin. To do this, your child should sit on the floor, keeping his or her hurt leg straight. One end of a bungee cord or piece of rubber tubing is hooked around a table leg. The other end is hitched around the child's toes. The child then scoots back just far enough to stretch the cord. Next, the child slowly bends the foot toward his or her body. When the child cannot bend the foot any closer, he or she slowly points the foot in the opposite direction (toward the table). This exercise (15 repetitions of "foot curling") should be done three times. The child should do this exercise routine twice daily.

When can my child play sports again?

With proper care, your child should feel better within two weeks to two months. Your child can start playing sports again only when the heel pain is gone. Your doctor will let you know when physical activity is safe.

Are there any problems linked with Sever disease?

No long-term problems have been linked with Sever disease. However, call your doctor if your child's heel pain does not get better or gets worse, or if you notice changes in skin color or swelling.

Can Sever disease be prevented?

Sever disease may be prevented by maintaining good flexibility while your child is growing. The stretching exercises can lower your child's risk for injuries during the growth spurt. Again, ask your doctor for advice. Good-quality shoes with firm support and a shock-absorbent sole will help. Your child should avoid excessive running on hard surfaces.

If your child has already recovered from Sever disease, stretching and putting ice on the heel after activity will help keep your child from getting this condition again.

This section provides a general overview on this topic and may not apply to everyone. To find out if this section applies to you and to get more information on this subject, talk to your family doctor.

Chapter 27

Turf Toe

Abstract

Injuries to the metatarsophalangeal (MTP) joint of the great toe have increased in incidence over the past 30 years following the introduction of artificial playing surfaces and the accompanying use of lighter footwear. Although most common in American football players, similar injuries can also occur in other sporting activities including soccer and dance, or following trauma to the great toe.

The mechanism of injury is typically hyperextension of the MTP joint, but injuries have also been reported secondary to valgus or varus stress, or rarely as a result of hyperflexion injury.[1,2] The abnormal forces applied to the first MTP joint at the time of injury, result in varying degrees of sprain or disruption of the supporting soft tissue structures, leading to the injury commonly referred to as turf toe. The extent of soft tissue disruption is influential in treatment planning and can be used to determine the prognosis for recovery.

This report will review the anatomy of the first MTP join, followed by a discussion of the mechanism of injury and the typical clinical presentation of an individual with turf toe. Finally, the role of imaging

"Turf Toe: Ligamentous Injury of the First Metatarsophalangeal Joint" is reprinted with permission from the Association of Military Surgeons of the United States, © 2004. This article originally appeared in *Military Medicine: International Journal of Association of Military Surgeons of the United States (AMSUS)*, Volume 169, Number 11, November 2004.

including radiography and magnetic resonance imaging, and standard treatment options for turf toe will be discussed.

Introduction

Turf toe is defined as a sprain of the soft tissue support structures of the metatarsophalangeal (MTP) joint of the great toe.[3] Bowers and Martin first coined the term in 1976[4] in a study that identified increasing numbers of MTP joint injuries at the University of West Virginia following the replacement of grass with artificial turf on its playing fields.

The most common mechanism of injury leading to turf toe is reported to be hyperextension of the MTP joint, however valgus, varus, and hyperflexion injuries have also been implicated as potential mechanisms.[3-8] In one study of sports-related injuries at a major university, injuries of the first MTP joint ranked third behind ankle and knee injuries for the total amount of lost playing time by athletes.[3] Although the number of lost days is less overall than that seen with knee and ankle injuries, the length of recovery for the individual athlete can be considerably longer following an injury to the first MTP joint.[1,9]

These facts underscore the need for establishing an accurate and timely diagnosis and conventional radiography and MR imaging can both play a significant role in confirming the clinical suspicion of injury as well as in defining the extent of injury and directing the appropriate treatment. There is currently no information in the literature regarding the incidence of turf toe among the active duty military population. However, one can assume that the incidence is similar to other young athletically active populations and the subject of MTP joint injuries is therefore worthy of review.

Discussion

The first MTP joint is a modified hinge joint that is inherently unstable. However, it derives significant stability from a complex array of soft tissue support structures, which include the capsule, collateral ligaments, plantar plate, as well as the flexor and extensor tendons, and two sesamoid bones.[10] The soft tissue support structures are very important in maintaining proper function of the first MTP joint as this joint bears the majority of a person's body weight (40–60 percent) during walking, with an increase in load bearing of up to two- to three-fold during running, and up to an eight-fold increase during jumping.[3,9,10] Injury to the supporting soft tissue structures can result in an inability to push off with the great toe, thus limiting the athlete's ability to run or jump.

The medial (tibial) and lateral (fibular) sesamoids are contained within the double tendon of the flexor hallucis brevis muscle, which originates on the cuboid and lateral cuneiform proximally and inserts distally on the proximal phalanx of the great toe via the plantar plate.[3,11] The abductor hallucis originates proximally on the calcaneus, while distally its tendon first attaches to the medial sesamoid and then continues on to insert along the medial aspect of the proximal phalanx via the plantar plate forming a portion of the medial joint capsule.[11] Laterally the adductor hallucis follows a similar anatomic pattern, inserting onto the base of the proximal phalanx by way of the lateral sesamoid.[3] The muscle is a bi-headed structure with the oblique head originating along the proximal portions of the lateral four metatarsals while the transverse head originates across the lateral four MTP joints.[11] The first MTP joint is also supported by fanshaped medial and lateral collateral ligaments, each consisting of two sub-parts, the metatarsophalangeal ligament and the metatarsosesamoid ligament.[3] The separate components of the collateral ligaments undergo varying degrees of stress as the joint progresses through its range of motion.[3] Along the plantar aspect of the first MTP joint is a thick fibrous structure referred to as the plantar plate. Distally, the plantar plate has a very strong attachment to the base of the proximal phalanx, while proximally its attachment to the metatarsal neck is relatively loose.[3] The joint's function is slightly more complex than a simple hinge joint with the two bones articulating in a sliding motion that results in compression of the articular surfaces when the joint is fully extended.

In approximately 85 percent of cases, turf toe results from a hyperextension injury of the first MTP joint, although other mechanisms of injury, including varus and valgus stress and rarely hyperflexion, have also been implicated. The incidence of turf toe has increased in American football players since the introduction of artificial turf and the typical injury occurs as follows. While the distal aspect of the player's foot is fixed on the ground with the toes dorsiflexed and the heel protruding into the air, another player falls across the back of the heel, thus driving the already extended joint into a hyperextended position beyond the range that the supporting structures can tolerate. During forced hyperextension, the medial and lateral sesamoids are pulled distally, thereby transferring increased load to the dorsal aspect of the metatarsal head. Depending upon the degree of increased load, the plantar complex beneath the metatarsal head undergoes partial or complete tearing.[7] Disruption of the plantar plate results in impaction of the articular surface of the proximal phalanx against the articular surface of the metatarsal head during full extension.[7]

Turf toe injuries are classified on the basis of severity.[3,7,12] Grade I injuries are the least severe and describe a strain of the capsule without loss of its functional integrity. The patient presents clinically with mild edema but no visible bruising. There is little change in the range of motion and the patient can continue to bear weight. Radiographs are normal and MR imaging may demonstrate mild surrounding soft tissue edema, however all of the soft tissue components of the capsule remain intact. The prognosis for full recovery is good and the patient can usually continue to play with only mild discomfort.[3,7] Grade I injuries may be treated with taping of the toe and the use of a stiff insole in the shoe.

Grade II injuries are more severe and represent partial thickness tearing of the plantar plate and capsular structures. These patients present clinically with ecchymosis and edema overlying the first MTP joint. Range of motion is restricted to a moderate degree, the patient experiences pain and may limp with weightbearing. The symptoms may progress over time and athletes with grade II injuries typically lose up to two weeks of athletic participation. Treatment of grade II injuries is usually conservative with pain control, elevation, rest, and icing of the joint. Motion of the joint may be permitted in several days as symptoms permit. Radiographs are typically normal and MR imaging will again demonstrate adjacent soft tissue edema. Fluid signal intensity may be seen extending partially through the plantar plate and capsular structures representing partial thickness disruption of these structures. The sesamoid bones typically remain in normal position.

Grade III injuries are the most severe and this grade of injury may be used to describe either chronic effects of a disrupted capsule,[12] or to describe an acute injury with complete disruption of the capsuloligamentous complex. In grade III injuries the plantar plate may be completely avulsed from the metatarsal neck and impaction of the metatarsal head may occur during full extension of the joint.[7] If there is a bipartite sesamoid, the component pieces may separate[3,12] or the sesamoid itself may fracture.[3] In severe injuries the sesamoids may diverge or migrate proximally.[3,13] These patients present with severe pain and tenderness to palpation and restricted range of motion. Marked edema and ecchymosis is usually present. The patient typically avoids weightbearing because of severe pain. The athlete will lose a minimum of four to six weeks of playing time and treatment may require prolonged immobilization or surgery.[7] Radiographs may demonstrate an associated capsular avulsion, compression fracture; sesamoid fracture, diastasis, or proximal migration. Comparison films with the contralateral foot or pre-injury radiographs may be helpful in detecting sesamoid abnormalities.[13] MR imaging is also capable of demonstrating each of these potential osseous abnormalities. In addition, MR imaging can demonstrate the extent of injury to each component of the capsuloligamentous structure, including the plantar plate, collateral ligaments, as well as the flexor and extensor tendons.[14] MR imaging can also demonstrate the integrity of the articular surface of the MTP joint.[7]

Radiography and MR imaging can be useful adjunctive tools in the evaluation of clinically suspected first MTP joint injuries. Specifically MR imaging can demonstrate the extent of soft tissue injury, which in turn can help direct proper treatment of the turf toe injury and can also help predict the length of recovery time that will be required for the athlete.

—by Ens. Lee R. Allen, MC, USNR;
Capt. Donald Flemming, MC, USN;
and Col. Timothy G. Sanders, MC, USAF

References

1. Coker, T.P., Arnold, J.A., Weber, D.L. Traumatic lesions of the metatarsophalangeal joint of the great toe in athletes. *The American Journal of Sports Medicine* 1978; 6: 326-334.

2. Massari, L., Ventre, T., Iiriilo, A. Atypical medial dislocation of the first metatarsophalangeal joint. *Foot and Ankle International* 1998; 19: 624-626.

3. Clanton, T.O. and Ford, J.J. Turf toe injury. *Clinics in Sports Medicine* 1994; 13: 731-741.

4. Bowers, K.D. and Martin, R.B. Turf-toe: A shoe-surface related football injury. *Medicine and Science in Sports* 1976; 8: 81-83.

5. Fabeck, L.G., Zekhini, C., Farokh, D., Descamps, P.Y., Delincc, P.E. Traumatic hallux valgus following rupture of the medial collateral ligament of the first metatarsophalangeal joint: A case report. *The Journal of Foot and Ankle Surgery* 2002; 41: 125-128.

6. Rodeo, S.A., O'Brien, S., Warren, R.F., Barnes, R., Wickiewicz, T.L., Dillingham, M.F. Turf-toe: An analysis of metatarsophalangeal joint sprains in professional football players. *The American Journal of Sports Medicine* 1990; 18:280-285.

7. Watson, T.S., Anderson, R.B., Davis, W.H. Periarticular injuries to the hallux metatarsophalangeal joint in athletes. *Foot and Ankle Clinics* 2000; 5: 687-713.

8. Frey, C., Andersen, G.D., Feder, K.S. Plantarflexion injury to the metatarsophalangeal joint ("sand toe"). *Foot and Ankle* 1996; 17: 576-581.

9. Clanton, T.O., Butler, J.E., Eggert, A. Injuries to the metatarsophalangeal joints in athletes. *Foot and Ankle* 1986;7:162-176.

10. Kubitz, E.R. Athletic injuries of the first metatarsophalangeal joint. *Journal of the American Podiatric Medical Association* 2003; 93: 325-332.

11. Thompson, J.C. *Netter's Concise Atlas of Orthopaedic Anatomy.* Icon Learning Systems LLC, Teterboro, New Jersey; 2002 pp 265-267.

12 Rodeo, S.A., Warren, R.F., O'Brien, S.J., Pavlov, H., Barnes, R., Hanks, G.A. Diastasis of bipartite sesamoids of the first metatarsophalangeal joint. *Foot and Ankle* 1993; 14: 425-434.

13. Graves, S.C., Prieskorn, D., Mann, R.A. Posttraumatic proximal migration of the first metatarsophalangeal joint sesamoids: A report of four cases. *Foot and Ankle* 1991; 12: 117-122.

14. Tewes, D.P., Fischer, D.A., Fritts, H.M., Guanche, C.A. MRI findings of acute turf toe: A case report and review of anatomy. *Clinical Orthopaedics and Related Research* 1994; 304: 200-203.

Chapter 28

Achilles Tendonitis

Introduction

Problems that affect the Achilles tendon are common among active middle aged people. These problems cause pain at the back of the calf, and may result in a rupture of the Achilles tendon in severe cases.

Anatomy

The Achilles tendon is a strong, fibrous band that connects the calf muscle to the heel. The calf is actually formed by two muscles, the underlying soleus and the thick outer gastrocnemius. Together, they form the gastroc-soleus muscle group. When they contract, they pull on the Achilles tendon causing your foot to point down and helping you raise up on your toes. This powerful muscle group helps when you sprint, jump, or climb. Several different problems can occur that affect the Achilles tendon, some rather minor and some quite severe.

Tendocalcaneal bursitis: A bursa is a fluid filled sac designed to limit friction between rubbing parts. These sacs, or bursae, are found in many places in the body. When a bursa becomes inflamed it is called a bursitis. Tendocalcaneal bursitis is an inflammation in the bursa behind the heel bone. This bursa limits friction where the thick fibrous Achilles tendon that runs down the back of the calf glides up and down behind the heel.

Achilles tendonitis: A violent strain can cause injury to the calf muscles or the Achilles tendon. This can happen during a strong contraction of the muscle, as when running or sprinting. Landing on the ground after a jump can force the foot upward, also causing injury. The strain can affect different portions of the muscles or tendon. For instance, the strain may occur in the belly of the muscle. Or it may happen where the muscles join the Achilles tendon (called the musculotendinous junction). Chronic overuse may contribute to changes in the Achilles tendon as well, leading to degeneration and thickening of the tendon.

Achilles tendon rupture: In severe cases, the force may even rupture the tendon. The classic example is the middle aged tennis player or weekend warrior who places too much stress on the tendon and experiences a rupture of the tendon. In some instances, the rupture may be preceded by a period of tendonitis which renders the tendon weaker than normal.

Causes

Problems with the Achilles tendon seems to occur in different ways. Initially, irritation of the outer covering of the tendon, called the paratenon, causes a peritendinitis. The word *peritendinitis* simply indicates that there is inflammation around the tendon. Inflammation of the tendocalcaneal bursa (described above) may also be present with the peritendinitis. Either of these conditions may be due to repeated overuse, or ill-fitting shoes that rub on the tendon or bursa.

As we age, a tendon is subject to degeneration within the substance of the tendon. The term *degeneration* means that wear and tear occurs in the tendon over time and leads to a situation where the tendon is weaker than normal. Degeneration in a tendon usually shows up as a loss of the normal arrangement of the fibers of the tendon. Tendons are made up of strands of a material called collagen (think of a tendon as similar to a nylon rope and the strands of collagen as the nylon strands). Some of the individual strands of the tendon become jumbled due to the degeneration, other fibers break, and the tendon loses strength. The healing process in the tendon causes the tendon to become thickened as scar tissue tries to repair the tendon. This process can continue to the extent that a nodule forms within the tendon. This condition is called tendinosis. The area of tendinosis in the tendon is weaker than normal tendon. The weakened, degenerative tendon sets the stage for the possibility of actual rupture of the Achilles tendon.

Symptoms

Tendocalcaneal bursitis usually begins with pain and irritation at the back of the heel. There may be visible redness and swelling in the area. The back of the shoe may further irritate the condition, making it difficult to tolerate shoewear. Achilles tendonitis usually occurs further up the leg, just above the heel bone itself. The Achilles tendon in this area may be noticeably thickened and tender to the touch. Pain is present with walking especially when pushing off on the toes. Finally, Achilles tendon rupture is usually an unmistakable event. Some bystanders may report actually hearing the snap, and the victim of a rupture usually describes a sensation like someone kicked me in the calf. Following rupture there may be swelling in the calf and there is usually no ability to raise up on the toes.

Diagnosis

Diagnosis is almost always by clinical history and physical examination. In cases where there is question whether or not the Achilles tendon has been ruptured, an MRI scan may be necessary to confirm the diagnosis, (but this is seldom the case.) The MRI (magnetic resonance imaging) machine uses magnetic waves rather than x-rays, to show the soft tissues of the body. With this machine, we are able to slice through the area we are interested in and see the tendons and ligaments very clearly. This test does not require any needles or special dye, and is painless.

Treatment

Non-surgical treatment for tendocalcaneal bursitis and Achilles tendonitis usually starts with combination of rest, anti-inflammatory medications such as aspirin or ibuprofen, and physical therapy measures. Several physical therapy treatment choices are available in the early stages of Achilles tendonitis or tendocalcaneal bursitis. The rehabilitation following rupture of the tendon is quite different.

Ice can be used in the first moments after this type of injury, and to calm an inflamed bursa. A bag of crushed or cubed ice held on to the ankle with an elastic wrap works well. Initially, this should be used for periods of 15 minutes every hour. A cold temperature whirlpool may be chosen for your condition. The cold water helps reduce swelling and pain, and the moving water in the whirlpool provides a massage action. In supervised physical therapy, your therapist may continue to treat with either an ice bag, cold pack, or ice massage.

An injury like this needs to be rested. This can be done by limiting activities like walking on the sore leg. A small (¼ inch) heel lift placed in your shoe can minimize stress by putting slack in the calf muscle and Achilles tendon. Be sure to place a similar sized lift in the other shoe to keep everything aligned.

Cortisone injection in this condition is not indicated, due to the increased risk of rupture of the tendon following injection.

Non-surgical treatment for an Achilles tendon rupture is somewhat controversial. It is clear that treatment with a cast will allow the vast majority of tendon ruptures to heal, but the incidence of re-rupture is increased in those patients treated with casting for eight weeks when compared with those undergoing surgery. In addition, the strength of the healed tendon is significantly less in patients who elect cast treatment. For these reasons, many orthopaedists feel that Achilles tendon ruptures in younger active patients should be surgically repaired.

Surgical treatment for Achilles tendonitis is not usually necessary for most patients. However, in some cases of persistent tendonitis/tendinosis a procedure called debulking of the Achilles tendon may be suggested to help treat the problem. This procedure is usually done through an incision on the back of the ankle near the Achilles tendon. The tendon is identified and any inflamed paratenon tissue (the covering of the tendon) is removed. The tendon is then split and the degenerative portion of the tendon is removed. The split tendon is then repaired and allowed to heal. It is unclear why, but removing the degenerative portion of the tendon seems to stimulate repair of the tendon to a more normal state.

Surgery may also be suggested if you have a ruptured Achilles tendon. Repair of the torn Achilles tendon is achieved by reattaching the two ends of the torn tendon. This procedure is usually done through an incision on the back of the ankle near the Achilles tendon. There are numerous ways that have been used to actually repair the tendon, but most all involve sewing the two ends of the tendon together in some fashion. There are some repair techniques that have been developed to minimize the size of the incision.

In the past, the complications of surgical repair of the Achilles tendon made surgeons think twice before suggesting surgery. The complications arose because the skin where the incision must be made is thin and has a poor blood supply. This can lead to an increase in the chance of the wound not healing and infection setting in. Now that this is better recognized, the complication rate is lower and surgery is recommended more often.

After surgery, you will most likely be placed in a cast, or brace, to protect the repair—and the skin incision. A cast or brace will probably be required for six to eight (6-8) weeks. Following removal of the cast, a shoe with a fairly high heel may be recommended for several weeks longer. Physical therapy will probably be recommended for regaining the motion of the ankle and the strength in the calf muscles.

Chapter 29

Sesamoiditis

Most bones in the human body are connected to each other at joints. But there are a few bones that are not connected to any other bone. Instead, they are connected only to tendons or are embedded in muscle. These are the sesamoids. The kneecap (patella) is the largest sesamoid. Two other very small sesamoids (about the size of a kernel of corn) are found in the underside of the forefoot near the great toe, one on the outer side of the foot and the other closer to the middle of the foot.

Sesamoids act like pulleys. They provide a smooth surface over which the tendons slide, thus increasing the ability of the tendons to transmit muscle forces. The sesamoids in the forefoot also assist with weight bearing and help elevate the bones of the great toe. Like other bones, sesamoids can break (fracture). Additionally, the tendons surrounding the sesamoids can become irritated or inflamed. This is called sesamoiditis and is a form of tendonitis. It is common among ballet dancers, runners, and baseball catchers.

Signs and Symptoms

- Pain is focused under the great toe on the ball of the foot. With sesamoiditis, pain may develop gradually; with a fracture, pain will be immediate.

Reproduced with permission from "Sesamoiditis," in Johnson, TR, (ed): *Your Orthopaedic Connection*. Rosemont, IL, American Academy of Orthopaedic Surgeons. Available at http://orthoinfo.aaos.org. Co-developed by the American Orthopaedic Foot and Ankle Society. Published December 2001.

- Swelling and bruising may or may not be present.

- You may experience difficulty and pain in bending and straightening the great toe.

Examination and Diagnosis

During the examination, the physician will look for tenderness at the sesamoid bones. Your doctor may manipulate the bone slightly or ask you to bend and straighten the toe. He or she may also bend the great toe up toward the top of the foot to see if the pain intensifies.

Your physician will request x-rays of the forefoot to ensure a proper diagnosis. In many people, the sesamoid bone nearer the center of the foot (the medial sesamoid) has two parts (bipartite). Because the edges of a bipartite medial sesamoid are generally smooth, and the edges of a fractured sesamoid are generally jagged, an x-ray is useful in making an appropriate diagnosis. Your physician may also request x-rays of the other foot to compare the bone structure. If the x-rays appear normal, the physician may request a bone scan.

Treatment

Treatment is generally nonoperative. However, if conservative measures fail, your physician may recommend surgery to remove the sesamoid bone.

Sesamoiditis

- Stop the activity causing the pain.

- Take aspirin or ibuprofen to relieve the pain.

- Rest and ice the sole of your feet. Do not apply ice directly to the skin, but use an ice pack or wrap the ice in a towel.

- Wear soft-soled, low-heeled shoes. Stiff-soled shoes like clogs may also be comfortable.

- Use a felt cushioning pad to relieve stress.

- Return to activity gradually, and continue to wear a cushioning pad of dense foam rubber under the sesamoids to support them. Avoid activities that put your weight on the balls of the feet.

- Tape the great toe so that it remains bent slightly downward (plantar flexion).

- Your doctor may recommend an injection of a steroid medication to reduce swelling.

- If symptoms persist, you may need to wear a removable short leg fracture brace for four to six weeks.

Fracture of the Sesamoid

- You will need to wear a stiff-soled shoe or a short, leg-fracture brace.

- Your physician may tape the joint to limit movement of the great toe.

- You may have to wear a J-shaped pad around the area of the sesamoid to relieve pressure as the fracture heals.

- Pain relievers such as aspirin or ibuprofen may be recommended.

- It may take several months for the discomfort to subside.

- Cushioning pads or other orthotic devices are often helpful as the fracture heals.

Chapter 30

Other Foot and Ankle Injuries

Chapter Contents

Section 30.1

Foot and Ankle Emergencies

Immediate Treatment

Foot and ankle emergencies happen every day. Broken bones, dislocations, sprains, contusions, infections, and other serious injuries can occur at any time. Early attention is vitally important. Whenever you sustain a foot or ankle injury, you should seek immediate treatment from a podiatric physician.

This advice is universal, even though there are lots of myths about foot and ankle injuries. Some of them follow:

Myths

"It can't be broken, because I can move it."

False: This widespread idea has kept many fractures from receiving proper treatment. The truth is that often you can walk with certain kinds of fractures. Some common examples: Breaks in the smaller, outer bone of the lower leg, small chip fractures of either the foot or ankle bones, and the often neglected fracture of the toe.

"If you break a toe, immediate care isn't necessary."

False: A toe fracture needs prompt attention. If x-rays reveal it to be a simple, displaced fracture, care by your podiatric physician usually can produce rapid relief. However, x-rays might identify a displaced or angulated break. In such cases, prompt realignment of the fracture by your podiatric physician will help prevent improper or incomplete healing. Often, fractures do not show up in the initial x-ray. It may be necessary to x-ray the foot a second time, seven to ten days later. Many patients develop post-fracture deformity of a toe, which in turn results in a deformed toe with a painful corn. A good general rule is: Seek prompt treatment for injury to foot bones.

"If you have a foot or ankle injury, soak it in hot water immediately."

False: Don't use heat or hot water on an area suspect for fracture, sprain, or dislocation. Heat promotes blood flow, causing greater swelling. More swelling means greater pressure on the nerves, which causes more pain. An ice bag wrapped in a towel has a contracting effect on blood vessels, produces a numbing sensation, and prevents swelling and pain. Your podiatric physician may make additional recommendations upon examination.

"Applying an elastic bandage to a severely sprained ankle is adequate treatment."

False: Ankle sprains often mean torn or severely overstretched ligaments, and they should receive immediate care. X-ray examination, immobilization by casting or splinting, and physiotherapy to ensure a normal recovery all may be indicated. Surgery may even be necessary.

"The terms **fracture, break,** *and* **crack** *are all different."*

False: All of those words are proper in describing a broken bone.

Before Seeing the Podiatrist

If an injury or accident does occur, the steps you can take to help yourself until you can reach your podiatric physician are easy to remember if you can recall the word "rice."

1. **Rest:** Restrict your activity and get off your foot/ankle.

2. **Ice:** Gently place a plastic bag of ice wrapped in a towel on the injured area in a 20-minute-on, 40-minute-off cycle.

3. **Compression:** Lightly wrap an Ace bandage around the area, taking care not to pull it too tight.

4. **Elevation:** To reduce swelling and pain, sit in a position that allows you to elevate the foot/ankle higher than your waist.

5. For bleeding cuts, cleanse well, apply pressure with gauze or a towel, and cover with a clean dressing. See your podiatrist as

soon as possible. It's best not to use any medication on the cut before you see the doctor.

6. Leave blisters unopened if they are not painful or in a weight-bearing area of the foot. A compression bandage placed over a blister can provide relief.

7. Foreign materials in the skin—such as slivers, splinters, and sand—can be removed carefully, but a deep foreign object, such as broken glass or a needle, must be removed professionally.

8. Treatment for an abrasion is similar to that of a burn, since raw skin is exposed to the air and can easily become infected. It is important to remove all foreign particles with thorough cleaning. Sterile bandages should be applied, along with an antibiotic cream or ointment.

Prevention

1. Wear the correct shoes for your particular activity.

2. Wear hiking shoes or boots in rough terrain.

3. Don't continue to wear any sports shoe if it is worn unevenly.

4. The toe box in "steel-toe" shoes should be deep enough to accommodate your toes comfortably.

5. Always wear hard-top shoes when operating a lawn mower or other grass-cutting equipment.

6. Don't walk barefoot on paved streets or sidewalks.

7. Watch out for slippery floors at home and at work. Clean up obviously dangerous spills immediately.

8. If you get up during the night, turn on a light. Many fractured toes and other foot injuries occur while attempting to find one's way in the dark.

Section 30.2

Chilblains and Frostbite

This section includes text from both "Chilblains," and "Frostbite," December 17, 2005. This information is reprinted with the permission from DermNet, the website of the New Zealand Dermatological Society. Visit www.dermnet.org.nz for patient information on numerous skin conditions and their treatment. © 2005 New Zealand Dermatological Society.

Chilblains

Chilblains are itchy and/or tender red or purple bumps that occur as a reaction to cold. The condition is also known as pernio and is a localized form of vasculitis.

Chilblains occur several hours after exposure to the cold in temperate humid climates. They are sometimes aggravated by sun exposure. Cold causes constriction of the small arteries and veins in the skin and rewarming results in leakage of blood into the tissues and swelling of the skin.

Chilblains are less common in countries where the cold is more extreme because the air is drier and people have specially designed living conditions and clothing. Children and the elderly are most often affected.

Chilblains are more likely to develop in those with poor peripheral circulation (i.e. blue-red mottled skin on the limbs).

Contributing Factors

- a familial tendency

- peripheral vascular disease due to diabetes, smoking, hyperlipidemia

- poor nutrition (e.g., anorexia nervosa)

- hormonal changes: chilblains can improve during pregnancy

- connective tissue disease (lupus erythematosus)

- bone marrow disorders

271

Common Sites for Chilblains

- backs and sides of the fingers and toes
- heels
- lower legs
- thighs, especially in horse riders
- wrists of babies
- over fatty lumps (lipomas)
- nose
- ears

Each chilblain comes up over a few hours as an itchy red swelling and subsides over the next 7-14 days. In severe cases blistering, pustules, scabs, and ulceration can occur. Occasionally the lesions may be ring-shaped. They may become thickened and persist for months.

In children recurrences each winter for a few years are common but complete recovery is usual. Chilblains in elderly people have a tendency to get worse every year unless precipitating factors are avoided.

Treatment

Unfortunately chilblains respond poorly to treatment. The following may be useful:

- A potent topical steroid applied accurately for a few days may relieve itch and swelling.
- Antibiotic ointment or oral antibiotics may be necessary for secondary infection.

Prevention

The hands and feet must not be allowed to get cold. Do not smoke! The following measures may help to keep you warm:

- Insulated and heated home and workplace—stop up all drafts.
- Warm clothing especially gloves, thick woolen socks, and comfortable protective footwear—keep the head and neck warm with hat and scarf.
- Before going outside, soak hands in warm water for several minutes to warm hands through then dry thoroughly.

- Exercise vigorously before going outside.

- Wear cotton-lined waterproof gloves for wet work.

- Apply sunscreen to exposed skin even on dull days.

- Take vasodilator medication such as nifedipine prescribed before the onset of cold weather and taken throughout winter. Side effects include flushing and headache.

Frostbite

What is frostbite?

Frostbite is a condition where the skin and underlying tissue actually freeze. It occurs when body parts, usually the extremities such as the toes, feet, fingers, ears, nose, and cheeks are exposed to extremely cold conditions. The condition rarely occurs in fit and healthy individuals in still air temperature above minus 10 degrees Celsius, but may do so at higher temperatures in high winds due to the wind-chill effect.

What causes frostbite?

Certain processes taking place in the body, in response to exposure to extreme cold, cause frostbite.

- Firstly, blood flow to the skin and extremities is slowed down as blood vessels constrict (narrow). This occurs so blood can be redirected to the vital organs to keep the body alive and warm. Ice crystals form in the tissues, the blood vessel walls are damaged, and the cells start to break down.

- Secondly, with continued exposure to the cold, as the extremities get colder and colder, the blood vessels dilate (widen) for a brief period before constricting again. This happens because the body is trying to preserve as much function in the extremities as possible. However, the blood returning to the extremities leaks out through the leaky blood vessels. This causes further damage to the tissues.

Who gets frostbite?

Certain groups of people are at greater risk of getting frostbite than others; these include the following:

273

- winter and high-altitude athletes (e.g., mountaineers and skiers)

- individuals stranded in extreme cold weather conditions

- soldiers, cold weather rescuers, and laborers working in cold environments

- homeless people

- very young and the very old people

- people with decreased blood flow to the extremities such as those with peripheral vascular disease or diabetes

- those taking certain drugs that constrict blood vessels (e.g., nicotine (smoking) or beta blockers)

What are the signs and symptoms?

The signs and symptoms of frostbite include coldness, firmness, stinging, burning, numbness, clumsiness, pain, throbbing, excessive sweating, pallor or blue skin discoloration, rotting skin, and gangrene. Frostbite has been classified under the following categories that relate to the degree of injury.

- **First-degree frostbite:** This is also called frost nip and occurs in people who live in very cold climates or do a lot of outdoor activity in winter. It involves the top layer of skin (epidermis) and presents as numbed skin that has turned white in color. The skin may feel stiff to touch, but the tissue underneath is still warm and soft. Blistering, infection, or scarring seldom occurs if frost nip is treated promptly.

- **Second-degree frostbite:** This is superficial frostbite and presents as white or blue skin that feels hard and frozen. Blisters usually form within 24 hours of injury and are filled with clear or milky fluid. The tissue underneath is still intact but medical treatment is required to prevent further damage.

- **Third-degree frostbite:** Deep frostbite appears as white, blotchy, and/or blue skin. The underlying skin tissue is damaged and feels hard and cold to touch. Blood-filled blisters form black thick scabs over a matter of weeks. Proper medical treatment by personnel trained to deal with severe frostbite is required to help prevent severe or permanent injury. Amputation may be required to prevent severe infection.

- **Fourth-degree frostbite:** Fourth degree frostbite is where full-thickness damage affects muscles, tendons, and bone, with resultant tissue loss.

What treatment is available?

Prior to reaching a place that can provide proper medical attention the following should take place.

- Shelter patient from the cold and move to a warmer place.

- Replace wet clothing with dry soft clothing to minimize further heat loss.

- Do not try to thaw frostbite unless in a warm place (warming and then re-exposing frozen parts to the cold cause permanent damage).

- Do not rub the affected area with warm hands or snow, apply direct heat such as heater, fire, or heating pad, as this can cause further injury.

- Warm the entire body, not just the frostbitten parts, by wrapping in blankets and protecting the frostbitten parts until a suitable place is reached to start the rewarming process.

Once the patient has reached an appropriate facility, the rewarming process can take place. Rewarming should be rapid to avoid further damage.

- An appropriate warming technique is the use of a whirlpool bath or tub of water at 40-42 degrees Celsius. Avoid warmer temperatures or dry heat because of the risk of thermal injury.

- Warm wet packs at the same temperature can be used if a water tub is not available.

- Rewarming or thawing usually takes about 20-40 minutes and is complete when tips of the affected area flush, the skin is soft and sensation returns.

- Apply dry, sterile dressings to the frostbitten areas and place between fingers and toes to keep them separated. Try to restrict movement of the affected areas as much as possible.

- Clean any dead tissue around clear blisters, but leave blood-filled blisters intact to reduce the risk of infection.

- Analgesics such as morphine sulphate may be administered for pain. The thawing out can be very painful.

Within days of the thawing process further blisters may form. These should settle after about a week but may leave behind dead blackened tissue that form scabs. If the frostbite is superficial, pink new skin will appear beneath the scab. If frostbite is deep, the end of the finger or toe will gradually separate off. In some cases surgery may be required to remove dead tissue. This is not usually performed until three to four weeks after the initial injury, as the full extent of damage to tissues is not usually complete until this time.

—by Vanessa Ngan, Staff Writer

Section 30.3

Trench Foot

"Disaster Recovery Fact Sheet: Trench Foot or Immersion Foot," U.S. Department of Health and Human Services, Centers for Disease Control and Prevention, September 9, 2005.

What is trench foot?

Trench foot, also known as immersion foot, occurs when the feet are wet for long periods of time. It can be quite painful, but it can be prevented and treated.

What are the symptoms of trench foot?

Symptoms of trench foot include a tingling and/or itching sensation, pain, swelling, cold and blotchy skin, numbness, and a prickly or heavy feeling in the foot. The foot may be red, dry, and painful after it becomes warm. Blisters may form, followed by skin and tissue dying and falling off. In severe cases, untreated trench foot can involve the toes, heel, or entire foot.

How is trench foot prevented and treated?

When possible, air-dry and elevate your feet, and exchange wet shoes and socks for dry ones to help prevent the development of trench foot.

Treatment for trench foot is similar to the treatment for frostbite. Take the following steps:

- Thoroughly clean and dry your feet.

- Put on clean, dry socks daily.

- Treat the affected part by applying warm packs or soaking in warm water (102° to 110° F) for approximately five minutes.

- When sleeping or resting, do not wear socks.

- Obtain medical assistance as soon as possible.

- If you have a foot wound, your foot may be more prone to infection. Check your feet at least once a day for infections or worsening of symptoms.

Section 30.4

Tarsal Tunnel Syndrome

Text in this section was written by David A. Cooke, MD, Diplomate, American Board of Internal Medicine. © 2007 Omnigraphics, Inc.

What is tarsal tunnel syndrome?

Tarsal tunnel syndrome is an uncommon foot condition caused by pressure on one or more of the nerves in the foot. It should be considered in anyone who complains of numbness, tingling, or pain in their toes or forefoot.

On the inner side of the ankle, there is an area known as the tarsal tunnel. The bones of the foot and ankle fit together in a way that creates a tunnel, with three walls of bone. The fourth wall, over the top, is created by the flexor retinaculum. The flexor retinaculum is a tough sheet of connective tissue that helps keep tendons from slipping out of place. Two large tendons pass through this tunnel, along with an artery and vein, and the tibial nerve. The tibial nerve branches into the medial and lateral plantar nerves within this tunnel.

Even in a normal person, this space is always relatively tight. If anything causes there to be less space than usual in the tunnel, it will create pressure on the tendons, vessels, and nerves that run through there. The nerves, the most fragile structures in the tunnel, become compressed.

Because the tibial nerve branches within the tunnel, there can be compression of the tibial nerve, the medial plantar nerve, the lateral plantar nerve, or all three. These nerves provide sensation to different portions of the sole of the foot. If they are compressed, the result is pain or numbness in the areas served by the nerves. When this occurs, tarsal tunnel syndrome is diagnosed.

What conditions can cause tarsal tunnel syndrome?

There are a wide variety of conditions that can cause tarsal tunnel syndrome. A fracture or dislocation of the foot or ankle may narrow the tunnel. Inflammation of the tendons in the tunnel, due to injury or autoimmune diseases such as rheumatoid arthritis, may cause them to swell, creating less space in the tunnel for the nerves. Individuals with diabetes are at increased risk for tarsal tunnel syndrome, due to the tendency of the diabetes to cause several types of nerve damage. Cysts or tumors in the tarsal tunnel will take up space, and compress the nerves. Varicose veins and bone spurs can also sometimes affect the tunnel. People with flat feet are at increased risk for tarsal tunnel syndrome. Sometimes, wearing poorly-designed shoes or unusual foot positioning can also narrow the tunnel. For example, wearing flat shoes (e.g. slippers, flip-flops) with no arch support can shift the bones in ways that cause tarsal tunnel syndrome. However, in about half of cases of tarsal tunnel syndrome, no specific cause be found.

How do I know if I have tarsal tunnel syndrome?

People with tarsal tunnel syndrome usually notice pain, tingling, burning, or numbness on the sole of their foot. This usually affects the toes and the forefoot, but may extend backwards towards the heel. Depending on exactly which nerve is being compressed, the symptoms may be felt on the inner side of the sole, the outer side of the sole, or the entire bottom of the foot. Pain tends to be worse with activity, and usually improves with rest.

If tarsal tunnel syndrome is suspected, an initial evaluation by a primary care physician is usually appropriate. It is important to distinguish tarsal tunnel syndrome from several other foot conditions which may cause similar symptoms, including peripheral neuropathy, Morton neuroma, and plantar fasciitis. The patient's description of the symptoms, as well as the physical exam, can usually narrow down the diagnosis.

Tarsal tunnel syndrome can be confirmed by a nerve conduction study (NCS), which tests the function of the involved nerves and can localize the site of injury. Magnetic resonance imaging (MRI) can help confirm the diagnosis, and can be useful for determining whether a space-occupying lesion such as a cyst or tumor is present.

What treatments are available?

Depending upon the physician's level of experience with the problem, the primary care physician may prescribe treatment, or refer to an orthopedist or podiatrist. Treatment of tarsal tunnel syndrome usually starts with simple measures. Avoiding walking barefoot, and wearing shoes with proper arch support and heel padding can help significantly. For some patients, a referral for shoe orthotics can also improve symptoms. Altering activities to avoid positions that narrow the tunnel can also be helpful. Nonsteroidal anti-inflammatory drugs (NSAIDs) are often prescribed to improve pain and reduce swelling. Temporary immobilization of the ankle in a brace may also be effective. Physical therapy is sometimes performed.

If initial treatment is not successful, additional approaches are available. Corticosteroid injections into the tunnel to reduce swelling and inflammation are sometimes performed, and will cure some cases of tarsal tunnel syndrome. However, persistent tarsal tunnel syndrome frequently requires surgical intervention.

Surgery for tarsal tunnel syndrome is usually performed by orthopedists or podiatrists. Usually, this involves a flexor retinaculum release procedure. The thick connective tissue that creates the roof of the tarsal tunnel is cut through, opening up the tunnel. If a space-occupying lesion is present, it is removed. The surgery releases pressure on the nerves, and allows them to heal.

With milder cases of tarsal tunnel syndrome, recovery is often complete. Surgery can provide full cures in up to 75 percent of patients. However, a substantial proportion of patients may continue to have tarsal tunnel syndromes, even following surgery. Further advances in the treatment of this disorder will be welcome.

Part Four

Deformities of the Foot and Ankle

Chapter 31

Foot Deformities

Hammer Toe

Definition: Hyperextension of the metatarsophalangeal (MTP) and distal interphalangeal (DIP) joints accompanied by flexion of the proximal interphalangeal (IP) joint.

Pathomechanics: Hammer toe can develop any time there is imbalance across the MTP joint. Multiple causes include plantarflexion of the metatarsals, forefoot valgus, hallux abductovalgus, toe extensor paralysis, interossei imbalance, and loss of lumbrical function.

Potential problems: High pressure over the dorsal surface of the proximal IP joint and plantar metatarsal heads.

Treatment: Extra depth shoe; spot stretch the dorsal aspect of the shoe over the problem area; or surgical correction of the deformity.

Claw Toe

Definition: Hyperextension of the MTP joint and flexion of the proximal and distal IP joints. Commonly associated with pes cavus. Usually involves all the toes.

"BPHC Foot Deformities—PT," U.S. Department of Health and Human Services, Health Resources and Services Administration, National Hansen's Disease Program (http://bphc.hrsa.gov/nhdp/foot-deformities-pt.htm. Accessed September 2006.

Pathomechanics: Instability of the MTP joint, leading to muscle imbalance and eventual extension of the MTP and flexion of the IP joints. Multiple causes include forefoot adductus, congenital plantar-flexed first ray, forefoot supinatus, pes cavus, and arthritis of the MTP joint.

Potential problems: High pressure over dorsum of proximal IP joints, plantar surface of metatarsal heads, and distal end of the toes.

Treatment: Extra depth shoe; toe pillow to relieve pressure over the distal toe; spot relief on the dorsum of the shoe; surgical correction of the deformity.

Drop Foot

Causes: Caused by weakness or paralysis of the ankle dorsiflexors. May be a result of peripheral neuropathy or trauma to the deep peroneal nerve.

Pathomechanics: The loss of ankle dorsiflexion can cause the patient to drag the toe during normal gait.

Potential problems: Toe ulceration secondary to repeated dragging of the toes, frequent falls, gastrocnemius tightness, and possible plantarflexion contracture. The plantar flexed position will increase forefoot pressure during gait.

Treatment: Ankle-foot orthosis; tendon transfer.

Charcot Foot

Definition: An insidious, non-infectious chronic destruction of bones and joints resulting in fractures, subluxations, and dislocations. Signs and symptoms include swelling, increased skin temperature, deformity, bony prominence, and unstable joints. Pain may or may not be present.

Pathomechanics: Neuropathic changes with resulting ligamentous laxity and joint dislocation. Lack of normal protective sensation allows damage to go unrecognized by the patient and with persistent activity, periarticular fractures result. As trauma continues, inflammation and bone absorption is promoted and bony deformity increases.

Potential problems: Fractures, loss of medial longitudinal arch, abnormal weight bearing pattern of the foot, and ulcerations.

Treatment: Early intervention and prevention is the best treatment. Use of skin temperature scanner is a very useful tool to assess possibility of a Charcot joint. Skin temperature elevation of greater than two degrees may indicate an acute process. If an acute Charcot foot is diagnosed, three months in a non-weight bearing cast is essential to allow adequate healing. Temperatures can then be re-assessed to ensure the acute process has halted. Very slow progression to ambulation is undertaken using a rigid rocker-bottom sole and custom inserts which are crucial in decreasing the stresses on the foot. Frequent temperature readings are taken and compared to the baseline. In acute dislocation, surgical correction may be possible if joint fragmentation has not occurred. In chronic cases, however, surgery is a last resort. Protective splinting, bracing, and/or footwear is the treatment of choice.

Hallux Limitus

Definition: Ankylosing of the first MTP joint.

Pathomechanics: A rigid hallux does not allow the normal toe extension necessary during the end stages of gait. This can be caused by hypermobility of the first ray associated with abnormal pronation and excessive calcaneal eversion. Other potential causes include degenerative joint disease of the first MTP, trauma, acute inflammation, and excessively long first metatarsal. Any process leading to bony changes in the first MTP joint can produce hallux limitus.

Potential problems: Increased weight bearing and ulceration at the 1st and 5th metatarsal heads.

Treatment: Rigid rocker-bottom shoe; custom insert with relief for the 1st hallux.

Rearfoot Varus

Pathomechanics: At heel strike, the lateral aspect of the heel comes in contact with the ground. Because of the varus position of the heel, excessive pronation is required to bring the medial heel to the floor. In response, supination occurs very quickly, preparing the foot for toe off and propulsion. A spin callus over the 2nd and 3rd metatarsal heads can result from this transition from excessive pronation back to supination.

Potential problems: Hypermobility may decrease stability of the 1st ray, increased sheer forces on the 2nd and 3rd metatarsal heads, lateral ankle sprains, plantar fasciitis, and posterior tibialis tendonitis.

Treatment: For the insensitive foot, use of a semi-rigid or rigid orthotic may be contraindicated. Use a softer, more accommodative orthotic with a medial wedge (not greater than four–six degrees) coupled with a shoe with good rearfoot control. When fabricating the orthotic for the patient with normal sensation, use of a semi-rigid material may be more advantageous.

Forefoot Varus (Compensated)

Pathomechanics: As heel strike occurs, the foot will attempt to get all the metatarsals on the ground to increase stability. Because of the varus position of the forefoot, excessive subtalar (rearfoot) pronation is required to achieve this goal. The excessive pronation leads to hypermobility at the midtarsal joint and eventual dorsiflexion of the 1st ray. The result is increased shear and loading of the 2nd and 3rd metatarsal heads. In addition, the full compensation of the forefoot varus will cause foot abduction relative to the line of progression. The medial aspect of the 1st ray then becomes a lever for push off and can develop heavy callus or breakdown.

Potential problems: Ulceration at the metatarsal heads and medial hallux, plantar fasciitis, hallux abductovalgus, medial knee pain secondary to excessive pronation and increased tibial rotation, piriformis tendonitis secondary to increased hip rotation, and calcaneal spurring secondary to traction force of the plantar fascia.

Treatment: Use a rigid to semi-rigid orthotic depending on activity level; Medial wedge with a maximum of eight degrees of correction; be conservative and it may be beneficial to add medial wedging slowly to allow accommodation. Deep heel seat is essential to control the calcaneus. Taping and other modalities are effective as well. When dealing with the insensitive foot, use of a softer, more accommodative material is advisable when fabricating the orthotic.

Forefoot Varus (Uncompensated)

Pathomechanics: The uncompensated forefoot varus lacks the subtalar joint pronation required to bring the foot flat on the floor. The calcaneus never everts past vertical and the weight bearing forces are concentrated on the lateral border of the forefoot through most of the gait cycle. As the foot moves toward terminal stance, the lower extremity pivots over the 5th metatarsal head in order to begin the weight shift to the opposite extremity. Heavy callus formation and eventual breakdown over the lateral border of the foot and 5th metatarsal head can result from this type of biomechanical position.

Potential problems: Stress fracture of the 5th metatarsal, fibular fracture, ankle sprains, and deep capsular pain, commonly known in children as "growing pains."

Treatment: Soft, accommodative orthotic with a shock absorbing shoe. Post only the medial forefoot (0-60 percent) and avoid posting the rearfoot. Would benefit from calcaneal mobilization into eversion.

Forefoot Valgus and/or Plantarflexed First Ray

Pathomechanics: Due to the plantar flexed position of the 1st ray, there is early and excessive loading of the medial aspect of the foot during the beginning of stance phase. As the foot moves from heel strike to mid-stance, compensatory supination occurs at the subtalar joint in order to disperse weight across the metatarsal heads. The increased loading of the lateral border of the foot is then closely followed by pronation as the heel rises and weight bearing moves again to the medial foot and eventually to the opposite extremity. This drastic and sudden movement of pronation to supination and back at the subtalar joint can lead to hypermobility problems and causes excessive shearing at the forefoot.

Potential problems: Lack of shock absorption, stress fracture of the 1st and 5th metatarsal heads, plantar fasciitis, hip and knee complications secondary to lack of shock absorption, and 1st ray metatarsalgia. Most symptoms are up the kinetic chain.

Treatment: Shock absorbing shoe; a soft and accommodative orthotic with maximum six degree valgus wedge (usually three–four degrees), with rigid plantarflexed 1st ray; can cut out the area of the 1st ray in the orthotic to allow the 1st ray to plantarflex.

Equinus

Definition: Anything less than ten degrees dorsiflexion with the knee fully extended.

Pathomechanics: Equinus causes compensatory pronation at the subtalar joint during the gait cycle. The long-term effect is to increase the mobility at the mid-tarsal joint. As terminal stance is reached during the gait cycle; this increased mobility causes a lack of stability at the 1st ray and thus an increased load at the 2nd and 3rd metatarsal heads.

Potential problems: Increased forefoot pressure and possible ulceration over the 2nd and 3rd metatarsal heads, metatarsalgia, hyperextension of the knee, and talonavicular pain.

Treatment: Stretching of the gastroc-soleus complex; semi-soft accommodative insert with a slight medial wedge under the forefoot to decrease the plantar flexion that occurs at the mid-tarsal joint.

Calcaneus

Definition: Continuous position of ankle dorsiflexion.

Pathomechanics: Heel remains in contact with the floor throughout the gait cycle.

Potential problems: Increased pressure over the heel area. Very difficult to heal once ulcerated.

Treatment: Accommodative orthotic with heel cup integrated into the insert to relieve heel pressure during weight bearing activities.

Chapter 32

Congenital and Genetic Abnormalities

Chapter Contents

Section 32.1

Clubfoot and Other Foot Deformities

Clubfoot is a word used to describe certain ankle and foot abnormalities usually present at birth. The defect can be mild or severe and it can involve one foot or both. The medical term for clubfoot is equinovarus. There also are a number of other milder foot deformities that may appear similar.

How common is clubfoot?

Clubfoot is one of the most common birth defects. Severe forms of clubfoot affect some 5,000 babies (about 1 in 735) born in the United States each year. Boys are affected with severe forms of clubfoot twice as often as girls. Mild foot deformities are even more common, with both sexes affected in approximately equal numbers.

How does clubfoot affect a child?

An affected foot points downward, with the toes turned inward and the bottom of the foot twisted inward. If both feet are "clubbed," the toes point toward each other instead of straight ahead. The foot bones, ankle joints, and muscles and ligaments of the foot may be abnormal. The heel cord often is very tight, making it impossible to bring the foot up to a normal position without a specialist's help.

Clubfoot is not painful and it doesn't bother the baby until he or she begins to stand and walk. Untreated, the ankle remains twisted and the foot can't move up and down as it normally would, creating an awkward gait.

If both feet are affected (as is true in about 50 percent of cases), the child walks on the balls of his feet or, if the feet are badly twisted, on the sides or even the top part of the feet instead of the soles. The part walked on may become infected, develop a large, hard callus, and the entire leg often is unable to grow as it should. Painful arthritic changes also develop.

If only one foot is affected, that foot and calf will be smaller than those on the other side.

What are some other common foot deformities?

Calcaneovalgus is the most common type of foot deformity. This causes the foot to be sharply angled at the heel, with the foot pointing up and outward. In many cases, the top of the foot can touch the shinbone. Usually, this mild foot deformity goes away without treatment, and there are no lasting effects.

Metatarsus adductus is another mild foot deformity in which the front part of the foot is turned inward. Although present at birth, this foot deformity may not be diagnosed until the baby is a month to a few months old. This condition causes the child to walk with a toe-in gait. Most affected children require no treatment, as the condition often resolves itself. However, more severe cases are treated to help the foot work better and to prevent later problems in fitting shoes.

How is clubfoot diagnosed?

Clubfoot and certain other foot abnormalities generally can be recognized during the newborn examination. Some doctors recommend x-rays of the foot to see if the bones in the foot are abnormally shaped. This helps determine if the baby has a true clubfoot, or the foot is turned inward due to problems such as abnormal positioning in the uterus. In the latter case, the child may outgrow the problem, although some may require treatment. Clubfoot sometimes is diagnosed before birth, during an ultrasound examination. Though the disorder cannot be treated before birth, parents have a chance to locate a good orthopaedic surgeon and learn about treatment options.

How are clubfoot and other foot deformities treated?

There are a number of treatments for clubfoot. Most involve some form of manipulation, casts, and often surgery. A baby with clubfoot should be treated by an orthopaedic surgeon who is experienced in dealing with clubfoot, and who can discuss the various treatment options with parents.

Generally, treatment for clubfoot is started soon after birth, often during the first week of life. In the most common method of treatment, the doctor turns the foot forward as far as it can go without pain, and puts a plaster cast on to hold it that way. Every week or two, the cast is changed to bring the foot closer to normal. After about six to twelve weeks of treatment, the doctor may x-ray the foot again to see if treatment is correcting the foot. If treatment is working, casting probably will be continued. It usually takes about three to six months of casting to straighten the foot.

However, in many cases, casting cannot sufficiently correct the foot and surgery is recommended. Often, the heel cord and other tendons, along with the joint capsules of the ankle and foot, are too tight to be stretched by a cast and the doctor must operate to lengthen and open them. At the time of surgery, the surgeon repositions the foot bones in the correct position. Surgery often is performed when the baby is about six months old, although some doctors recommend surgery earlier or later, depending upon how well the foot is correcting and the doctor's personal experience.

Following surgery, the foot will need casting for another six to twelve weeks. This may be followed by full-time or nighttime use of braces for varying periods of time. A child whose clubfoot was corrected with casting alone also may need braces for varying periods of time. Because clubfoot has a tendency to recur during the first seven years of life, the child will require checkups for many years.

Most babies with calcaneovalgus and metatarsus adductus do not need treatment. The vast majority of cases of calcaneovalgus improve within the first 12 months, and resolve during the first year of walking. Parents sometimes are taught gentle stretching exercises to hasten improvement. Most cases of metatarsus adductus also resolve without treatment by age three. However, when the foot stays firmly in the abnormal position (i.e., the doctor has trouble moving the foot into normal position), treatment is recommended. This may include exercises, corrective shoes, or casting. When the foot is rigid, treatment should begin prior to eight months of age for the best results. Surgery occasionally may be necessary for rigid metatarsus adductus.

With early expert treatment, most children with even severe clubfoot can grow up to wear regular shoes, take part in sports, and lead full, active lives. However, the affected foot and leg generally do not completely catch up in growth with the unaffected leg. The difference is slight—leg length usually varies by an inch or less, and shoe size varies between one and two sizes. Untreated, a severe clubfoot stays twisted and grows that way.

What causes clubfoot and other foot deformities?

In most occurrences, the exact cause of clubfoot isn't known. In the past, it was thought that the baby's feet were twisted or cramped because of the way the baby lay in its mother's womb. This is true of some foot deformities that correct themselves after birth (including calcaneovalgus and mild metatarsus adductus). Many scientists think clubfoot (equinovarus) starts early in pregnancy, probably around the 10th to 12th weeks of gestation.

Clubfoot is caused by a combination of heredity and other factors that may affect prenatal growth, such as infection, drugs, disease, or other factors in the uterine or outside environment. One recent study suggests that women who smoke during pregnancy may increase their risk of having a baby with clubfoot, especially if they have a family history of clubfoot. Compared to women with no family history of clubfoot who did not smoke, smokers with no family history of clubfoot had a 34 percent increased risk; smokers with a family history of clubfoot had a 20-fold increased risk. Nonsmokers with a family history of clubfoot had a six times greater risk of having an affected baby compared to nonsmokers without a family history of clubfoot.

Although most children with clubfoot have no other birth defects, occasionally other defects do occur. In a minority of cases, clubfoot occurs as part of a syndrome which includes a number of birth defects. Children with spina bifida (open spine) sometimes have a form of clubfoot. This is caused by damaged spinal nerves that affect the legs. In other cases, feet that are normal at birth may become twisted as a result of muscle or nerve diseases.

Can clubfoot be prevented?

Although the disabling effects of clubfoot often may be prevented through early treatment, there is no method of preventing the defect at this time. However, women should refrain from smoking, which may reduce their risk of having an affected baby, especially if they have a family history of clubfoot. (Smoking also increases the risk of having a low-birthweight or premature baby, as well as other pregnancy complications.) Genetic counseling can help parents understand the odds with each pregnancy for having a child with clubfoot. Generally, if a child has an isolated clubfoot (no other birth defects present), the recurrence risks in another pregnancy are low (about 3 percent).

What research is being done?

Researchers are seeking a better understanding of the genetic and environmental factors that may contribute to clubfoot. Researchers also are studying how an unborn baby's muscles, bones, and nerves grow, for insight into the cause and prevention of clubfoot and other birth defects. The March of Dimes supports many studies on fetal muscle, nerve, and bone development and the genetic and environmental factors that may influence them.

Refere

Honein, [M.A. ...] ng, and clubfoot: an indi[...] *merican Journal of Epide[...]* 658-665.

Lochmi[...] diopathic talipes equinov[...] volume 79, 1998, pages 9[...]

Ponseti, I. [...], in *Iowa Health Book: O*[...]al of Iowa, January 199[...]

Spokan[...]rnational Shrine Headqu[...]

Sulliva[...]instein, S. (eds.): *Lovell and Winter's Pediatric Orthopaedics, 4th Edition*. Philadelphia, J.B. Lippincott Company, 1996, pages 1077-1135.

Section 32.2

Intoeing (Pigeon Toes)

One of the most common developmental problems in children is the occurrence of intoeing/out-toeing. If you have noticed that your child's feet turn in (or out), this condition is often considered normal and, with time, your child's feet will return to the normal position without the need for treatment.

What is intoeing/out-toeing?

Out-toeing usually occurs during the first 12 months due to the hip positioning while in the uterus. Out-toeing will resolve without any form of treatment.

Intoeing develops from one of three areas: the foot, the knee, or at the hip.

The Foot—Metatarsus Adductus: This is the most common cause of intoeing from birth to two years of age and is believed to be caused by positioning in the uterus, or family history. If the foot is flexible and can be gently pulled into the correct position, no treatment is necessary, If the foot is rigid and your child is under eight months of age, your physician may recommend casting.

The Knee—Tibial Torsion: This is noticed most commonly during the second year of life after the child has started walking. The shin bone (tibia) is slightly twisted or rotated causing the foot to turn in. This may be due to the position while in the uterus, or a positive family history.

The Hip—Femoral Anteversion: Children between the ages of one and six may walk with their knee caps pointing inward. This is caused by an internal rotation of the thigh bone (femur). Usually this occurs more often in girls.

Often, many children will have a little of two or three of these causes leading to their intoeing. Bowing of the legs may be associated with this.

What is the treatment for intoeing/out-toeing?

Observation is the best treatment for out-toeing and intoeing. You can take pictures of your child standing, at yearly intervals, and then compare the progression of the straightening process.

Very rarely is another form of treatment necessary. Only if, for some reason, your child does not "grow out of this condition" by the age of eight will surgical options be considered.

What are some answers to commonly asked questions?

- Your child's intoeing is a common developmental condition.

- Bracing, twister cables, and corrective shoes are not necessary. Many years ago, it was believed that these treatments helped correct intoeing, but years of studies have shown them not to be effective.

- Falling is a part of the learning to walk process and is not exclusively caused by intoeing.

- Intoeing should not affect your child's abilities to walk, run, play, or lead a normal life.

All information provided in this section is for informational purposes only and should not be relied upon for medical diagnosis, prognosis, or treatment for any specific condition or individual. Always seek the advice of your physician or other health care provider with any questions you may have regarding a medical condition. The information found here is not meant to substitute for the advice of a qualified physician. If you have, or think you have, a medical emergency, dial 911 or call your doctor or local emergency services agency immediately.

Section 32.3

Metatarsus Adductus

Alternative names: Metatarsus varus; Forefoot varus

Definition: Metatarsus adductus is a foot deformity characterized by an inward bending of the front half of the foot.

Causes, Incidence, and Risk Factors

Metatarsus adductus is thought to occur as a result of the infant's position inside the uterus. It can occur when the feet are bent inward, toward the midline, at the instep.

This is a relatively common disease affecting about one out of every 1,000 to 2,000 live births. Risk factors may include a condition called oligohydramnios where the mother does not produce enough amniotic fluid in the uterus.

Symptoms

- The front of the foot is bent inward (toward the midline) at the instep.

- The back of the foot and the ankles are normal. With a clubfoot, which is a different deformity, the foot will be pointed down and the ankle turned in as well.

Signs and Tests

Physical examination is sufficient to diagnose metatarsus adductus.

Treatment

Treatment depends on the severity of the deformity. Most children with metatarsus adductus can correct the deformity with normal use of their feet as they develop. These cases do not require any treatment.

For children who cannot do this, but who have an affected foot that can be easily manipulated to normal positioning, stretching exercises are all that is needed.

Rarely, this disease causes a rigid deformity that cannot be corrected with simple manipulation. In these cases, casting and even surgery may be required. Other diagnoses may need to be considered in these children. A pediatric orthopaedic surgeon should be involved in treating more severe deformities.

Expectations (Prognosis)

Prognosis is excellent with nearly all patients attaining a normal appearing, fully functional foot.

Complications

Developmental dislocation of the hip may be associated with a small number of infants with metatarsus adductus.

Calling Your Health Care Provider

Call your health care provider if you are concerned about the appearance or flexibility of your infant's feet.

Section 32.4

Pes Planus (Flat Feet)

Alternative names: Pes planovalgus; Flat feet; Fallen arches; Pronation of feet

Definition: Pes planus is a condition where the arch or instep of the foot collapses and comes in contact with the ground. In some individuals, this arch never develops.

Causes, Incidence, and Risk Factors

Flat feet are a common condition. In infants and toddlers, the longitudinal arch is not developed and flat feet are normal. The arch develops in childhood, and by adulthood, most people have developed normal arches.

When flat feet persist, the majority are considered variations of normal. Most feet are flexible and an arch appears when the person stands on his or her toes. Stiff, inflexible, or painful flat feet may be associated with other conditions and require attention.

Painful flat feet in children may be caused by a condition called tarsal coalition. In tarsal coalition, two or more of the bones in the foot fuse together, limiting motion and often leading to a flat foot.

Most flat feet do not cause pain or other problems. Flat feet may be associated with pronation, a leaning inward of the ankle bones toward the center line. Shoes of children who pronate, when placed side by side, will lean toward each other (after they have been worn long enough for the foot position to remodel their shape).

Foot pain, ankle pain, or lower leg pain (especially in children) may be a result of flat feet and should be evaluated by a health care provider.

Symptoms

- absence of longitudinal arch of foot when standing

- foot pain
- heel tilts away from the midline of the body more than usual

Signs and Tests

Examination of the foot is sufficient for the health care provider to make the diagnosis of flat foot. However, the underlying cause must be determined. If an arch develops when the patient stands on their toes, then the flat foot is called flexible and no treatment or further workup is necessary.

If there is pain associated with the foot or if the arch does not develop with toe-standing, x-rays are necessary. If a tarsal coalition is suspected, a CT scan is often ordered. If a posterior tibial tendon injury is suspected, your health care provider may recommend an MRI.

Treatment

Flexible flat feet that are painless do not require treatment. If pain due to flexible flat feet occurs, an orthotic (arch supporting insert in the shoe) can bring relief. With the increased interest in running, many shoe stores carry shoes for normal feet and pronated feet. The shoes designed for pronated feet make long distance running easier and less tiring as they correct for the positional abnormality.

Rigid or painful flat feet require the evaluation of a health care provider. The exact treatment depends on the cause of the flat feet. For tarsal coalition, treatment starts with rest and possibly casting.

If this fails to improve the pain, surgery may be necessary to either resect the fused bone or actually completely fuse several bones in a corrected position. For problems with the posterior tibial tendon, treatment may start with rest, antiinflammatory medications, and shoe inserts or ankle braces.

In more advanced cases, surgery may be necessary to clean the tendon, repair the tendon, or actually fuse some of the joints of the foot in a corrected position in very advanced cases.

Expectations (Prognosis)

Most cases of flat feet are painless and no problems are to be expected. The prognosis of painful flat feet again depends on the cause of the condition. Usually treatment is successful, regardless of the cause.

If a fusion is required then there is some loss of ankle motion, especially turning the foot inward and outward, but otherwise patients with fusions report tremendous improvement in pain and function.

Complications

Flat feet are not really associated with any complications except pain. Some causes of flat feet can be successfully treated without surgery if caught early, but occasionally, surgery is the last option to relieve pain.

While usually successful, surgery sometimes does not result in satisfactory results for all patients. Some have persistent pain and other possible surgical complications include infection and failure of fused bones to heal.

Calling Your Health Care Provider

Call your health care provider if you experience persistent pain in your feet or your child complains of foot pain or lower leg pain.

Prevention

Most cases are not preventable.

Section 32.5

Accessory Navicular

Not everyone has the same number of bones in his feet. It is not uncommon for both the hands and the feet to contain extra small accessory bones, or ossicles, that sometimes cause problems.

This text will help you understand:

- where the accessory navicular is located;
- why the extra bone can cause problems;
- how doctors treat the condition.

Where is the accessory navicular located?

The navicular bone of the foot is one of the small bones on the midfoot. The bone is located at the instep, the arch at the middle of the foot. One of the larger tendons of the foot, called the posterior tibial tendon, attaches to the navicular before continuing under the foot and into the forefoot. This tendon is a tough band of tissue that helps hold up the arch of the foot. If there is an accessory navicular, it is located in the instep where the posterior tibial tendon attaches to the real navicular bone.

The accessory navicular is a congenital anomaly, meaning that you are born with the extra bone. As the skeleton completely matures, the navicular and the accessory navicular never completely grow, or fuse, into one solid bone. The two bones are joined by fibrous tissue or cartilage. Girls seem to be more likely to have an accessory navicular than boys.

How does an accessory navicular cause problems?

Just having an accessory navicular bone is not necessarily a bad thing. Not all people with these accessory bones have symptoms.

Symptoms arise when the accessory navicular is overly large or when an injury disrupts the fibrous tissue between the navicular and the accessory navicular. A very large accessory navicular can cause a bump on the instep that rubs on your shoe causing pain.

An injury to the fibrous tissue connecting the two bones can cause something similar to a fracture. The injury allows movement to occur between the navicular and the accessory bone and is thought to be the cause of pain. The fibrous tissue is prone to poor healing and may continue to cause pain. Because the posterior tibial tendon attaches to the accessory navicular, it constantly pulls on the bone, creating even more motion between the fragments with each step.

What does the condition feel like?

The primary reason an accessory navicular becomes a problem is pain. There is no need to do anything with an accessory navicular that is not causing pain. The pain is usually at the instep area and can be pinpointed over the small bump in the instep. Walking can be painful when the problem is aggravated. As stated earlier, the condition is more common in girls. The problem commonly becomes symptomatic in the teenage years.

How do doctors identify the problem?

The diagnosis begins with a complete history and physical examination by your surgeon. Usually the condition is suggested by the history and the tenderness over the area of the navicular. X-rays will usually be required to allow the surgeon to see the accessory navicular. Generally no other tests are required.

What can be done for a painful accessory navicular?

The treatment for a symptomatic accessory navicular can be divided into nonsurgical treatment and surgical treatment. In the vast majority of cases, treatment usually begins with nonsurgical measures. Surgery usually is only considered when all nonsurgical measures have failed to control your problem and the pain becomes intolerable.

Nonsurgical Treatment: If the foot becomes painful following a twisting type of injury and an x-ray reveals the presence of an accessory navicular bone, your doctor may recommend a period of immobilization in a cast or splint. This will rest the foot and perhaps allow the disruption between the navicular and accessory navicular to heal.

Your doctor may prescribe antiinflammatory medication. Sometimes an arch support can relieve the stress on the fragment and decrease the symptoms. If the pain subsides and the fragment becomes asymptomatic, further treatment may not be necessary.

Surgery: If all nonsurgical measures fail and the fragment continues to be painful, surgery may be recommended.

The most common procedure used to treat the symptomatic accessory navicular is the Kidner procedure. A small incision is made in the instep of the foot over the accessory navicular. The accessory navicular is then detached from the posterior tibial tendon and removed from the foot. The posterior tibial tendon is reattached to the remaining normal navicular. Following the procedure, the skin incision is closed with stitches, and a bulky bandage and splint are applied to the foot and ankle.

What should I expect from treatment?

Nonsurgical Rehabilitation: Patients with a painful accessory navicular may benefit with four to six physical therapy treatments. Your therapist may design a series of stretching exercises to try and ease tension on the posterior tibial tendon. A shoe insert, or orthotic, may be used to support the arch and protect the sore area.

This approach may allow you to resume normal walking immediately, but you should probably cut back on more vigorous activities for several weeks to allow the inflammation and pain to subside.

Treatments directed to the painful area help control pain and swelling. Examples include ultrasound, moist heat, and soft-tissue massage. Therapy sessions sometimes include iontophoresis, which uses a mild electrical current to push antiinflammatory medicine to the sore area.

After Surgery: You may need to use crutches for several days after surgery. Your stitches will be removed in 10 to 14 days (unless they are the absorbable type, which will not need to be taken out).You should be safe to be released to full activity in about six weeks.

Chapter 33

Bunions and Treatments for Bunion Pain

Chapter Contents

Section 33.1

Bunions (Hallux Valgus)

Description

One of the more common conditions treated by podiatric surgeons is the painful bunion. Patients with this condition will usually complain of pain when wearing certain shoes, especially snug fitting dress shoes, or with physical activity, such as walking or running. Bunions are most commonly treated by conservative means. This may involve shoe gear modification, padding, and orthoses. When this fails to provide adequate relief, surgery is often recommended. There are several surgical procedures to correct bunions. Selection of the most appropriate procedure for each patient requires knowledge of the level of deformity, review of the x-rays, and an open discussion of the goals of the surgical procedure. Almost all surgical procedures require cutting and repositioning the first metatarsal. In the case of mild to moderate bunion deformities the bone cut is most often performed at the neck of the metatarsal (near the joint).

Cause of Bunion Deformity

The classic bunion, medically known as hallux abductovalgus or HAV, is a bump on the side of the great toe joint. This bump represents an actual deviation of the 1st metatarsal and often an overgrowth of bone on the metatarsal head. In addition, there is also deviation of the great toe toward the second toe. In severe cases, the great toe can either lie above or below the second toe. Shoes are often blamed for creating these problems. This, however, is inaccurate. It has been noted that primitive tribes where going barefoot is the norm will also develop bunions. Bunions develop from abnormal foot structure and mechanics (e.g. excessive pronation), which place an undue load on the 1st metatarsal. This leads to stretching of supporting soft tissue structures such as joint capsules and ligaments with the end result being gradual deviation of the 1st metatarsal. As the deformity increases, there is an abnormal pull of certain tendons, which leads to the drifting of the great toe toward the 2nd toe. At this stage, there is also adaptation of the joint itself that occurs.

Symptoms Related to Bunion Deformity

The most common symptoms associated with this condition are pain on the side of the foot. Shoes will typically aggravate bunions. Stiff leather shoes or shoes with a tapered toe box are the prime offenders. This is why bunion pain is most common in women whose shoes have a pointed toe box. The bunion site will often be slightly swollen and red from the constant rubbing and irritation of a shoe. Occasionally, corns can develop between the 1st and 2nd toe from the pressure the toes rubbing against each other. On rare occasions, the joint itself can be acutely inflamed from the development of a sac of fluid over the bunion called a bursa. This is designed to protect and cushion the bone. However, it can become acutely inflamed, a condition referred to as bursitis.

Treatment of Bunion Deformity

Early treatment of bunions is centered on providing symptomatic relief. Switching to a shoe with a rounder, deeper toe box and made of a softer, more pliable leather will often provide immediate relief. The use of pads and cushions to reduce the pressure over the bone can also be helpful for mild bunion deformities. Functional foot orthotics, by controlling abnormal pronation, reduces the deforming forces leading to bunions in the first place. These may help reduce pain in mild bunion deformities and slow the progression of the deformity. When these conservative measures fail to provide adequate relief, surgical correction is indicated. The choice of surgical procedures (bunionectomy) is based on a biomechanical and radiographic examination of the foot. Because there is actual bone displacement and joint adaptation, most successful bunionectomies require cutting and realigning the 1st metatarsal (an osteotomy). Simply "shaving the bump" is often inadequate in providing long-term relief of symptoms and, in some cases, can actually cause the bunion to progress faster. The most common procedure performed for the correction of bunions is the 1st metatarsal neck osteotomy, near the level of the joint. This refers to the anatomical site on the 1st metatarsal where the actual bone cut is made. Other procedures are performed in the shaft of the metatarsal bone (see procedures performed in the shaft of the metatarsal) and still other procedures are selected by the surgeon that are performed in the base of the metatarsal bone (see surgeries performed in the base of the metatarsal).

You may view animations for the following bunion surgical procedures by following the links online at http://www.podiatrynetwork .com/r_bunions.cfm:

- Head Osteotomy
- Long Arm V
- Lapidus

Section 33.2

Bunion Surgery: Distal Head Procedures

"Bunion Surgery—Distal Head Procedures,"
by Kenneth Oglesby, DPM, and John Giurini, DPM. © 2005
PodiatryNetwork.com. All rights reserved. Reprinted with permission.

Description

First metatarsal neck osteotomies are known by various names based on the individual who first described the procedure (e.g. Austin, Reverdin-Green, Kalish-Austin). Regardless of the procedure, the goal of all these procedures is the same—remove the bump and realign the joint. The first part of all bunion procedures involves removing the bump of bone from the side of the 1st metatarsal head. This is performed in a manner so as not to damage the viable part of the joint and not to leave any irregularities of bone that can cause future irritation in shoes. Once this is completed, the podiatric surgeon will create an osteotomy (bone cut) through the first metatarsal that will allow shifting the bone and realigning the joint. Depending on the type of osteotomy, the actual shape of the bone cut can vary. In the case of the Austin bunionectomy, the bone cut is V-shaped with the "V" sitting on its side and the tip of the "V" pointing toward the joint. When this cut is completed, the head of the metatarsal and joint is shifted toward the 2nd toe. In this way the bone and joint are repositioned in a more normal position. The Reverdin-Green osteotomy is made in a similar location, but is trapezoidal in shape rather than V-shaped. Both these procedures are stable bone cuts and provide good correction of mild to moderate deformities. The Kalish-Austin bunionectomy is a modification of the Austin bunionectomy. It also is a V-shaped bone cut, but is typically used for greater degrees of bunion deformities.

Because bone is cut and repositioned, it is often preferred to fixate or hold the bone in place with some external device. In the case of the Austin and Reverdin-Green osteotomies, this is most often accomplished by the use of a stainless steel pin across the bone cut. This prevents accidental displacement and loss of correction. Over the past five years, it has become increasing more advantageous to use small stainless steel or titanium screws to provide compression of the bone and to hold the bone in position. This is the main advantage of the Kalish-Austin bunionectomy. By using the screws, bone will heal faster and will allow for earlier ambulation. The screws are typically left in permanently unless they cause irritation of the soft tissues, while the pins are generally removed in the office setting in three to four weeks following the day of surgery. The surgery is generally preformed as an outpatient in a hospital or outpatient surgery center. Some surgeons will perform this procedure in their office. Anesthesia is the choice of the surgeon made in consultation with the patient and anesthesiologist. Anesthesia may be a general anesthesia, twilight anesthesia, or a local anesthesia.

Postoperative Care

The postoperative course and rehabilitation following bunion surgery depends on the procedure and can vary amongst podiatric surgeons. Patients have varying levels of postoperative pain, but quite often the pain is significantly less than what the patient anticipates. A period of total non-weight bearing with crutches may be recommended in the first three to five days. In many instances, the surgeon may allow the patient bear full weight in a postoperative surgical shoe. In all cases patients are instructed to limit their activities and to elevate their feet above their heart during the first three to five days. After this, a resumption of gradual weight bearing with a special surgical shoe is begun. Walking without the postoperative shoe is strictly prohibited. In cases where a pin is used, return to full weight bearing with a stiff soled walking shoe is allowed after the pin has been removed, generally in three to four weeks following the bunion surgery. Screws provide increased stability when used to fixate bone cuts and most patients can return to full weight bearing and regular shoes in three to four weeks following the surgery. The postoperative and rehabilitative course is improved by the use of ice and elevation of the extremity as much as possible. One of the most important aspects of the postoperative treatment is early motion of the joint to prevent joint stiffness. In most cases, range-of-motion exercises are begun almost immediately following surgery. No matter what form of bone fixation is used, pins or screws, bone healing will take six to eight weeks or longer. During this period of time, it is important that the patient not walk without shoes or in thin-soled shoes or sandals. Should the patient risk walking without an adequately supportive shoe, they risk re-fracturing the bone and increase the duration of excessive swelling during the healing phase.

Possible Complications

Complications following bunion surgery are uncommon, but may include infection, suture reaction, delayed or nonunion of the osteotomy, irritation from the pin or screws, stiff joint, or recurrence of the deformity. Recurrence of the deformity can be halted or slowed with the use of functional foot orthotics. It is important to realize that surgery does not correct the cause of the bunion deformity. Functional foot orthotics, however, do address the cause of the deformity and their use is strongly encouraged following bunion surgery. A rare complication is the overcorrection of the bunion deformity. This condition, called hallux varus, may require additional surgery for its correction.

This text should serve as a guideline for patients who are contemplating bunion surgery. The most commonly performed procedures for treatment of bunions have been discussed here. Procedures are selected based on surgeon's experience and preference. Patients are encouraged to discuss the surgery, the postoperative course, and possible complications with their podiatric surgeon openly before consenting to surgical intervention.

Section 33.3

Bunion Surgery: Shaft Procedures

"Bunion Surgery—Shaft Procedures,"
by Matthew Rockett, DPM. © 2005 PodiatryNetwork.com.
All rights reserved. Reprinted with permission.

Description

Hallux valgus or bunion deformities have many different surgical techniques for their correction. One group of procedures that your surgeon may use is the shaft osteotomies. These osteotomies are different from the head osteotomies and also the procedures performed at the base of the metatarsal or at the metatarsocuneiform joint, because they are performed in the middle of the first metatarsal.

The shaft osteotomies were designed to use internal fixation (screws) and to correct larger deformities. In most of these cases, your surgeon will use two screws to fixate the osteotomy. The osteotomy is longer than the head procedures and has more inherent stability because of more bone contact. Also these procedures can correct larger deformities than the head procedures and about the same deformities as the base procedures.

There are two basic shaft osteotomy procedures that your doctor may talk to you about: The Z bunionectomy or the offset V bunionectomy. These osteotomies are very similar and are used interchangeably, based on different patient characteristics, by most surgeons that perform these procedures. The decision to use these procedures over other procedures is typically surgeon preference. In most cases, these procedures are used for patients with mild to severe structural bunions without hypermobility. In older patients with poor bone stock, the surgeon may opt for other procedures.

What Is the Post-Operative Course?

Typically, the patient is allowed to bear weight immediately after surgery in a surgical shoe. Some doctors may have you use crutches for one to two weeks or use a slipper cast. This is surgeon's preference.

It is not unusual for the front part of your foot to look bruised after the surgery. So at the first dressing change, do not be surprised if your toes and the top of your foot are bruised. This will dissipate in three to six weeks. At two weeks after surgery, the sutures are typically removed and at three weeks most patients are advanced into a surgical shoe. After the first or second week, your surgeon may have you start range-of-motion exercises of your big toe joint. It is important that you follow your doctor's instructions on all range-of-motion exercises to help return motion to the operative foot. As with all surgery on the foot and ankle, the limiting factor to advance into different shoe gear is swelling. This swelling can last from six months to one year after surgery. Typically most patients returned to pre-operative dress shoes in six to eight weeks after surgery.

With any surgery, complications are possible. Every procedure has unique complications and your surgeon will discuss these with you before surgery. Make sure that you ask any questions that you have about the surgery with your surgeon.

Section 33.4

Keller Bunionectomy

"Keller Bunionectomy," by John Giurini, DPM. © 2005
PodiatryNetwork.com. All rights reserved. Reprinted with permission.

Description

Pain or discomfort in the great toe joint is a common occurrence amongst people seeking podiatric treatment. There are numerous reasons why people may experience pain or discomfort in this region. Pain in this area may be due to a restriction of motion, a condition referred to as hallux limitus or rigidus. This condition can lead to jamming of the joint and potential degenerative joint disease or arthritis. Ironically, this will lead to even further stiffening of the joint and pain with walking. Bunions or hallux abductovalgus deformities can also cause pain in the great toe joint. After years of this abnormal alignment of the joint arthritic changes can occur causing even more pain. Prior injury to the joint can lead to the development of traumatic arthritis. This is another potential cause of pain in the great toe joint. Patients with diabetes may develop an altogether different problem related to this lack of motion. In the presence of peripheral neuropathy (lack of painful sensation), these patients can develop skin breakdown and ulceration.

As you can see, there are numerous causes for a painful joint. There are also numerous options, conservative and surgical, to treat these conditions. A Keller arthroplasty is a surgical procedure designed to eliminate pain and discomfort in this joint. It is typically reserved for cases of severe arthritis, previous failed surgeries, diabetic ulcerations, or certain types of bunion deformities.

Indications for Surgery

As with all surgical procedures there are certain criteria that are followed in choosing one procedure over another for any individual patient. In the case of the Keller arthroplasty, it is most commonly reserved for patients over the age of 55 with limited athletic activity. These patients are best able to tolerate the alteration in toe function created by this procedure. There should also be a moderate to severe amount of pain on movement of the joint, either passively or with walking, that is not relieved by shoe gear, orthotics, or other non-surgical means. X-rays are helpful to evaluate the condition of the bone and joint. These may show joint space narrowing, bone spurs, or joint deterioration. As with any surgery, it is important that the patient have a clear understanding of all available options. They should also be aware of what to expect after surgery.

The Surgical Procedure

The procedure itself is fairly straightforward. An incision is made over the great toe joint. Once the joint is exposed, a small portion of bone is removed from the base of the proximal phalanx. This allows for an increase in motion in the joint and a reduction in pain. The defect created by the removal of the bone will fill in with soft tissue, creating a "false joint." Some surgeons may choose to place a pin across the joint to maintain the position of the toe and to allow for scarring. The pin is usually left in place for three to four weeks. The soft tissue structures are then reattached and the wound is closed. The patient is then placed in a surgical shoe. Casting is not necessary and limited ambulation is usually allowed following this procedure.

What to Expect after Surgery

The postoperative recuperation usually involves use of the surgical shoe for two to three weeks. Limited ambulation may be allowed. If a pin was inserted, this is usually removed after three to four weeks. Because the pin exits out the tip of the great toe, it can usually be removed in the office. It does not require a second surgical procedure. Once the pin is removed, the patient can get the foot wet, increase their weightbearing activities, begin range-of-motion exercises, and gradually advance to sneakers. Most people can return to their usual shoe gear and activity at six weeks.

The most common postoperative concerns are prolonged swelling. It is not unusual for some degree of swelling to persist beyond three months. This will typically resolve on its own. Occasionally, the use of a compression sock will expedite resolution of the swelling. Also, an orthotic device may be helpful to allow for more efficient transfer of weight during ambulation and more even distribution of weightbearing forces. All in all, when the preoperative criteria are met, this procedure can provide a significant degree of relief from a painful great toe joint.

Chapter 34

Tailor's Bunion (Bunionette)

A bunionette is similar to a bunion, but it develops on the outside of the foot. It is sometimes referred to as a tailor's bunion because tailors once sat cross-legged all day with the outside edge of their feet rubbing on the ground. This produced a pressure area and callus at the bottom of the fifth toe.

This text will help you understand:

- where a bunionette develops;

- why a bunionette causes problems;

- what can be done to treat a bunionette.

Where does a bunionette develop?

A bunionette occurs over the area of the foot where the small toe connects to the foot. This area is called the metatarsophalangeal joint, or MTP joint. The metatarsals are the long bones of the foot. The phalanges are the small bones in each toe. The big toe has two phalanges, and the other toes have three phalanges each.

How does a bunionette develop?

Today a bunionette is most likely caused by an abnormal bump over the end of the fifth metatarsal (the metatarsal head) rubbing on shoes that are too narrow. Some people's feet widen as they grow older, until the foot splays. This can cause a bunion on one side of the foot and a bunionette on the other if they continue to wear shoes that are too narrow. The constant pressure produces a callus and a thickening of the tissues over the bump, leading to a painful knob on the outside of the foot.

Many problems that occur in the feet are the result of abnormal pressure or rubbing. One way of understanding what happens in the foot as a result of abnormal pressure is to view the foot simply. Essentially a foot is made up of hard bone covered by soft tissue that we then put a shoe on top of. Most of the symptoms that develop over time are because the skin and soft tissue are caught between the hard bone on the inside and the hard shoe on the outside.

Any prominence, or bump, in the bone will make the situation even worse over the bump. Skin responds to constant rubbing and pressure by forming a callus. The soft tissues underneath the skin respond to the constant pressure and rubbing by growing thicker. Both the thick callus and the thick soft tissues under it are irritated and painful. The answer to decreasing the pain is to remove the pressure. The pressure can be reduced from the outside by changing the pressure from the shoes. The pressure can be reduced from the inside by surgically removing any bony prominence.

What do bunionettes feel like?

The symptoms of a bunionette include pain and difficulty buying shoes that will not cause pain around the deformity. The swelling in the area causes a visible bump that some people find unsightly.

How do doctors identify a bunionette?

The diagnosis of a bunionette is usually obvious on physical examination. X-rays may help to see if the foot has splayed and will help decide what needs to be done if surgery is necessary later.

What can be done for a bunionette?

Nonsurgical Treatment: Treatment initially is directed at obtaining proper shoes that will accommodate the width of the forefoot. Pads over the area of the bunionette may help relieve some of the pressure and reduce pain. These pads are usually sold in drug and grocery stores. They are small and round with a hole in the middle, like a small doughnut.

Surgery: If all else fails, surgery may be recommended to reduce the deformity. Surgery usually involves removing the prominence of bone underneath the bunion to relieve pressure. Surgery may also be done to realign the fifth metatarsal if the foot has splayed.

Bunionette Removal: To remove the prominence, the surgeon makes a small incision in the skin over the bump. The bump is then removed with a small chisel, and the bone edges are smoothed. Once enough bone has been removed, the skin is closed with small stitches.

Distal Osteotomy: If your doctor decides that the angle of the metatarsal is too great, the fifth metatarsal bone may be cut and re-aligned. This is called an osteotomy. Once the surgeon has performed the osteotomy, the bones are realigned and held in position with metal pins. The metal pins remain in place while the bones heal.

What should I expect after treatment?

Nonsurgical Rehabilitation: Patients with a painful bunionette may benefit from four to six physical therapy treatments. Your therapist can offer ideas of shoes that have a wide forefoot, or toe box. The added space in this part of the shoe keeps the metatarsals from getting squeezed inside the shoe. A special pad can also be placed over the bunionette. These simple changes to your footwear may allow you to resume normal walking immediately, but you should probably cut back on more vigorous activities for several weeks to allow the inflammation and pain to subside.

Treatments directed to the painful area help control pain and swelling. Examples include ultrasound, moist heat, and soft-tissue massage. Therapy sessions sometimes include iontophoresis, which uses a mild electrical current to push anti-inflammatory medicine to the sore area. This treatment is especially helpful for patients who can't tolerate injections.

After Surgery: Patients are usually fitted with a post-op shoe. This shoe has a stiff, wooden sole that protects the toes by keeping the foot from bending. Any pins are usually removed after the bone begins to mend (usually three or four weeks).

You will probably need crutches briefly after surgery, and a therapist may be consulted to help you use your crutches. You will probably wear a bandage or dressing for about a week following the procedure. The stitches are generally removed in 10 to 14 days. However, if your surgeon chose to use sutures that dissolve, you won't need to have the stitches taken out.

During your follow-up visits, x-rays will probably be taken so that the surgeon can follow the healing of the bones and determine how much correction has been achieved.

Chapter 35

Hammer Toe

Definition: Hammer toe is a deformity of the toe in which the end of the toe is bent downward.

Causes, Incidence, and Risk Factors

Hammer toe usually affects the second toe, although it may also affect the other toes. The toe assumes a claw-like position. The condition may occur as a result of pressure from a bunion. A corn on the top of a toe and a callus on the sole of the foot develop, which make walking painful. A high foot arch may also develop.

The condition may be congenital (present at birth) or acquired by wearing short, narrow shoes. The condition also occurs in children who continue to wear shoes they have outgrown.

The rare case in which all toes seem to be involved may indicate a problem with the nerves or spinal cord.

Symptoms

- claw-like deformity of a toe
- corn formation on the top of a toe
- callus formation on the sole of the foot

"Hammer Toe," © 2006 A.D.A.M., Inc. Reprinted with permission. Updated November 22, 2004 by Benjamin D. Roye, MD, MPH.

- foot pain—pain in the joint where the great toe joins the foot (MTP joint)

Signs and Tests

A physical examination of the foot confirms the presence of hammer toe.

Treatment

Mild hammer toe in children can be treated with foot manipulation and splinting the affected toe. Properly-sized footwear or wide toe-box shoes usually provide comfort and can reduce aggravation of hammer toes. The protruding joint can be protected with corn pads or felt pads, corrective footwear, or other foot devices. Exercises may be helpful.

Severe hammer toe requires an operation to straighten the joint. The surgery may involve cutting or transferring tendons or fusing the joints of the toe together.

Expectations (Prognosis)

If the condition is treated early, surgery can often be avoided. Treatment will reduce the associated pain and difficulty with walking.

Complications

- foot deformity
- posture changes caused by difficulty in walking

Calling Your Health Care Provider

Call for an appointment with your health care provider if hammer toe is present, for instructions on the best treatment. Also call for an appointment if pain gets worse or difficulty walking occurs.

Prevention

Avoid wearing shoes that are too short or narrow. Check children's shoe sizes frequently, especially during periods of rapid growth.

Chapter 36

Claw Toe

People often blame the common foot deformity claw toe on wearing shoes that squeeze your toes, such as shoes that are too short or high heels. However, claw toe also is often the result of nerve damage caused by diseases like diabetes or alcoholism, which can weaken the muscles in your foot. Having claw toe means your toes "claw," digging down into the soles of your shoes and creating painful calluses. Claw toe gets worse without treatment and may become a permanent deformity over time.

Symptoms

- Your toes are bent upward (extension) from the joints at the ball of the foot.

- Your toes are bent downward (flexion) at the middle joints toward the sole of your shoe.

- Sometimes your toes also bend downward at the top joints, curling under the foot.

- Corns may develop over the top of the toe or under the ball of the foot.

Reproduced with permission from "Claw Toe," in Johnson, TR, (ed): *Your Orthopaedic Connection*. Rosemont, IL, American Academy of Orthopaedic Surgeons. Available at http://orthoinfo.aaos.org. Co-developed by the American Orthopaedic Foot and Ankle Society. Published March 2002.

Evaluation

If you have symptoms of a claw toe, see your doctor for evaluation. You may need certain tests to rule out neurological disorders that can weaken your foot muscles, creating imbalances that bend your toes. Trauma and inflammation can also cause claw toe deformity.

Treatment

Claw toe deformities are usually flexible at first, but they harden into place over time. If you have claw toe in early stages, your doctor may recommend a splint or tape to hold your toes in correct position. Additional advice is as follows:

- Wear shoes with soft, roomy toe boxes and avoid tight shoes and high-heels.

- Use your hands to stretch your toes and toe joints toward their normal positions.

- Exercise your toes by using them to pick up marbles or crumple a towel laid flat on the floor.

If you have claw toe in later stages and your toes are fixed in position:

- a special pad can redistribute your weight and relieve pressure on the ball of your foot.

- try special "in depth" shoes that have an extra 3/8" depth in the toe box.

- ask a shoe repair shop to stretch a small pocket in the toe box to accommodate the deformity.

If these treatments do not help, you may need surgery to correct the problem.

Part Five

Health Conditions that Affect the Feet

Chapter 37

Pregnancy and Your Feet

Definition

Pregnancy triggers many different changes in a woman's body. Many women have common complaints throughout their pregnancy. One of these complaints, often overlooked, is foot pain. Due to the natural weight gain during pregnancy, a woman's center of gravity is completely altered. This causes a new weight-bearing stance and added pressure to the knees and feet.

Two of the most common foot problems experienced by pregnant woman are overpronation and edema. These problems can lead to pain at the heel, arch, or the ball of foot. Many women may also experience leg cramping and varicose veins due to weight gain. Because of this, it is important for all pregnant women to learn more about foot health during their pregnancy to help make this nine-month period more comfortable for them.

Cause

Overpronation and edema are very common foot problems experienced during pregnancy.

Overpronation, also referred to as flatfeet, is caused when a person's arch flattens out upon weight bearing and their feet roll inward when walking. This can create extreme stress or inflammation on the plantar fascia, the fibrous band of tissue that runs from the heel to the forefoot.

Overpronation can make walking very painful and can increase strain on the feet, calves, and/or back. The reason many pregnant women suffer from overpronation is the added pressure on the body as a result of weight gain. Overpronation is also very prominent in people who have flexible, flatfeet or in people who are obese.

Edema, also referred to as swelling in the feet, normally occurs in the latter part of pregnancy. Edema results from the extra blood accumulated during pregnancy. The enlarging uterus puts pressure on the blood vessels in the pelvis and legs causing circulation to slow down and blood to pool in the lower extremities. The total water fluid in the body remains the same as before pregnancy, however, it becomes displaced. When feet are swollen, they can become purplish in color. Sometimes extra water is retained during pregnancy, adding to the swelling. If there is swelling in the face or hands, a doctor should be contacted immediately.

Treatment and Prevention

There are effective ways to treat both overpronation and edema during pregnancy.

Overpronation can be treated conservatively with "ready-made" orthotics. These orthotics should be designed with appropriate arch support and medial rearfoot posting to correct the overpronation. Proper fitting footwear is also very important in treating overpronation. Choose comfortable footwear that provides extra support and shock absorption.

It is important to treat overpronation for pain relief, but also to prevent other foot conditions from developing such as plantar fasciitis, heel spurs, metatarsalgia, posttibial tendonitis, and/or bunions.

Edema in the feet can be minimized by the following methods:

- Elevate your feet as often as possible. If you have to sit for long periods of time, place a small stool by your feet to elevate them.

- Wear proper fitting footwear. Footwear that is too narrow or short will constrict circulation.

- Have your feet measured several times throughout your pregnancy. They will probably change sizes.

- Wear seamless socks that do not constrict circulation.

- If you are driving for a long period of time, take regular breaks to stretch your legs to promote circulation.

- Exercise regularly to promote overall health; walking is the best exercise.

- Drink plenty of water to keep the body hydrated. This helps the body retain less fluid.

- Eat a well-balanced diet and avoid foods high in salt that can cause water retention.

Swelling is normally similar in both feet. If swelling is not symmetrical in both feet, this may be a sign of a vascular problem and a doctor should be contacted immediately.

If any problems persist, consult your doctor.

Chapter 38

Foot, Leg, and Ankle Swelling

Alternative names: Swelling of the ankles—feet—legs; Ankle swelling; Foot swelling; Leg swelling; Edema—peripheral, Peripheral edema

Definition: Abnormal buildup of fluid in the ankles, feet, and legs is called peripheral edema.

Considerations

Painless swelling of the feet and ankles is a common problem, particularly in older people. It may affect both legs and may include the calves or even the thighs. Because of the effect of gravity, swelling is particularly noticeable in these locations.

Common Causes

Foot, leg, and ankle swelling is common with the following situations:

- prolonged standing
- long airplane flights or automobile rides
- menstrual periods (for some women)

- pregnancy—excessive swelling may be a sign of preeclampsia, a serious condition sometimes called toxemia, that includes high blood pressure and swelling
- being overweight
- increased age
- injury or trauma to your ankle or foot

Swollen legs may be a sign of heart failure, kidney failure, or liver failure. In these conditions, there is too much fluid in the body.

Other conditions that can cause swelling to one or both legs include:

- blood clot;
- leg infection;
- venous insufficiency (when the veins in your legs are unable to adequately pump blood back to the heart);
- varicose veins;
- burns (including sunburn);
- insect bite or sting;
- starvation or malnutrition;
- surgery to your leg or foot.

Certain medications may also cause your legs to swell:

- hormones like estrogen (in birth control pills or hormone replacement therapy) and testosterone
- a group of blood pressure lowering drugs called calcium channel blockers (such as nifedipine, amlodipine, diltiazem, felodipine, and verapamil)
- steroids
- antidepressants, including MAO inhibitors (such as phenelzine and tranylcypromine) and tricyclics (such as nortriptyline, desipramine, and amitriptyline)

Home Care

- Elevate your legs above your heart while lying down.
- Exercise your legs. This helps pump fluid from your legs back to your heart.

- Wear support stockings (sold at most drug and medical supply stores).
- Try to follow a low-salt diet, which may reduce fluid retention and swelling.

Call Your Health Care Provider

Call 911 if:

- you feel short of breath;
- you have chest pain, especially if it feels like pressure or tightness.

Call your doctor right away if:

- you have decreased urine output;
- you have a history of liver disease and now have swelling in your legs or abdomen;
- your swollen foot or leg is red or warm to the touch;
- you have a fever;
- you are pregnant and have more than just mild swelling or have a sudden increase in swelling.

Also call your doctor if self care measures do not help or swelling worsens.

What to Expect at Your Health Care Provider's Office

Your doctor will take a medical history and conduct a thorough physical examination, with special attention to your heart, lungs, abdomen, legs, and feet.

Your doctor will ask questions like the following:

- What specific body parts swell? Your ankles, feet, legs? Above the knee or below?
- Do you have swelling at all times or is it worse in the morning or the evening?
- What makes your swelling better?
- What makes your swelling worse?
- Does the swelling get better when you elevate your legs?
- What other symptoms do you have?

Diagnostic tests that may be performed include the following:

- blood tests such as a CBC or blood chemistry
- ECG
- chest x-ray or extremity x-ray
- urinalysis

The specific treatment will be directed at whatever underlying cause is found. Diuretics may be prescribed. These are effective in reducing the swelling but have some side effects. Home treatment for benign causes of leg swelling should be tried before drug therapy under medical supervision.

Prevention

Avoid sitting or standing without moving for prolonged periods of time. When flying, stretch your legs often and get up to walk when possible. When driving, stop to stretch and walk every hour or so. Avoid wearing restrictive clothing or garters around your thighs. Exercise regularly. Lose weight if you need to.

References

Cho, S. Peripheral edema. *Am J Med.* 2002; 113(7): 580-586.

Schroeder, B.M. ACOG practice bulletin on diagnosing and managing preeclampsia and eclampsia. American College of Obstetricians and Gynecologists. *Am Fam Physician.* 2002; 66(2): 330-331.

Chapter 39

Diabetes

Chapter Contents

Section 39.1

Foot Health and Diabetes

This document is part of the "Working Together to Manage Diabetes," program of the National Diabetes Education Program, a joint initiative of the National Institutes of Health and the Centers for Disease Control and Prevention, National Institute of Diabetes and Digestive and Kidney Diseases, 2004. Available online at http://www.ndep.nih.gov/diabetes/WTMD.

Prevalence of Foot Symptoms and Complications

Early manifestations of diabetes may present initially in the foot. Foot symptoms increase the risk for comorbid complications, of which nontraumatic lower-extremity amputations (LEAs) are the greatest concern. According to 1997 hospital discharge data, diabetes accounted for approximately 87,720 LEAs in the United States, representing 67 percent of all LEAs. Between 1980 and 2001, the number of diabetes-related hospital discharges with LEA increased from an average of 33,000 to 82,000 per year. LEA rates were highest among men, non-Hispanics/Latinos, African Americans, and the elderly.

One study found that 80 percent of nontraumatic LEAs are preceded by a foot ulceration, which provides a portal for infection. According to the Behavioral Risk Factor Surveillance System (BRFSS) data, approximately 12 percent of U.S. adults with diabetes had a history of foot ulcer, a risk factor for LEA. Another report identified minor trauma, ulceration, and faulty wound healing as precursors to 73 percent of LEAs, often in combination with gangrene and infection. Other risk factors include the presence of sensory peripheral neuropathy, altered biomechanics, elevated pressure on the sole of the foot, and limited joint mobility.

People with diabetes who have neuropathy are 1.7 times more likely to develop a foot ulceration; in persons with both neuropathy and foot deformity, the risk is 12 times greater; in those who also have a history of pathology (prior amputation or ulceration), the risk is 36 times greater.

People with diabetes who have increased risk for lower-extremity ulceration and amputation are males, people with diabetes for more

334

than ten years, people who use tobacco, and those with a history of poor glycemic control or the presence of cardiac, retinal, or renal complications.

Foot Evaluation in People with Diabetes

The podiatrist uses the following considerations in evaluating the feet of people with diabetes to assess the risk for complications.

- **Neuropathy:** The presence of subjective tingling, burning, numbness, or the sensation of bugs crawling on skin may indicate peripheral sensory neuropathy. On clinical examination, this condition can be detected with an instrument known as a Semmes-Weinstein 5.07 (10 gram) monofilament.

- **Vasculopathy:** Cramping of calf muscles when walking ("charley horse") that requires frequent rest periods suggests intermittent claudication. This condition, often caused by insufficient blood supply to the region beneath the knee, indicates the presence of early or moderate occlusion of the arteries that is common to the lower extremities of people with diabetes. Intense cramping and aching in the toes only at night indicates "rest pain," which is usually relieved by hanging the feet over the side of the bed and by walking. This symptom signifies the end-stage blood vessel disorder and tissue ischemia that precedes diabetic gangrene. Although poor blood supply is not a risk factor for developing ulceration, it is a significant risk factor for amputation.

- **Dermatological conditions:** Corns and calluses (hyperkeratotic lesions) of the feet result from elevated mechanical pressure and shearing of the skin. They often precede breakdown of skin and lead to blisters or ulceration. Superficial lacerations and fissures, or maceration (softening) between the toes or on the heel, all can serve as portals for infection. Corns, calluses, and bleeding beneath the nail may signify the presence of sensory neuropathy.

- **Musculoskeletal symptoms:** Structural changes in the diabetic foot may develop in conjunction with muscle-tendon imbalances as a result of motor neuropathy. These deformities include the presence of hammer toes, bunions, high-arched foot, or flatfoot—all of which increase the potential for focal irritation of the foot in the shoe.

- **Lifestyle and family history:** People with diabetes who smoke are four times more likely than nondiabetic smokers to develop lower-extremity vascular disease. Poor diet and low physical activity levels worsen long-term control of blood glucose and increase the risk of progression of disorders of the peripheral nervous system and/or blood vessels. A family history of cerebrovascular accidents and coronary artery disease may indicate a risk of developing lower-extremity arterial complications. Inherited foot types may predispose to biomechanical deformities that lead to problems with skin breakdown.

Comprehensive Foot Examination

A comprehensive foot examination (including checking pulses, checking sensation, evaluating general foot structure, and evaluating skin and nails for abnormalities) helps determine the person's category of risk for developing foot complications. Persons with diabetes who are at high risk have one or more of the following characteristics:

- loss of protective sensation
- absent pedal pulses
- foot deformity
- history of foot ulcers, or
- prior amputation

Low-risk individuals have none of these characteristics. Assessment of risk status identifies people who need more intensive care and evaluation. Further patient education, early intervention, and special footwear if indicated can prevent ulcers and ultimately LEAs.

Section 39.2

Diabetic Neuropathies: The Nerve Damage of Diabetes

National Diabetes Information Clearinghouse, a service of the National Institute of Diabetes and Digestive and Kidney Diseases, National Institutes of Health, NIH Publication No. 02-3185, May 2002.

Diabetic neuropathies are a family of nerve disorders caused by diabetes. People with diabetes can, over time, have damage to nerves throughout the body. Neuropathies lead to numbness and sometimes pain and weakness in the hands, arms, feet, and legs. Problems may also occur in every organ system, including the digestive tract, heart, and sex organs. People with diabetes can develop nerve problems at any time, but the longer a person has diabetes, the greater the risk.

An estimated 50 percent of those with diabetes have some form of neuropathy, but not all with neuropathy have symptoms. The highest rates of neuropathy are among people who have had the disease for at least 25 years.

Diabetic neuropathy also appears to be more common in people who have had problems controlling their blood glucose levels, in those with high levels of blood fat and blood pressure, in overweight people, and in people over the age of 40. The most common type is peripheral neuropathy, also called distal symmetric neuropathy, which affects the arms and legs.

Causes

The causes are probably different for different varieties of diabetic neuropathy. Researchers are studying the effect of glucose on nerves to find out exactly how prolonged exposure to high glucose causes neuropathy. Nerve damage is likely due to a combination of factors:

- **metabolic factors,** such as high blood glucose, long duration of diabetes, possibly low levels of insulin, and abnormal blood fat levels

- **neurovascular factors,** leading to damage to the blood vessels that carry oxygen and nutrients to the nerves

- **autoimmune factors** that cause inflammation in nerves
- **mechanical injury** to nerves, such as carpal tunnel syndrome
- **inherited traits** that increase susceptibility to nerve disease
- **lifestyle factors** such as smoking or alcohol use

Symptoms

Symptoms depend on the type of neuropathy and which nerves are affected. Some people have no symptoms at all. For others, numbness, tingling, or pain in the feet is often the first sign. A person can experience both pain and numbness. Often, symptoms are minor at first, and since most nerve damage occurs over several years, mild cases may go unnoticed for a long time. Symptoms may involve the sensory or motor nervous system, as well as the involuntary (autonomic) nervous system. In some people, mainly those with focal neuropathy, the onset of pain may be sudden and severe.

Symptoms may include the following:

- numbness, tingling, or pain in the toes, feet, legs, hands, arms, and fingers
- wasting of the muscles of the feet or hands
- indigestion, nausea, or vomiting
- diarrhea or constipation
- dizziness or faintness due to a drop in postural blood pressure
- problems with urination
- erectile dysfunction (impotence) or vaginal dryness
- weakness

In addition, the following symptoms are not due to neuropathy but nevertheless often accompany it:

- weight loss
- depression

Types of Diabetic Neuropathy

Diabetic neuropathies can be classified as peripheral, autonomic, proximal, and focal. Each affects different parts of the body in different ways.

- **Peripheral neuropathy** causes either pain or loss of feeling in the toes, feet, legs, hands, and arms.

- **Autonomic neuropathy** causes changes in digestion, bowel and bladder function, sexual response, and perspiration. It can also affect the nerves that serve the heart and control blood pressure. Autonomic neuropathy can also cause hypoglycemia (low blood sugar) unawareness, a condition in which people no longer experience the warning signs of hypoglycemia.

- **Proximal neuropathy** causes pain in the thighs, hips, or buttocks and leads to weakness in the legs

- **Focal neuropathy** results in the sudden weakness of one nerve, or a group of nerves, causing muscle weakness or pain. Any nerve in the body may be affected.

Neuropathy Affects Nerves throughout the Body

Peripheral Neuropathy

- toes
- feet
- legs
- hands
- arms

Autonomic Neuropathy

- heart and blood vessels
- digestive system
- urinary tract
- sex organs
- sweat glands
- eyes

Proximal Neuropathy

- thighs
- hips
- buttocks

Focal Neuropathy

- eyes
- facial muscles
- ears
- pelvis and lower back
- thighs
- abdomen

Peripheral Neuropathy

This type of neuropathy damages nerves in the arms and legs. The feet and legs are likely to be affected before the hands and arms. Many people with diabetes have signs of neuropathy upon examination but have no symptoms at all. Symptoms of peripheral neuropathy may include the following:

- numbness or insensitivity to pain or temperature
- a tingling, burning, or prickling sensation
- sharp pains or cramps
- extreme sensitivity to touch, even a light touch
- loss of balance and coordination

These symptoms are often worse at night.

Peripheral neuropathy may also cause muscle weakness and loss of reflexes, especially at the ankle, leading to changes in gait (walking). Foot deformities, such as hammer toes and the collapse of the midfoot, may occur. Blisters and sores may appear on numb areas of the foot because pressure or injury goes unnoticed. If foot injuries are not treated promptly, the infection may spread to the bone, and the foot may then have to be amputated. Some experts estimate that half of all such amputations are preventable if minor problems are caught and treated in time.

Autonomic Neuropathy

Autonomic neuropathy affects the nerves that control the heart, regulate blood pressure, and control blood glucose levels. It also affects other internal organs, causing problems with digestion, respiratory function, urination, sexual response, and vision. In addition, the system that restores blood glucose levels to normal after a hypoglycemic episode may be affected, resulting in loss of the warning signs of hypoglycemia such as sweating and palpitations.

Unawareness of Hypoglycemia

Normally, symptoms such as shakiness occur as blood glucose levels drop below 70 mg/dL. In people with autonomic neuropathy, symptoms may not occur, making hypoglycemia difficult to recognize.

However, other problems can also cause hypoglycemia unawareness so this does not always indicate nerve damage.

Heart and Circulatory System

The heart and circulatory system are part of the cardiovascular system, which controls blood circulation. Damage to nerves in the cardiovascular system interferes with the body's ability to adjust blood pressure and heart rate. As a result, blood pressure may drop sharply after sitting or standing, causing a person to feel light-headed—or even to faint. Damage to the nerves that control heart rate can mean that it stays high, instead of rising and falling in response to normal body functions and exercise.

Digestive System

Nerve damage to the digestive system most commonly causes constipation. Damage can also cause the stomach to empty too slowly, a condition called gastroparesis. Severe gastroparesis can lead to persistent nausea and vomiting, bloating, and loss of appetite. Gastroparesis can make blood glucose levels fluctuate widely as well, due to abnormal food digestion.

Nerve damage to the esophagus may make swallowing difficult, while nerve damage to the bowels can cause constipation alternating with frequent, uncontrolled diarrhea, especially at night. Problems with the digestive system may lead to weight loss.

Urinary Tract and Sex Organs

Autonomic neuropathy most often affects the organs that control urination and sexual function. Nerve damage can prevent the bladder from emptying completely, allowing bacteria to grow in the bladder and kidneys and causing urinary tract infections. When the nerves of the bladder are damaged, urinary incontinence may result because a person may not be able to sense when the bladder is full or control the muscles that release urine.

Neuropathy can also gradually decrease sexual response in men and women, although the sex drive is unchanged. A man may be unable to have erections or may reach sexual climax without ejaculating normally. A woman may have difficulty with lubrication, arousal, or orgasm.

Sweat Glands

Autonomic neuropathy can affect the nerves that control sweating. When nerve damage prevents the sweat glands from working properly, the body cannot regulate its temperature properly. Nerve damage can also cause profuse sweating at night or while eating.

Eyes

Finally, autonomic neuropathy can affect the pupils of the eyes, making them less responsive to changes in light. As a result, a person may not be able to see well when the light is turned on in a dark room or may have trouble driving at night.

Proximal Neuropathy

Proximal neuropathy, sometimes called lumbosacral plexus neuropathy, femoral neuropathy, or diabetic amyotrophy, starts with pain in either the thighs, hips, buttocks, or legs, usually on one side of the body. This type of neuropathy is more common in those with type 2 diabetes and in older people. It causes weakness in the legs, manifested by an inability to go from a sitting to a standing position without help. Treatment for weakness or pain is usually needed. The length of the recovery period varies, depending on the type of nerve damage.

Focal Neuropathy

Occasionally, diabetic neuropathy appears suddenly and affects specific nerves, most often in the head, torso, or leg. Focal neuropathy may cause:

- inability to focus the eye;
- double vision;
- aching behind one eye;

- paralysis on one side of the face (Bell palsy);
- severe pain in the lower back or pelvis;
- pain in the front of a thigh;
- pain in the chest, stomach, or flank;
- pain on the outside of the shin or inside the foot;
- chest or abdominal pain that is sometimes mistaken for heart disease, heart attack, or appendicitis.

Focal neuropathy is painful and unpredictable and occurs most often in older people. However, it tends to improve by itself over weeks or months and does not cause long-term damage.

People with diabetes also tend to develop nerve compressions, also called entrapment syndromes. One of the most common is carpal tunnel syndrome, which causes numbness and tingling of the hand and sometimes muscle weakness or pain. Other nerves susceptible to entrapment may cause pain on the outside of the shin or the inside of the foot.

Preventing Diabetic Neuropathy

The best way to prevent neuropathy is to keep your blood glucose levels as close to the normal range as possible. Maintaining safe blood glucose levels protects nerves throughout your body.

For additional information on preventing diabetes complications, including neuropathy, see the *Prevent Diabetes Problems* series, available from the National Diabetes Information Clearinghouse at 800-860-8747.

Diagnosis

Neuropathy is diagnosed on the basis of symptoms and a physical exam. During the exam, the doctor may check blood pressure and heart rate, muscle strength, reflexes, and sensitivity to position, vibration, temperature, or a light touch.

The doctor may also do other tests to help determine the type and extent of nerve damage.

- A comprehensive foot exam assesses skin, circulation, and sensation. The test can be done during a routine office visit. To assess protective sensation or feeling in the foot, a nylon monofilament (similar to a bristle on a hairbrush) attached to a wand is used to touch the foot. Those who cannot sense pressure from the monofilament have lost protective sensation and are at risk for developing foot sores that may not heal properly. Other tests include checking reflexes and assessing vibration perception, which is more sensitive than touch pressure.

- Nerve conduction studies check the transmission of electrical current through a nerve. With this test, an image of the nerve conducting an electrical signal is projected onto a screen. Nerve impulses that seem slower or weaker than usual indicate possible damage. This test allows the doctor to assess the condition of all the nerves in the arms and legs.

- Electromyography (EMG) shows how well muscles respond to electrical signals transmitted by nearby nerves. The electrical activity of the muscle is displayed on a screen. A response that is slower or weaker than usual suggests damage to the nerve or muscle. This test is often done at the same time as nerve conduction studies.

- Quantitative sensory testing (QST) uses the response to stimuli, such as pressure, vibration, and temperature, to check for neuropathy. QST is increasingly used to recognize sensation loss and excessive irritability of nerves.

- A check of heart rate variability shows how the heart responds to deep breathing and to changes in blood pressure and posture.

- Ultrasound uses sound waves to produce an image of internal organs. An ultrasound of the bladder and other parts of the urinary tract, for example, can show how these organs preserve a normal structure and whether the bladder empties completely after urination.

- Nerve or skin biopsy involves removing a sample of nerve or skin tissue for examination by microscope. This test is most often used in research settings.

Treatment

The first step is to bring blood glucose levels within the normal range to prevent further nerve damage. Blood glucose monitoring, meal planning, exercise, and oral drugs or insulin injections are needed to control blood glucose levels. Although symptoms may get worse when blood glucose is first brought under control, over time, maintaining lower blood glucose levels helps lessen neuropathic symptoms. Importantly, good blood glucose control may also help prevent or delay the onset of further problems.

Additional treatment depends on the type of nerve problem and symptom, as described in the following sections.

Foot Care

People with neuropathy need to take special care of their feet. The nerves to the feet are the longest in the body and are the ones most often affected by neuropathy. Loss of sensation in the feet means that sores or injuries may not be noticed and may become ulcerated or infected. Circulation problems also increase the risk of foot ulcers.

More than half of all lower limb amputations in the United States occur in people with diabetes—86,000 amputations per year. Doctors estimate that nearly half of the amputations caused by neuropathy and poor circulation could have been prevented by careful foot care. Here are the steps to follow:

- Clean your feet daily, using warm—not hot—water and a mild soap. Avoid soaking your feet. Dry them with a soft towel; dry carefully between your toes.

- Inspect your feet and toes every day for cuts, blisters, redness, swelling, calluses, or other problems. Use a mirror (laying a mirror on the floor works well) or get help from someone else if you cannot see the bottoms of your feet. Notify your health care provider of any problems.

- Moisturize your feet with lotion, but avoid getting it between your toes.

- After a bath or shower, file corns and calluses gently with a pumice stone.

- Each week or when needed, cut your toenails to the shape of your toes and file the edges with an emery board.

- Always wear shoes or slippers to protect your feet from injuries. Prevent skin irritation by wearing thick, soft, seamless socks.

- Wear shoes that fit well and allow your toes to move. Break in new shoes gradually by wearing them for only an hour at a time at first.

345

- Before putting your shoes on, look them over carefully and feel the insides with your hand to make sure they have no tears, sharp edges, or objects in them that might injure your feet.

- If you need help taking care of your feet, make an appointment to see a foot doctor, also called a podiatrist.

For additional information on foot care, see the listing for the National Diabetes Information Clearinghouse in Chapter 48, A Directory of Foot and Ankle Health Resources.

Pain Relief

To relieve pain, burning, tingling, or numbness, the doctor may suggest aspirin, acetaminophen, or nonsteroidal anti-inflammatory drugs (NSAIDs) such as ibuprofen. (People with renal disease should use NSAIDs only under a doctor's supervision.) A topical cream called capsaicin is another option. Tricyclic antidepressant medications such as amitriptyline, imipramine, and nortriptyline, or anticonvulsant medications such as carbamazepine or gabapentin may relieve pain in some people. Codeine may be prescribed for a short time to relieve severe pain. Also, mexiletine, used to regulate heartbeat, has been effective in treating pain in several clinical trials.

Other pain treatments include transcutaneous electronic nerve stimulation (TENS), which uses small amounts of electricity to block pain signals, as well as hypnosis, relaxation training, biofeedback, and acupuncture. Walking regularly or using elastic stockings may also help leg pain.

Gastrointestinal Problems

To relieve mild symptoms of gastroparesis—indigestion, belching, nausea, or vomiting—doctors suggest eating small, frequent meals, avoiding fats, and eating less fiber. When symptoms are severe, the doctor may prescribe erythromycin to speed digestion, metoclopramide to speed digestion and help relieve nausea, or other drugs to help regulate digestion or reduce stomach acid secretion.

To relieve diarrhea or other bowel problems, the doctor may prescribe an antibiotic such as tetracycline, or other medications as appropriate.

Dizziness and Weakness

Sitting or standing slowly may help prevent the lightheadedness, dizziness, or fainting associated with blood pressure and circulation problems. Raising the head of the bed or wearing elastic stockings may also help. Some people may benefit from increased salt in the diet and treatment with salt-retaining hormones. Others may benefit from high blood pressure medications. Physical therapy can help when muscle weakness or loss of coordination is a problem.

Urinary and Sexual Problems

To clear up a urinary tract infection, the doctor will probably prescribe an antibiotic. Drinking plenty of fluids will help prevent another infection. People who have incontinence should try to urinate at regular intervals (every three hours, for example) since they may not be able to tell when their bladder is full.

To treat erectile dysfunction in men, the doctor will first do tests to rule out a hormonal cause. Several methods are available to treat erectile dysfunction caused by neuropathy, including taking oral drugs, using a mechanical vacuum device, or injecting a drug called a vasodilator into the penis before sex. The vacuum and vasodilator raise blood flow to the penis, making it easier to have and maintain an erection. Another option is to surgically implant an inflatable or semi-rigid device in the penis. A constriction ring or penile sling may be helpful.

Vaginal lubricants may be useful for women when neuropathy causes vaginal dryness. To treat problems with arousal and orgasm, the doctor may refer the woman to a gynecologist.

Points to Remember

- Diabetic neuropathies are nerve disorders caused by many of the abnormalities common to diabetes, such as high blood glucose.

- Neuropathy can affect nerves throughout the body, causing numbness and sometimes pain in the hands, arms, feet, or legs, and problems with the digestive tract, heart, and sex organs.

- Treatment first involves bringing blood glucose levels within the normal range. Good blood glucose control may help prevent or delay the onset of further problems.

- Foot care is another important part of treatment. People with neuropathy need to inspect their feet daily for any injuries. Untreated injuries increase the risk of infected foot sores and amputation.

- Treatment also includes pain relief and other medications as needed, depending on the type of nerve damage.

- Smoking significantly increases the risk of foot problems and amputation. If you smoke, ask your health care provider for help in quitting.

Hope through Research

The National Institute of Diabetes and Digestive and Kidney Diseases (NIDDK) and the National Institute of Neurological Disorders and Stroke (NINDS) conduct and support research to help people with diabetes, including studies related to diabetic neuropathy. A complete listing of clinical research studies can be found at http://www.Clinical Trials.gov.

Section 39.3

Prevent Diabetes Problems: Keep Feet and Skin Healthy

"Prevent Diabetes Problems: Keep Your Feet and Skin Healthy," National Diabetes Information Clearinghouse, a service of the National Institute of Diabetes and Digestive and Kidney Diseases, National Institutes of Health, NIH Publication No. 06-4282, March 2006.

What are diabetes problems?

Too much glucose (sugar) in the blood for a long time can cause diabetes problems. This high blood glucose (also called blood sugar) can damage many parts of the body, such as the heart, blood vessels, eyes, and kidneys. Heart and blood vessel disease can lead to heart attacks and strokes. You can do a lot to prevent or slow down diabetes problems.

This section is about feet and skin problems caused by diabetes. You will learn the things you can do each day and during each year to stay healthy and prevent diabetes problems.

What should I do each day to stay healthy with diabetes?

- Follow the healthy eating plan that you and your doctor or dietitian have worked out.

- Be active a total of 30 minutes most days. Ask your doctor what activities are best for you.

- Take your medicines as directed.

- Check your blood glucose every day. Each time you check your blood glucose, write the number in your record book.

- Check your feet every day for cuts, blisters, sores, swelling, redness, or sore toenails.

- Brush and floss your teeth every day.

- Control your blood pressure and cholesterol.

- Don't smoke.

How can diabetes hurt my feet?

High blood glucose from diabetes causes two problems that can hurt your feet:

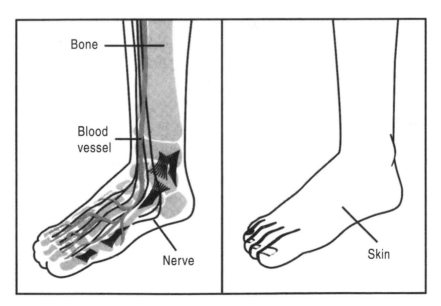

Figure 39.1. High blood glucose can cause feet and skin problems.

1. **Nerve damage:** One problem is damage to nerves in your legs and feet. With damaged nerves, you might not feel pain, heat, or cold in your legs and feet. A sore or cut on your foot may get worse because you do not know it is there. This lack of feeling is caused by nerve damage, also called diabetic neuropathy (ne-ROP-uh-thee). It can lead to a large sore or infection.

2. **Poor blood flow:** The second problem happens when not enough blood flows to your legs and feet. Poor blood flow makes it hard for a sore or infection to heal. This problem is called peripheral (puh-RIF-uh-rul) vascular disease. Smoking when you have diabetes makes blood flow problems much worse.

These two problems can work together to cause a foot problem. For example, you get a blister from shoes that do not fit. You do not feel the pain from the blister because you have nerve damage in your foot. Next, the blister gets infected. If blood glucose is high, the extra glucose feeds the germs. Germs grow and the infection gets worse. Poor blood flow to your legs and feet can slow down healing. Once in a while a bad infection never heals. The infection might cause gangrene (GANG-green). If a person has gangrene, the skin and tissue around the sore die. The area becomes black and smelly.

To keep gangrene from spreading, a doctor may have to do surgery to cut off a toe, foot, or part of a leg. Cutting off a body part is called an amputation (amp-yoo-TAY-shun).

What can I do to take care of my feet?

*   Wash your feet in warm water every day. Make sure the water is not too hot by testing the temperature with your elbow. Do not soak your feet. Dry your feet well, especially between your toes

*   Look at your feet every day to check for cuts, sores, blisters, redness, calluses, or other problems. Checking every day is even more important if you have nerve damage or poor blood flow. If you cannot bend over or pull your feet up to check them, use a mirror. If you cannot see well, ask someone else to check your feet.

*   If your skin is dry, rub lotion on your feet after you wash and dry them. Do not put lotion between your toes

*   File corns and calluses gently with an emery board or pumice stone. Do this after your bath or shower.

- Cut your toenails once a week or when needed. Cut toenails when they are soft from washing. Cut them to the shape of the toe and not too short. File the edges with an emery board.

- Always wear shoes or slippers to protect your feet from injuries.

- Always wear socks or stockings to avoid blisters. Do not wear socks or knee-high stockings that are too tight below your knee.

- Wear shoes that fit well. Shop for shoes at the end of the day when your feet are bigger. Break in shoes slowly. Wear them one to two hours each day for the first one to two weeks.

- Before putting your shoes on, feel the insides to make sure they have no sharp edges or objects that might injure your feet.

How can I get my doctor to help me take care of my feet?

- Tell your doctor right away about any foot problems.

- Ask your doctor to look at your feet at each diabetes checkup. To make sure your doctor checks your feet, take off your shoes and socks before your doctor comes into the room.

- Ask your doctor to check how well the nerves in your feet sense feeling.

- Ask your doctor to check how well blood is flowing to your legs and feet.

- Ask your doctor to show you the best way to trim your toenails. Ask what lotion or cream to use on your legs and feet.

- If you cannot cut your toenails or you have a foot problem, ask your doctor to send you to a foot doctor. A doctor who cares for feet is called a podiatrist (puh-DY-uh-trist).

What are common diabetes foot problems?

Anyone can have corns, blisters, and athlete's foot. If you have diabetes and your blood glucose stays high, these foot problems can lead to infections.

Corns and **calluses** are thick layers of skin caused by too much rubbing or pressure on the same spot. Corns and calluses can become infected.

Blisters can form if shoes always rub the same spot. Wearing shoes that do not fit or wearing shoes without socks can cause blisters. Blisters can become infected.

Ingrown toenails happen when an edge of the nail grows into the skin. The skin can get red and infected. Ingrown toenails can happen if you cut into the corners of your toenails when you trim them. If toenail

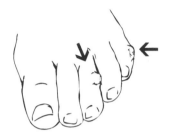

Figure 39.2. Corn and callus.

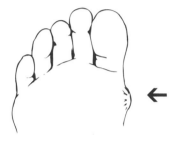

Figure 39.3. Blister.

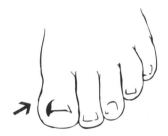

Figure 39.4. Ingrown toenail

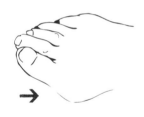

Figure 39.5. Bunion.

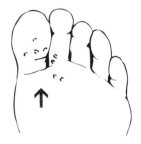

Figure 39.6. Plantar warts.

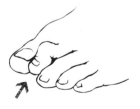

Figure 39.7. Hammer toe.

edges are sharp, smooth them with an emery board. You can also get an ingrown toenail if your shoes are too tight.

A **bunion** forms when your big toe slants toward the small toes and the place between the bones near the base of your big toe grows big. This spot can get red, sore, and infected. Bunions can form on one or both feet. Pointy shoes may cause bunions. Bunions often run in the family. Surgery can remove bunions.

Plantar warts are caused by a virus. The warts usually form on the bottoms of the feet.

Hammer toes form when a foot muscle gets weak. The weakness may be from diabetic nerve damage. The weakened muscle makes the tendons in the foot shorter and makes the toes curl under the feet. You may get sores on the bottoms of your feet and on the tops of your toes. The feet can change their shape. Hammer toes can cause problems with walking and finding shoes that fit well. Hammer toes can run in the family. Wearing shoes that are too short can also cause hammer toes.

Dry and cracked skin can happen because the nerves in your legs and feet do not get the message to keep your skin soft and moist. Dry skin can become cracked and allow germs to enter. If your blood glucose is high, it feeds the germs and makes the infection worse.

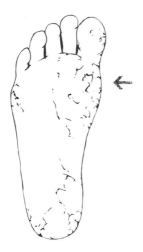

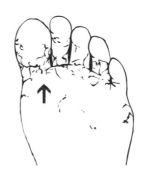

Figure 39.8. *Dry and cracked skin.*   **Figure 39.9.** *Athlete's foot.*

Athlete's foot is a fungus that causes redness and cracking of the skin. It is itchy. The cracks between the toes allow germs to get under the skin. If your blood glucose is high, it feeds the germs and makes the infection worse. The infection can spread to the toenails and make them thick, yellow, and hard to cut.

All of these foot problems can be taken care of. Tell your doctor about any foot problem as soon as you see it.

How can special shoes help my feet?

Special shoes can be made to fit softly around your sore feet or feet that have changed shape. These special shoes help protect your feet. Medicare and other health insurance programs may pay for special shoes. Talk to your doctor about how and where to get them. [See Chapter 46, Podiatric Patients and Financial Concerns, for more information.]

How can diabetes hurt my skin?

Diabetes can hurt your skin in two ways:

1. If your blood glucose is high, your body loses fluid. With less fluid in your body, your skin can get dry. Dry skin can be itchy, causing you to scratch and make it sore. Also, dry skin can crack. Cracks allow germs to enter and cause infection. If your blood glucose is high, it feeds germs and makes infections worse. Skin can get dry on your legs, feet, elbows, and other places on your body.

2. Nerve damage can decrease the amount you sweat. Sweating helps keep your skin soft and moist. Decreased sweating in your feet and legs can cause dry skin.

What can I do to take care of my skin?

*   After you wash with a mild soap, make sure you rinse and dry yourself well. Check places where water can hide, such as under the arms, under the breasts, between the legs, and between the toes.

*   Keep your skin moist by using a lotion or cream after you wash. Ask your doctor to suggest one.

*   Drink lots of fluids, such as water, to keep your skin moist and healthy.

- Wear all-cotton underwear. Cotton allows air to move around your body better.

- Check your skin after you wash. Make sure you have no dry, red, or sore spots that might lead to an infection.

- Tell your doctor about any skin problems.

Where can I go for more information?

- **Diabetes teachers** (nurses, dietitians, pharmacists, and other health professionals): To find a diabetes teacher near you, call the American Association of Diabetes Educators toll-free at 800-TEAMUP4 (800-832-6874), or look on the internet at http://www.diabeteseducator.org and click on "Find an Educator."

- **Dietitians:** To find a dietitian near you, call the American Dietetic Association toll-free at 800-366-1655, or look on the internet at http://www.eatright.org and click on "Find a Nutrition Professional."

- **Government:** The National Institute of Arthritis and Musculoskeletal and Skin Diseases (NIAMS) is part of the National Institutes of Health. To learn more about feet and skin problems, write or call the National Institute of Arthritis and Musculoskeletal and Skin Diseases Information Clearinghouse, 1 AMS Circle, Bethesda, MD 20892-3675, 877-226-4267 (toll-free); or see http://www.niams.nih.gov on the internet.

- **The "Prevent Diabetes Problems" Series:** The "Prevent Diabetes Problems" series includes seven booklets that can help you learn more about how to prevent diabetes problems. For free single copies of these booklets, write, call, fax, or e-mail the National Diabetes Information Clearinghouse: Contact information can be found in Chapter 48, "A Directory of Foot and Ankle Health Resources."

Section 39.4

Prevention and Early Intervention for Diabetes Foot Problems

Excerpted from *Feet Can Last a Lifetime: A Health Care Provider's Guide to Preventing Diabetes Foot Problems*, National Diabetes Education Program, a joint initiative of the National Institutes of Health and the Centers for Disease Control and Prevention, National Institute of Diabetes and Digestive and Kidney Diseases, November 2000. Available online at http://www.ndep.nih.gov/diabetes/pubs/Feet_HCGuide.pdf.

National Goals for Diabetes Foot Care

During their lifetime, 15 percent of people with diabetes will experience a foot ulcer and between 14 and 24 percent of those with a foot ulcer will require amputation. National Hospital Discharge Survey data for 1996 indicate that 86,000 people with diabetes underwent one or more lower-extremity amputations. Diabetes is the leading cause of amputation of the lower limbs. Yet it is clear that at least half of these amputations might be prevented through simple but effective foot care practices.

Healthy People 2010, the U.S. Department of Health and Human Services' report that specifies health objectives for the nation, calls for the following:

- an increase in the proportion of people with diabetes aged 18 years and older who have at least an annual foot examination (baseline 55 percent, target 75 percent)

- a decrease in foot ulcers due to diabetes (baseline and target figures are "developmental")

- a decrease in lower extremity amputations due to diabetes (baseline 11 per 1,000, target 5 per 1,000 per year). This objective is based on the estimate that at least 50 percent of the amputations that occur each year in people with diabetes can be prevented through screening for high risk patients and the provision of proper foot care.

Ethnic Groups at Higher Risk for Amputation

Analysis of a statewide California hospital discharge database indicated that in 1991, the age-adjusted incidence of diabetes-related lower extremity amputations per 10,000 people with diabetes was 95.3 in African Americans, 56.0 in non-Hispanic whites, and 44.4 in Hispanics. Amputations were 1.72 and 2.17 times more likely in African Americans compared with non-Hispanic whites and Hispanics, respectively. Hispanics had a higher proportion of amputations (82.7 percent) associated with diabetes as opposed to other causes of amputation, than did African Americans (61.6 percent) or non-Hispanic whites (56.8 percent).

Age-adjusted amputation rates in south Texas in 1993 were 60.68 per 10,000 for non-Hispanic whites, 94.08 for Mexican Americans, and 146.59 for African Americans. The incidence of amputations for Pima Indians in Arizona was 24.1 per 1,000 person-years compared to 6.5 per 1,000 person-years for the overall U.S. population with diabetes. Increased awareness and identification of diabetes-related foot disease is especially important in these high-risk ethnic groups.

The President's Initiative to Eliminate Racial and Ethnic Disparities in Health is focused on eliminating serious disparities in health access and outcomes experienced by racial and ethnic minority populations in six areas of health. Diabetes is one of the targeted areas. A near-term goal for this initiative is to reduce lower extremity amputation rates among African Americans with diabetes by 40 percent.

Frequency of Foot Examinations

Foot examinations, both by people with diabetes and their health care providers, are critical preventive actions. In the 1989 National Health Interview Survey (NHIS), 52 percent of all people with diabetes stated that they checked their feet at least daily, but 22 percent stated that they never checked their feet. More self-exams were reported by insulin-treated individuals than those who did not use insulin.

Estimates of the frequency of provider-performed annual foot examinations vary. Data from the Centers for Disease Control's Behavioral Risk Factor Surveillance System (BRFSS) indicate that 55 percent of adults with diabetes ages 18 years and older reported having at least an annual foot examination by a health care provider in 1998 (mean value from 39 states). BRFSS data from 1995 to 1998 indicate that 86.3 percent of people with diabetes had seen a physician or other health care provider for diabetes care in the previous 12 months; 67.7 percent of adults with diabetes reported having had their feet examined in the previous 12 months. In an earlier nationwide survey, primary care physicians reported performing semi-annual foot examinations for 66 percent of patients with type 1 diabetes and for 52 percent of patients with type 2 diabetes.

Personal and Financial Costs

Diabetes foot disease is a major burden for both the individual and the health care system and may increase as the population ages. The total annual cost for the more than 86,000 amputations is over $1.1 billion dollars. This cost does not include surgeons' fees, rehabilitation costs, prostheses, time lost from work, and disability payments. Regarding quality of life, a study of patients with diabetes showed that those with foot ulcers scored significantly lower than those without foot ulcers in all eight areas of a measure of physical and social function.

Foot disease is the most common complication of diabetes leading to hospitalization. In 1995, foot disease accounted for 6 percent of hospital discharges listing diabetes and lower extremity ulcers, and in 1995 the average hospital stay was 13.7 days. The average hospital reimbursement from Medicare for a lower-extremity amputation in 1992 was $10,969, and from private insurers it was $26,940. At the same time, rehabilitation was reimbursed at a rate of $7,000 to $21,000.

Prevalence estimates for ulcers in diabetes patient populations vary. Fifteen percent of all patients with diabetes in a population-based study in southern Wisconsin experienced ulcers or sores on the foot or ankle. The prevalence increased with age, especially in patients who were aged 30 or under at diagnosis of diabetes. In a large staff-model health maintenance organization, the incidence, outcomes and costs of treatment for foot ulcers were studied over two years in a group of patients with diabetes. In this population, the incidence was nearly 2 percent per year and the direct medical care cost for a 40- to 65-year-old male with a new foot ulcer was $27,987 over the two years after diagnosis.

After an amputation, the chance of another amputation of the same extremity or of the opposite extremity within five years is as high as 50 percent. The five-year mortality rate after lower extremity amputation ranges from 39 to 68 percent.

Risk Factors for Lower Extremity Amputation (LEA)

Peripheral neuropathy, peripheral vascular disease, and prior foot ulcer are independently associated with risk of LEA. A 1996 study of

Pima Indians with diabetes confirmed this finding and included the presence of foot deformity as another independent risk factor. The presence of plantar callus also is highly predictive of subsequent ulceration in patients with diabetic neuropathy and is more predictive of ulceration than increased plantar foot pressures.

Hyperglycemia is an additional risk factor. In a 1996 study, Finnish researchers determined risk factors for amputation in 1,044 middle-aged patients with type 2 diabetes who were followed for up to seven years. Because the incidence of amputation was similar in both sexes (5.6 percent men and 5.3 percent women), all statistical analyses were carried out combining men and women. This study found that high fasting plasma glucose levels at baseline, high HbA1c, and the duration of diabetes were independently associated with a two-fold risk of amputation. Signs of peripheral neuropathy, bilateral absence of vibration sense and bilateral absence of Achilles tendon reflexes, were two times more frequent in patients with amputation than in patients without amputation.

The Diabetes Control and Complications Trial (DCCT), a ten-year clinical study that concluded in 1993, demonstrated that keeping blood glucose levels as close to normal as possible slows significantly the onset and progression of eye, kidney, and nerve diseases caused by diabetes. The study showed that any sustained lowering of the blood glucose helps, even if the person has a history of poor control. A follow-up study indicated that the reduction in risk for microvascular changes persisted for at least four years after the DCCT ended, despite increasing blood glucose levels. The United Kingdom Prospective Diabetes Study reported that type 2 patients randomized to intensive blood glucose control with sulfonylureas or insulin had a significantly lower prevalence of neuropathy at 9 and 15 years than patients randomized to conventional therapy.

Evidence for a relationship between use of tobacco and/or alcohol and ulcers or amputation is variable. Cigarette smoking, however, is a major risk factor for microvascular and macrovascular disease and is likely to contribute to diabetes foot disease. People with foot and ankle neuropathy are more likely to have gait abnormalities, postural instability, and sway, and are 15 times more likely to suffer some type of injury during ambulation than those without neuropathy.

The most important risk factors for diabetes foot problems, however, are peripheral neuropathy and peripheral vascular disease, as noted by Shaw and Boulton. There also is a complex interplay between these abnormalities and a considerable number of other contributory factors such as limited mobility, altered foot pressures, glycemic control, ethnic background, and more. The authors stress, however, that identification of patients at high risk for ulceration is simple and preventive care should focus on patient education.

Causal Pathways for Lower Extremity Amputations (LEAs)

A study of the causal pathways for LEAs in patients with diabetes identified the most common sequences of events. Seventy-three percent of the amputations in study subjects were a result of the causal sequence of minor trauma, cutaneous ulceration, and wound-healing failure. Estimates of the cumulative proportions of various causes indicated that 86 percent of amputations were attributed to initial minor trauma causing tissue injury.

Precipitating or Pivotal Events

In the causal pathway study noted above, foot trauma was caused by shoe-related repetitive pressure leading to cutaneous ulceration in 36 percent of all cases, accidental cuts or wounds in 8 percent, thermal trauma (frostbite or burns) in 8 percent, and decubitus ulceration in 8 percent. Similarly, another study found that in one-third of diabetic amputees with peripheral arterial disease, the initial lesion was self-induced. The most common cause of self-injury was ill-fitting new shoes; the second most common cause was cutting toenails improperly. Other investigators identified external precipitating factors in 84 percent of study patients with foot ulcers. The most common factors were ill-fitting shoes/socks, acute mechanical trauma, stress ulcer, and paronychia.

Tools to Identify High Risk Feet

The importance of identifying individuals at risk for foot ulceration and LEA and the need for preventive foot care practices for both the provider and the patient are significant. Identifying patients' risk category for foot ulceration helps to determine the frequency needed for provider foot examinations, the level of emphasis on self-care of the feet, and patient responsibilities.

Several simple tools have been developed to identify people at high risk for ulceration. These tools include a patient report and a clinical examination to quantify loss of peripheral sensation (using a monofilament or vibration perception threshold testing), and to detect the presence of foot deformities, peripheral vascular disease, and prior foot ulcers. The largest study to use the Semmes-Weinstein 5.07 (10-gram) monofilament is the Strong Heart Study of 3,638 American Indians living in Arizona, North and South Dakota, and Oklahoma. Use of these measures has been shown to predict subsequent ulceration and amputation.

In one study, during annual patient examinations, researchers recorded the presence of a foot deformity, history of lower extremity ulceration or amputation, and the ability to perceive the Semmes-Weinstein 5.07 (10-gram) monofilament at eight sites on the plantar surface of each foot. Based on the findings, subjects were classified as sensate or insensate and placed in one of four risk categories. Insensitivity to the monofilament occurred in 68 (19 percent) of the patients screened. Over a 32-month follow-up period, 41 of these patients developed ulcerations and 14 amputations occurred.

The recommended number of monofilament applications needed to assess the risk for ulceration varies. One study shows that an 8-site 5.07 (10-gram) monofilament examination (four sites per foot) can be completed in 40 seconds and has 90 to 95 percent of the sensitivity of a 16-point examination. The four-site-per-foot examination specifies two of the touch sites—the first and third metatarsal heads. For the other two sites, the authors suggest any toes or other metatarsal heads. All sites should be free of calluses. Another study suggests that reasonable sensitivity and specificity (80 and 86 percent, respectively) to detect patients with an insensate foot can be achieved when the plantar aspect of either the first or fifth metatarsal head cannot feel a 5.07 (10-gram) monofilament.

A self-administered sensory test with a 5.07 (10-gram) monofilament may be useful to identify high risk feet. In a study that compared patient and provider sensory test findings for 145 subjects, 68 percent of patients self-tested without the assistance of another person, and patient/provider disagreement with findings occurred in 12 percent of cases. Sensory loss, previously undetected by providers, was found in 16 percent of patients. Self-administered tests provided patients an opportunity to become more active team members and resulted in early detection of insensate feet. The authors caution that self-testing should not replace regular foot evaluation by a health care provider.

Education Reduces Lower Extremity Abnormalities

In a randomized, controlled study, researchers provided intervention patients with foot care education, behavioral contracts, and telephone and postcard prompts. The researchers placed foot care prompts on the medical record and provided practice guidelines and flow sheets to clinicians assigned to those patients. Results showed that primary care physicians in the intervention group conducted more examinations of lower extremities, identified those at risk for amputation, and referred more patients for specialized foot care. Patients in the intervention group received more patient education, made more changes in appropriate self-care behaviors, and had fewer short-term foot problems than patients in the control group.

Ollendorf and others developed a model to estimate the economic benefits of amputation prevention strategies targeted at individuals with a history of foot ulcer over a period of three years. Estimates were based on an average lifetime cost of $48,152 for lower extremity amputation. For an estimated 679 individuals during the first year, the total potential economic benefits of strategies to reduce amputation risk ranged from two to three million dollars over three years ($2,900 to $4,442 per person with a history of foot ulcer). Benefits were highest for patient/provider educational interventions, followed by therapeutic shoe coverage, and multidisciplinary care.

Multidisciplinary team care can be a cost-effective method for foot screening, preventive care, and treatment of active ulcers. One study of team care for high risk patients with a history of foot ulcers found a two-year foot ulcer incidence rate of 30 percent in the intervention group compared with 58 percent in the standard treatment group. The team involved physicians, nurses, podiatrists, and shoe specialists.

A study of 639 patients in a rural primary care clinic showed significant reductions in lower extremity amputations. This prospective study of American Indians with diabetes, compared three consecutive two- to three-year time periods: a "standard care" period during which patients received foot care at the discretion of the primary care provider; a "public health" period during which patients were screened for foot problems and high risk individuals received foot care education and protective footwear; and a "stepped care" period during which comprehensive guidelines for foot management were adapted to their practice and implemented by a six-person primary care team.

The average annual amputation incidence per 1,000 diabetic person-years was 29 in the first period, 21 in the second, and 15 in the third, an overall 48 percent reduction.

A study was conducted at six Veterans Affairs Medical Centers to determine how accurately and reproducibly primary care providers could carry out a screening examination (including use of a monofilament) for foot ulcer risk among patients with diabetes. Forty primary care providers (including non-physicians) examined 147 patients; two primary care providers examined each patient; and a foot care specialist also examined 88 patients. The results showed that the foot examination was reproducible among primary care providers and accurate when compared with a foot care specialist, except in the assessment of foot deformity and pedal pulses. When training providers to conduct foot exams, particular attention to these skills may be important.

Components of Effective Self-Management

Findings from several studies indicate effective components of patient education that contribute to successful patient outcomes. These include giving detailed foot care recommendations, requesting patient commitment to self-care, demonstrating and practicing foot care procedures, and communicating a persistent message that foot complications can be avoided by self-care. In comparing the effectiveness of intensive versus conventional education, researchers found that patients in the intensive group showed greater improvement in foot care knowledge, better compliance with the recommended foot care routine, improved satisfaction with foot care, and greater reduction in the number of foot problems requiring treatment.

Foot care recommendations and demonstrations should include: washing, drying, and inspecting the feet; applying an emollient; cutting toenails; treating minor foot problems; selecting suitable footwear; dealing with temperature extremes; and contacting the physician if problems do not resolve quickly.

Lubricating the feet may be a simple yet very important way to help prevent foot ulcers. Over a one-year period, study patients who infrequently lubricated their feet were 3.1 times more likely to have a foot lesion than those who frequently lubricated their feet.

Patients with high risk feet should inspect them twice a day. Those with peripheral neuropathy, vascular disease, or eye disease should not attempt to cut their own toenails as this can lead to serious self-inflicted injury.

It is important for a health care provider or diabetes educator to review with the patient all written take-home instructions for self-care of the feet. In a program for African Americans, patients reported that the most useful parts of a take-home packet were the patient instruction booklet, the large hand mirror, and the foot care knowledge self-test with explanations of the answers.

Researchers found that the frequency of desired self-care behaviors improved when patients were given specific instructions stated as precisely as possible such as "dry between toes," "file calluses," and "never go barefoot" rather than more general instructions such as "avoid injury to your feet." Patients should never be allowed to walk on open plantar ulcers since continuous application of mechanical load will prevent healing. Walking aids, footwear modifications, or other interventions must be used to relieve weight.

Step-by-step guidelines have been published to assist providers to conduct patient education workshops on foot care including how to attract participants, promote the workshop, develop the agenda, identify appropriate speakers, and conduct a post-workshop evaluation.

Provider Foot Care Practices

A documented annual comprehensive foot examination is included in a set of national quality improvement measures for diabetes care as part of the Diabetes Quality Improvement Project (DQIP). Numerous public agencies (the Department of Defense, the Health Care Financing Administration (HCFA), the Indian Health Service, and the Veterans Health Administration), and private groups (the American Diabetes Association Provider Recognition Program and the National Committee for Quality Assurance) are using some or all of this set of eight DQIP performance measures. HCFA is responsible for Medicare and managed care plans that serve Medicare beneficiaries, as well as Medicaid programs. DQIP measures are likely to increase the frequency of documented annual foot exams by health care providers.

A study of provider practices found that clinicians were likely to prescribe preventive foot care behaviors when they were aware of a patient's high risk for LEA as evidenced by prior history of foot ulcer. Clinician awareness of two other major risk factors (peripheral neuropathy or peripheral vascular disease), however, did not increase preventive care practices. The study's authors concluded that physicians and patients need periodic reminders to identify patients in all high risk categories for ulcer or amputation and to schedule visits for foot care and education in self-care. To prevent unnecessary progression of foot problems, proactive communication is recommended between foot care specialists and providers less familiar with diabetes foot care management, as well as timely referral from primary care providers to specialists as necessary.

Self-Care Limitations in the Elderly

Barriers to carrying out daily foot care noted by elderly study subjects included lack of motivation, forgetfulness, vision problems, joint and knee problems, and family responsibilities. The ability of elderly people to identify foot lesions was investigated further in a matched comparison, controlled study. Findings showed that 43 percent of patients with a history of foot ulcers could not reach and remove simulated lesions on their toes; over 50 percent of the older subjects reported difficulty trimming their toe nails; and only 14 percent had sufficient joint flexibility to allow inspection of the plantar aspect of the foot. It can be concluded that elderly people who are unable to perform daily self-care of the feet would benefit more from regular foot care given by others than from intensive education.

Exercise

In people with diabetes, regular exercise can lower blood glucose, improve insulin sensitivity, raise HDL cholesterol, improve blood flow and heart muscle strength, enhance fibrinolysis, control weight, increase muscle mass, and provide an overall sense of well-being. Because of these effects, regular exercise may also delay the onset of neuropathy and atherosclerosis. People who have had type 1 diabetes for more than ten years, or type 2 diabetes for more than five years, should be screened for medical risk prior to beginning an exercise program. While the presence of neuropathy does not rule out exercise, care should be taken not to worsen soft tissue and joint injury or cause foot ulcers or bone injury. Stretching muscles before exercise is important to prevent ligament strain. Swimming or bicycling are recommended forms of exercise because they avoid abrasion to the feet. Attention to the construction and fit of footwear is essential.

Repetitive Stress and Special Footwear

People with intact sensation respond to repetitive stress that occurs during walking either by shifting the pressure to another part of the foot, by modifying the way the foot meets the ground, by resting, or by checking their shoes for problems. With the loss of peripheral sensation, however, many people with diabetes have no indication of lower extremity pain, pressure, or trauma and do not take measures to modify repetitive pressures. Lack of feeling makes shoe-fitting assistance essential.

Properly-constructed and well-fitting shoes and shoe inserts can minimize localized stresses by redistributing forces during walking. Besides helping patients keep feet healthy, shoes and orthoses also can help prevent diabetes complications. Investigators in a recent study found that after healing of the initial ulcer, re-ulceration occurred after one year in 58 percent of patients who resumed wearing their own footwear, compared to 28 percent of those who wore therapeutic footwear.

Shoe color can contribute to thermal injury of the insensate foot when shoes are worn in the sun for a prolonged period (two to three hours). One study showed that after 30 minutes of exposure to radiant heat, the mean increase in temperature was between 7.8 and 13.6 degrees Fahrenheit greater in a black leather walking shoe than in a similar white shoe.

Another study compared the prevalence and severity of foot deformities and the development of ulceration in people with diabetes after a great toe amputation. Due to altered pressure distribution, the foot with great toe amputation developed more frequent and more severe deformities of the lesser toes and metatarsophalangeal joints compared to the other intact foot. Because these patients were at high risk for subsequent ulceration, the use of special inserts and footwear to protect the feet was highly recommended.

Footwear and the Medicare Shoe Benefit

Professionally fitted shoes and prescription footwear are an important part of the overall treatment of the insensate foot because they aid in preventing limb loss. Footwear should relieve areas of excessive pressure, reduce shock and shear, and accommodate, stabilize, and support deformities. The type of footwear provided will depend on the patient's foot structure, activity level, gait, and footwear preference.

Shoes should be long enough and have room in the toe area and over the instep. Shoes with laces or Velcro allow adjustment for edema and deformities. Most people with early neuropathic changes can wear cushioned commercial footwear such as walking or athletic shoes. When used in conjunction with an off-the-shelf soft accommodative insole (Plastazote/urethane viscoelastic), comfort shoes and athletic footwear were as effective as prescribed depth shoes in reducing certain metatarsal and great toe pressures. Some people, however, may need the pressure areas redistributed with custom orthotics that often require prescribed depth footwear.

Custom-molded shoes, depth shoes, inserts, and shoe modifications can be fitted and furnished by a podiatrist, orthopedic foot surgeon, orthotist, or pedorthist. Depth-inlay shoes provide more room for toe deformities and for the insertion of customized insoles. Extra-wide shoes provide more room for bunions and other abnormalities. Rocker sole shoes reduce pressure under metatarsal heads and toes. They are particularly useful for reducing the risk of ulceration in patients with a stiff and rigid first metatarsal joint.

Since 1993, the Medicare footwear benefit has made special footwear available to more patients than ever before. To obtain coverage, patients must have physician certification that they are at high risk for ulceration or amputation, receive a written footwear prescription from a podiatrist or other qualified physician, and obtain the footwear from a qualified provider or supplier who will then file the appropriate claim forms. Utilization of the Medicare benefit was low in 1995 for three states studied—Washington, Alaska, and Idaho. Altogether, less than 1 percent of beneficiaries with diabetes meeting the appropriate criteria for the footwear benefit had a therapeutic footwear claim. Clearly, there is an opportunity to increase awareness of the availability of this benefit and how to obtain reimbursement.

Conclusion

The staggering human and economic costs of diabetes foot disease may be reduced significantly with increased practice of several simple preventive care measures designed to prevent foot ulcers and lower extremity amputations. Routine annual foot exams to identify high risk feet facilitate early interventions to help reduce the incidence of the most common precipitating events including injury and footwear-related trauma to the insensitive foot. The key elements of preventive care include: annual examination of the feet by health care providers to determine risk factors for ulceration; subsequent examination of high risk feet at each patient visit; patient education about daily self-care of the feet; use of proper footwear; and careful glucose management. National recommendations and objectives support the application of these practices based on the strong and time-tested evidence for the prevention of lower extremity ulcers and amputations. These national objectives can serve as a galvanizing call to action for policy makers, health care providers, and people with diabetes to make diabetes foot care and prevention a high priority.

Section 39.5

Achilles Tendon Surgery Helps Prevent Diabetic Foot Ulcers

Diabetic patients frustrated by hard-to-heal, infection-prone ulcers on their feet could benefit from a common, minimally invasive surgical procedure to relieve tightness in their Achilles tendons, the American College of Foot and Ankle Surgeons (ACFAS) reported recently.

The Achilles is the largest tendon in the human body, connecting the calf muscles to the heel bone. As we age, the tendon naturally tightens. However, diabetes exacerbates the process as increased blood sugar levels deposit glucose in the collagen of the tendon, greatly reducing its elasticity and making stretching almost impossible.

"A tight Achilles inhibits ankle movement, forcing diabetic patients to place excessive pressure on the front of the foot," said J. Christopher Moore, DPM, AACFAS, an Asheville, NC based foot and ankle surgeon. "Pressure normally absorbed by the ankle has to go somewhere else and the forefoot gets most of it, heightening risk for ulcer development underneath the toe joints."

Foot sores or ulcers are a common complication of diabetes. They result from sensation loss or neuropathy, which deprives diabetes patients of their ability to feel pressure or pain in the lower extremities. Therefore, according to the ACFAS consumer website, FootPhysicians.com, even the slightest cut, blister, or wound can develop into a diabetic foot ulcer. Such wounds can cause tissue and bone infections and can result in loss of a toe, a foot, a leg, or even a life.

Moore said published research has shown that surgery to lengthen the Achilles tendon in a diabetes patient can help prevent ulcer recurrence. "Our goal always is to close the wound as quickly as possible to avoid infection, and we're becoming more aware that preventing ulcer recurrence in patients with advanced diabetes is best achieved by a minimally invasive procedure to lengthen a tight Achilles tendon," said Moore.

Lengthening occurs by making three small, pinpoint cuts to loosen and stretch the tendon. This helps restore ankle flexibility and relieves forefoot pressure. The procedure allows diabetes patients who keep their blood sugar under control to walk more normally and may lower their risk for redeveloping foot ulcers.

"I have seen diabetic patients whose foot ulcers heal, yet continue to recur because the untreated Achilles tendon problem is the root cause," said Moore. He advises diabetic patients who have developed foot ulcers to see a foot and ankle surgeon to determine if the Achilles tendons surgery is appropriate for them.

Chapter 40

Neuromuscular Diseases

Chapter Contents

Section 40.1

Charcot-Marie-Tooth Disease

"Charcot-Marie-Tooth Disease Fact Sheet," National Institute of Neurological Disorders and Stroke, National Institutes of Health (NINDS), NIH Publication No. 02-4897, April 26, 2006. NINDS health-related material is provided for information purposes only and does not necessarily represent endorsement by or an official position of the National Institute of Neurological Disorders and Stroke or any other federal agency. Advice on the treatment or care of an individual patient should be obtained through consultation with a physician who has examined that patient or is familiar with that patient's medical history.

What is Charcot-Marie-Tooth disease?

Charcot-Marie-Tooth disease (CMT) is one of the most common inherited neurological disorders, affecting approximately 1 in 2,500 people in the United States. The disease is named for the three physicians who first identified it in 1886—Jean-Martin Charcot and Pierre Marie in Paris, France, and Howard Henry Tooth in Cambridge, England. CMT, also known as hereditary motor and sensory neuropathy (HMSN) or peroneal muscular atrophy, comprises a group of disorders that affect peripheral nerves. The peripheral nerves lie outside the brain and spinal cord and supply the muscles and sensory organs in the limbs. Disorders that affect the peripheral nerves are called peripheral neuropathies.

What are the symptoms of Charcot-Marie-Tooth disease?

The neuropathy of CMT affects both motor and sensory nerves. A typical feature includes weakness of the foot and lower leg muscles, which may result in foot drop and a high-stepped gait with frequent tripping or falls. Foot deformities, such as high arches and hammer toes (a condition in which the middle joint of a toe bends upwards) are also characteristic due to weakness of the small muscles in the feet. In addition, the lower legs may take on an "inverted champagne bottle" appearance due to the loss of muscle bulk. Later in the disease, weakness and muscle atrophy may occur in the hands, resulting in difficulty with fine motor skills.

Onset of symptoms is most often in adolescence or early adulthood, however presentation may be delayed until mid-adulthood. The severity of symptoms is quite variable in different patients and some people may never realize they have the disorder. Progression of symptoms is very gradual. CMT is not fatal and people with most forms of CMT have a normal life expectancy.

What are the types of Charcot-Marie-Tooth disease?

There are many forms of CMT disease. The principal types include CMT1, CMT2, CMT3, CMT4, and CMTX. CMT1 is the most frequent and results from abnormalities in the myelin sheath. There are three main types of CMT1. CMT1A is an autosomal dominant disease resulting from a duplication of the gene on chromosome 17 that carries the instructions for producing the peripheral myelin protein-22 (*PMP-22*). The *PMP-22* protein is a critical component of the myelin sheath. An overabundance of this gene causes the structure and function of the myelin sheath to be abnormal. Patients experience weakness and atrophy of the muscles of the lower legs beginning in adolescence; later they experience hand weakness and sensory loss. Interestingly, a different neuropathy distinct from CMT1A called hereditary neuropathy with predisposition to pressure palsy (HNPP) is caused by a deletion of one of the *PMP-22* genes. In this case abnormally low levels of the *PMP-22* gene result in episodic, recurrent, demyelinating neuropathy. CMT1B is an autosomal dominant disease caused by mutations in the gene that carries the instructions for manufacturing the myelin protein zero (*P0*) which is another critical component of the myelin sheath. Most of these mutations are point mutations, meaning a mistake occurs in only one letter of the DNA genetic code. To date, scientists have identified more than 30 different point mutations in the *P0* gene. As a result of abnormalities in *P0*, CMT1B produces symptoms similar to those found in CMT1A. The gene defect that causes CMT1C, which also has symptoms similar to those found in CMT1A, has not yet been identified.

CMT2 is less common than CMT1 and results from abnormalities in the axon of the peripheral nerve cell rather than the myelin sheath. Recently a mutation was identified in the gene that codes for the kinesin family member 1B-beta protein in families with CMT2A. Kinesins are proteins that act as motors to help power the transport of materials along the train tracks (microtubules) of the cell. Another recent finding is a mutation in the neurofilament-light gene, identified in a Russian family with CMT2E. Neurofilaments are structural proteins that help maintain the normal shape of a cell. Genes that cause other forms of CMT2 have not yet been identified.

CMT3 or Dejerine-Sottas disease is a severe demyelinating neuropathy that begins in infancy. Infants have severe muscle atrophy, weakness, and sensory problems. This rare disorder can be caused by a specific point mutation in the *P0* gene or a point mutation in the *PMP-22* gene.

CMT4 comprises several different subtypes of autosomal recessive demyelinating motor and sensory neuropathies. Each neuropathy subtype is caused by a different genetic mutation, may affect a particular ethnic population, and produces distinct physiologic or clinical characteristics. Patients with CMT4 generally develop symptoms of leg weakness in childhood and by adolescence they may not be able to walk. The gene abnormalities responsible for CMT4 have yet to be identified.

CMTX is an X-linked dominant disease and is caused by a point mutation in the *connexin-32* gene on the X chromosome. The *connexin-32* protein is expressed in Schwann cells—cells that wrap around nerve axons, making up a single segment of the myelin sheath. This protein may be involved in Schwann cell communication with the axon. Males who inherit one mutated gene from their mothers show moderate to severe symptoms of the disease beginning in late childhood or adolescence (the Y chromosome that males inherit from their fathers does not have the *connexin-32* gene). Females who inherit one mutated gene from one parent and one normal gene from the other parent may develop mild symptoms in adolescence or later or may not develop symptoms of the disease at all.

What causes Charcot-Marie-Tooth disease?

A nerve cell communicates information to distant targets by sending electrical signals down a long, thin part of the cell called the axon. In order to increase the speed at which these electrical signals travel, the axon is insulated by myelin, which is produced by another type of cell called the Schwann cell. Myelin twists around the axon like a jelly-roll cake and prevents dissipation of the electrical signals. Without an intact axon and myelin sheath, peripheral nerve cells are unable to activate target muscles or relay sensory information from the limbs back to the brain.

CMT is caused by mutations in genes that produce proteins involved in the structure and function of either the peripheral nerve axon or the myelin sheath. Although different proteins are abnormal

374

in different forms of CMT disease, all of the mutations affect the normal function of the peripheral nerves. Consequently, these nerves slowly degenerate and lose the ability to communicate with their distant targets. The degeneration of motor nerves results in muscle weakness and atrophy in the extremities (arms, legs, hands, or feet), and the degeneration of sensory nerves results in a reduced ability to feel heat, cold, and pain.

The gene mutations in CMT disease are usually inherited. Each of us normally possesses two copies of every gene, one inherited from each parent. Some forms of CMT are inherited in an autosomal dominant fashion, which means that only one copy of the abnormal gene is needed to cause the disease. Other forms of CMT are inherited in an autosomal recessive fashion, which means that both copies of the abnormal gene must be present to cause the disease. Still other forms of CMT are inherited in an X-linked fashion, which means that the abnormal gene is located on the X chromosome. The X and Y chromosomes determine an individual's sex. Individuals with two X chromosomes are female and individuals with one X and one Y chromosome are male. In rare cases the gene mutation causing CMT disease is a new mutation which occurs spontaneously in the patient's genetic material and has not been passed down through the family.

How is Charcot-Marie-Tooth disease diagnosed?

Diagnosis of CMT begins with a standard patient history, family history, and neurological examination. Patients will be asked about the nature and duration of their symptoms and whether other family members have the disease. During the neurological examination a physician will look for evidence of muscle weakness in the arms, legs, hands, and feet, decreased muscle bulk, reduced tendon reflexes, and sensory loss. Doctors look for evidence of foot deformities, such as high arches, hammer toes, inverted heel, or flat feet. Other orthopedic problems, such as mild scoliosis or hip dysplasia, may also be present. A specific sign that may be found in patients with CMT1 is nerve enlargement that may be felt or even seen through the skin. These enlarged nerves, called hypertrophic nerves, are caused by abnormally thickened myelin sheaths.

If CMT is suspected, the physician may order electrodiagnostic tests for the patient. This testing consists of two parts: nerve conduction studies and electromyography (EMG). During nerve conduction studies, electrodes are placed on the skin over a peripheral motor or sensory nerve. These electrodes produce a small electric shock that may cause mild discomfort. This electrical impulse stimulates sensory and motor nerves and provides quantifiable information that the doctor can use to arrive at a diagnosis. EMG involves inserting a needle electrode through the skin to measure the bioelectrical activity of muscles. Specific abnormalities in the readings signify axon degeneration. EMG may be useful in further characterizing the distribution and severity of peripheral nerve involvement.

If all other tests seem to suggest that a patient has CMT, a neurologist may perform a nerve biopsy to confirm the diagnosis. A nerve biopsy involves removing a small piece of peripheral nerve through an incision in the skin. This is most often done by removing a piece of the nerve that runs down the calf of the leg. The nerve is then examined under a microscope. Patients with CMT1 typically show signs of abnormal myelination. Specifically, "onion bulb" formations may be seen which represent axons surrounded by layers of demyelinating and remyelinating Schwann cells. Patients with CMT2 usually show signs of axon degeneration.

Genetic testing is available for some types of CMT and may soon be available for other types; such testing can be used to confirm a diagnosis. In addition, genetic counseling is available to parents who fear that they may pass mutant genes to their children.

How is Charcot-Marie-Tooth disease treated?

There is no cure for CMT, but physical therapy, occupational therapy, braces and other orthopedic devices, and even orthopedic surgery can help patients cope with the disabling symptoms of the disease.

Physical and occupational therapy, the preferred treatment for CMT, involves muscle strength training, muscle and ligament stretching, stamina training, and moderate aerobic exercise. Most therapists recommend a specialized treatment program designed with the approval of the patient's physician to fit individual abilities and needs. Therapists also suggest entering into a treatment program early; muscle strengthening may delay or reduce muscle atrophy, so strength training is most useful if it begins before nerve degeneration and muscle weakness progress to the point of disability.

Stretching may prevent or reduce joint deformities that result from uneven muscle pull on bones. Exercises to help build stamina or increase endurance will help prevent the fatigue that results from performing everyday activities that require strength and mobility. Moderate aerobic activity can help to maintain cardiovascular fitness and overall health. Most therapists recommend low-impact or no-impact exercises, such as biking or swimming, rather than activities such as walking or jogging, which may put stress on fragile muscles and joints.

Many CMT patients require ankle braces and other orthopedic devices to maintain everyday mobility and prevent injury. Ankle braces can help prevent ankle sprains by providing support and stability during activities such as walking or climbing stairs. High-top shoes or boots can also give the patient support for weak ankles. Thumb splints can help with hand weakness and loss of fine motor skills. Assistive devices should be used before disability sets in because the devices may prevent muscle strain and reduce muscle weakening. Some CMT patients may decide to have orthopedic surgery to reverse foot and joint deformities.

What research is being done?

The National Institute of Neurological Disorders and Stroke (NINDS) supports research on CMT and other peripheral neuropathies in an effort to learn how to better treat, prevent, and even cure these disorders. Ongoing research includes efforts to identify more of the mutant genes and proteins that cause the various disease subtypes, efforts to discover the mechanisms of nerve degeneration and muscle atrophy with the hope of developing interventions to stop or slow down these debilitating processes, and efforts to find therapies to reverse nerve degeneration and muscle atrophy.

One promising area of research involves gene therapy experiments. Research with cell cultures and animal models has shown that it is possible to deliver genes to Schwann cells and muscle. Another area of research involves the use of trophic factors or nerve growth factors, such as the hormone androgen, to prevent nerve degeneration.

Section 40.2

Charcot Foot:
The Diagnostic Dilemma

Charcot neuropathy is a progressive deterioration of weight-bearing joints, usually in the foot or ankle. Historically, neuropathy of the knee was most frequently caused by syphilis, and neuropathy of the shoulder was usually caused by syringomyelia. Today, the Charcot foot occurs most often in patients with diabetic neuropathy; other predisposing conditions include alcoholic neuropathy, sensory loss caused by cerebral palsy or leprosy, and congenital insensitivity to pain. In 1868, Charcot identified neuropathic joints with an unusual pattern of bone destruction in patients with tabes dorsalis. The first description of neuroarthropathy occurring with diabetes mellitus was published in 1936.

Pathogenesis

Two theories (neurotraumatic and neurovascular) explain the pathogenesis of Charcot foot.[1] The neurotraumatic theory attributes bony destruction to the loss of pain sensation and proprioception combined with repetitive and mechanical trauma to the foot. The neurovascular theory suggests that joint destruction is secondary to an autonomically stimulated vascular reflex that causes hyperemia and periarticular osteopenia with contributory trauma. Intrinsic muscle imbalance with increased heel and plantar forces can produce eccentric loading of the foot, propagating microfractures, ligament laxity, and progression to bony destruction.

As many as 50 percent of patients with Charcot foot remember a precipitating, minor traumatic event (such as an ankle sprain or previous foot procedure); however, multiple cases of spontaneous Charcot joint changes, including patients with foot infections, support hyperemia as the cause.[2]

Epidemiology

Neuropathic arthropathy is prevalent in 0.8 to 7.5 percent of diabetic patients with neuropathy; 9 to 35 percent of these affected patients have bilateral involvement.[3,4] The higher prevalences occur in referral-based practices. Most patients with neuropathic arthropathy have had poorly controlled diabetes mellitus for 15 to 20 years.

The tarsometatarsal (Lisfranc) joint is the most common site for arthropathy, with initial involvement usually occurring on the medial column of the foot. The distribution of neuropathic arthropathy is 70 percent at the midfoot and 15 percent at the forefoot or rearfoot; it is usually contained in one area. Nearly 50 percent of patients with neuropathy had an associated plantar ulcer.[4]

Classification

Neuropathic arthropathy is either atrophic or hypertrophic. The atrophic form is usually localized to the forefoot and causes osteolysis of the distal metatarsals. The metatarsal heads and shafts have a radiographic deformity that resembles a pencil point or "sucked candy cane." The hypertrophic type usually occurs at the midfoot, rearfoot, or ankle, and is traditionally defined according to the Eichenholtz classification system.[5] The first stage is the developmental, or fragmentation, stage (acute Charcot) and is characterized by periarticular fracture and joint dislocation leading to an unstable, deformed foot. Patients in the coalescence stage (subacute Charcot) present with resorption of bone debris. The consolidation, or reparative, stage (chronic Charcot) is associated with re-stabilization of the foot with fusion of the involved fragments. This leads to the return of a stable, although deformed, foot. An updated version of the Eichenholtz classification system[6] identifies a prefragmentation (or acute inflammatory) stage zero. This is the stage when early diagnosis and intervention are critical to prevent long-range sequelae.[7-9] This updated version of the classification system also more closely relates clinical findings to treatment options.

Diagnosis

Approximately 50 percent of patients with Charcot foot remember a precipitating, minor traumatic event, and about 25 percent of patients ultimately develop similar changes on the contralateral foot.[9] In patients with diabetes and neuropathy, Charcot joint can develop very rapidly after a minor trauma.

Because trauma is not a prerequisite for Charcot foot, a patient with diabetes and neuropathy, erythema, edema, increased temperature of the foot, and normal radiographs most likely has an acute Charcot process. These patients are afebrile, have stable insulin requirements and normal white blood cell counts, and often have no break in skin integrity. These are all conditions that make infection unlikely.

Brodsky[7,10] described a test to distinguish a Charcot process from infection in patients with associated plantar ulcers. With the patient supine, the involved lower extremity is elevated for five to ten minutes. If swelling and rubor dissipate, the diagnosis of a Charcot process is supported. If the swelling and rubor persist, an infectious process is likely.

Evidence of neuropathy is determined by decreased or absent sensation to pinprick, light touch, or vibration. Decreased or absent protective sensation of the foot can be confirmed quite quickly using a Semmes-Weinstein 10-g (also known as 5.07-gauge) monofilament wire. The 10-g monofilament correlates with the threshold of protective sensation. If the patient cannot feel the monofilament (when it is applied with just enough pressure to bend the monofilament) on at least four of ten sites, the test is abnormal, and the patient is considered to be at risk for ulcer formation.[11] Another study[12] has shown that testing only four sites on each foot provides information as accurate as that obtained by using eight sites or more. The test can be performed quickly and is sensitive and specific for identifying loss of protective sensation.[13]

Evaluation

In evaluating the patient who presents with an apparent soft tissue infection or a plantar ulcer, the physician should first determine whether probing to bone is possible. A study[14] showed that in patients with diabetes mellitus, probing to bone is strongly correlated with osteomyelitis. Comparison bilateral weight-bearing radiographs, which are critical in determining instability, should then be obtained; however, not all experts agree that comparison views are necessary.[15] If there is no radiographic evidence of osteomyelitis but the patient is neuropathic, indium-111 leukocyte scanning or magnetic resonance imaging (MRI) is warranted.[16] Indium scanning is highly specific for infection. MRI is extremely sensitive, but the presence of an osteoarthropathy can lead to false-positive results. A variety of other laboratory studies are also typically performed. A high erythrocyte sedimentation rate is frequently found in patients with osteomyelitis, but this test has an extremely low sensitivity. Measurement of the white blood cell count may not help distinguish Charcot changes from osteomyelitis.[16] Thus, differentiating Charcot from Charcot with infection remains difficult. Synovial and bone biopsies might be necessary for a definitive diagnosis. After determining that bone changes are charcoid, the patient's deformity is staged. If a neuropathic ulcer is present, it is graded using the Wagner classification[17] or an equivalent grading system.

Treatment

Total Contact Casting

Most cases of acute Charcot foot can be treated nonsurgically with pressure-relieving methods such as total contact casting (TCC), which is believed to be the gold standard of treatment. TCC was developed in the 1950s. Most of the cast padding is eliminated for exact conformity to the lower extremity, with the goal of evenly distributing forces across the plantar surface of the foot. A tubular stockinette with low-density foam or one-quarter inch felt is applied over the tibial crest and malleoli, and around the metatarsal heads with one layer of synthetic padding. A three-layer inner plaster shell is followed by a fiberglass outer shell.[13]

The first cast is changed after one week because of the rapid reduction of edema that occurs as a result of TCC and restricted, protected weight bearing. Changing the cast prevents shearing between cast and skin. Follow-up casts are changed at two- to four-week intervals until erythema and edema have resolved, the temperature of the affected limb has decreased and is similar to that of the contralateral limb, and stabilization has been established on radiographic findings.

The presence of a Wagner grade 3 (or higher) ulcer necessitates incision, drainage, and antibiotic therapy, with resolution of any abscess before application of the TCC. Periodic ulcer evaluation should be performed along with debridement at the time of cast changes.

After the initial radiographs, surveillance films should be taken at four- to six-week intervals (or more often if there is an acute change). It is quite common for the lower extremity to be confined in a TCC for up to four months, with conversion to a Charcot restraint orthotic walker (CROW) after the active phase of the condition is complete, as evidenced by temperature normalization and radiographic stability. Protective foot gear with orthotics will later be needed.

TCC with guarded ambulation will lower the risk of developing a contralateral Charcot process compared with strict nonweight-bearing with crutches. Sella and Barrette[8] found that 25 percent of patients in the early stages of Charcot with joint diastasis and subluxation who were treated with TCC did not develop foot deformity (severe fragmentation and collapse). TCC also has been associated with improved ulcer healing in noninfected plantar ulcers in patients with diabetes.[18]

Prefabricated Pneumatic Walking Brace

An alternative to TCC is a prefabricated pneumatic walking brace (PPWB), which has been found to decrease forefoot and midfoot plantar pressure in the treatment of neuropathic plantar ulceration.[19] Benefits include easier wound surveillance, ease of application, and the ability to use several types of dressings. Use of the PPWB is limited in patients who have severe foot deformity or who are noncompliant.

Further Treatments

After swelling and erythema resolve and radiographic stability has been achieved, the TCC is changed to either a CROW, an ankle foot orthosis, or a patellar tendon-bearing brace, depending on residual anterior edema. If anterior edema persists, the CROW full-enclosure system is used. This device is used for six months to two years, until a stable foot is obtained. Patients can then be fitted for extra-depth shoes with custom insoles or orthotics to accommodate any residual deformity. Return to conventional foot gear may not be possible in all cases.

The primary care physician may be the first to evaluate minor lower extremity trauma in a neuropathic patient. If the radiographic findings are normal, a one- to two-month period of immobilization with protected weight bearing, followed by supportive shoe wear, is advisable.[9] This treatment can usually prevent breakdown of the foot. Diagnosis of a charcoid process is delayed in as many as 25 percent of patients,[10] but early recognition can prevent amputation.

Surgical Treatment

Patients with a consolidated (stable chronic) Charcot foot with a residual exostosis or recurrent or nonhealing ulcer may require an exostosectomy. In patients whose subluxation produces a markedly unstable extremity, a joint stabilization procedure performed by a foot and ankle specialist may be required.

Proposed Treatments

Other treatments for the Charcot process have included electrical bone stimulation or low-intensity ultrasonography during the acute phase to enhance healing. Although pilot studies of electrical bone stimulation show promise, it has not been labeled by the U.S. Food and Drug Administration for the treatment of Charcot foot.[20] Another study found that use of a bisphosphonate (pamidronate) resulted in decreased erythema, decreased temperature, and decreased Charcot activity.[21] Additional controlled studies are needed to further evaluate the effectiveness of these treatments.

Final Comment

Primary care physicians must consider the diagnosis of Charcot syndrome in any neuropathic patient with erythema, edema, and elevated temperature regardless of local or systemic signs of infection. In the patient with diabetes and lower extremity neuropathy, any minor injury requires careful observation because of the tendency of the limb to proceed to a Charcot process. Early identification and treatment of the Charcot process helps prevent deformity and decreased function of the lower extremity, as well as possible subsequent amputation. Physicians should continually educate their patients about the proper care of a neuropathic foot and the use of orthotic devices or custom footwear. The patient with a history of a Charcot process should be seen regularly, with close attention given to erythema, edema, or increased temperature in the foot or ankle.

—by Todd C. Sommer, DO, DPM and Thomas H. Lee, MD

References

1. Brower, A.C., Allman, R.M. Pathogenesis of the neurotrophic joint: neurotraumatic vs. neurovascular. *Radiology* 1981; 139: 349-54.

2. Schon, L.C., Easley, M.E., Weinfeld, S.B. Charcot neuroarthropathy of the foot and ankle. *Clin Orthop* 1998; 349:116-31.

3. Armstrong, D.G., Todd, W.F., Lavery, L.A., Harkless, L.B., Bushman, T.R. The natural history of acute Charcot's arthropathy in the diabetic foot specialty clinic. *Diabet Med* 1997; 14:357-63.

4. Harrelson, J.M. The diabetic foot: *Charcot arthropathy. Instr Course Lect* 1993; 42:141-6.

5. Eichenholtz, S.N. *Charcot joints.* Springfield, IL: Thomas, 1966.

6. Kelikian, A.S. *Operative treatment of the foot and ankle.* Stamford, CT: Appleton & Lange, 1999: 153.

7. Brodsky, J.W. Outpatient diagnosis and care of the diabetic foot. *Instr Course Lect* 1993; 42:121-39.

8. Sella, E.J., Barrette, C. Staging of Charcot neuroarthropathy along the medial column of the foot in the diabetic patient. *J Foot Ankle Surg* 1999; 38:34-40.

9. Caputo, G.M, Ulbrecht, J., Cavanagh, P.R., Juliano, P. The Charcot foot in diabetes: six key points. *Am Fam Physician* 1998; 57:2705-10.

10. Brodsky, J.W. The diabetic foot. In Mann, R.A., Coughlin, M.J., eds. *Surgery of the foot and ankle. 6th ed.* St. Louis: Mosby, 1993.

11. Armstrong, D.G., Lavery, L.A., Vela, S.A., Quebedeaux, T.L., Fleischli, J.G. Choosing a practical screening instrument to identify patients at risk for diabetic foot ulceration. *Arch Intern Med* 1998; 158:289-92.

12. Smieja, M., Hunt, D.L., Edelman, D., Etchells, E., Cornuz, J., Simel, D.L. Clinical examination for the detection of protective sensation in the feet of diabetic patients. International Cooperative Group for Clinical Examination Research. *J Gen Intern Med* 1999; 14:418-24.

13. Myerson, M., Papa, J., Eaton, K., Wilson, K. The total-contact cast for management of neuropathic plantar ulceration of the foot. *J Bone Joint Surg* [Am] 1992; 74:261-9.

14. Grayson, M.L., Gibbons, G.W., Balogh, K., Levin, E., Karchmer, A.W. Probing to bone in infected pedal ulcers. A clinical sign of underlying osteomyelitis in diabetic patients. *JAMA* 1995; 273:721-3.

15. Schon, L.C., Marks, R.M. The management of neuroarthropathic fracture-dislocations in the diabetic patient. *Orthop Clin North Am* 1995; 26:375-92.

16. Lipsky, B.A. Osteomyelitis of the foot in diabetic patients. *Clin Infect Dis* 1997; 25:1318-26.

17. Wagner, F.W. The diabetic foot. *Orthopedics* 1987; 10:163-72.

18. Mason, J., O'Keeffe, C., Hutchinson, A., McIntosh, A., Young, R., Booth, A. A systematic review of foot ulcer in patients with type 2 diabetes mellitus. II: treatment. *Diabet Med* 1999; 16:889-909.

19. Baumhauer, J.F., Wervey, R., McWilliams, J., Harris, G.F., Shereff, M.J. A comparison study of plantar foot pressure in a standardized shoe, total contact cast, and prefabricated pneumatic walking brace. *Foot Ankle Int* 1997; 18:26-33.

20. Strauss, E., Gonya, G. Adjunct low intensity ultrasound in Charcot neuroarthropathy. *Clin Orthop* 1998; 349:132-8.

21. Selby, P.L., Young, M.J., Boulton, A.J. Bisphosphonates: a new treatment for diabetic Charcot neuroarthropathy. *Diabet Med* 1994; 11:28-31.

Section 40.3

Insensate Dysvascular Feet

Introduction

When studying the causes and prevention of foot ulceration, one must first consider the risk factors involved. The primary factor is peripheral neuropathy, which interferes with normal transmission of signals in peripheral nerves. Most health care professionals are now acutely aware of sensory neuropathy, in which loss of protective sensation results in damage to the feet.

Diabetes mellitus is the disease most often linked in the developed world with damage to the feet due to loss of protective sensation. In much of the developing world, insensitivity due to Hansen disease—formerly known as leprosy—is more frequent. Another fairly common cause of insensate feet, seen worldwide, is alcoholism.

Other forms of neuropathy, however, such as motor and autonomic neuropathy, can also play a significant role. Most commonly, motor neuropathy leads to a paralysis of the foot's intrinsic muscles, resulting in dorsal subluxation or clawing of the toes. As the toes subluxate dorsally, the plantar fat pad, which normally protects the metatarsal head area, moves distally, leaving thinner skin (which is poorly suited for force dispersion) under the metatarsal heads. Motor neuropathy may also weaken the foot dorsiflexors, leading to a loss of controlled descent of the forefoot following heel strike at the beginning of the stance phase of gait. Combined with loss of metatarsal head padding, the resultant slapping gait can cause rapid damage to the skin of the plantar forefoot.

Autonomic neuropathy causes dryness of the skin due to lack of normal sweat production. This condition may lead to fissuring of the skin, creating portals of entry for bacteria. Poor management of diabetes, resulting in chronic hyperglycemia, leads to glycosylation of collagen with diminished capacity to heal wounds.

Smoking is another risk factor of real significance. In the short term, vessels constrict, and over a longer period of time, smoking can enhance development of atherosclerosis. On a daily basis, healing is also impaired by the blood's decreased ability to deliver oxygen to tissues. (Carbon monoxide binds sites on hemoglobin, which normally carry oxygen.)

Development of foot ulceration is also related to the duration of diabetes. In a study of 119 diabetics in our clinic [Patient-Family Education Clinic at the University of Miami School of Medicine], those with ulcers had diabetes for an average of 16 years, while those without ulcers had diabetes only 11 years. The age at which patients developed ulcers was striking, averaging only 54 years. It is a major challenge to restore function to individuals at the height of their productive years. There were no significant differences in age, race, or type of diabetes (i.e., insulin-dependent or noninsulin-dependent) among those who developed ulcers and those who did not.

We used a biothesiometer to obtain the vibratory perception threshold (VPT) as a measure of sensory loss. Overall, those with a VPT greater than the normal upper limit of 25 had a ten-fold increased risk of having ulceration compared with those patients with readings of less than 25. If the reading was more than 43, there was a thirty-fold increase in risk. In our series, the average VPT of patients with ulcers was 40. Those without ulcers averaged 23.5.[1]

It is sometimes thought ulceration must be related to lack of circulation. However, we determined the Doppler ischemic index at the ankle in 58 patients with ulcers and 42 without and found no significant difference.

Acute Management

To manage any disease process, lesions should be classified by a method that has therapeutic significance. For this reason, we triage our insensate foot lesions by the method of Meggitt and Wagner.[2] Grade 0 is represented by a callused area over a bony prominence with no evidence of skin breakdown. Nonetheless, these insensitive feet are at risk. As local pressure builds up on skin squeezed between a prominent bone internally and the unyielding floor and hard callus externally, a superficial ulceration or Grade 1 lesion occurs. If weight relief and modified shoewear are not obtained, a Grade 2 lesion will supervene.

Grade 2 ulcers are deep, penetrating to tendon or joint capsule, but do not enter the joint. The next stage is a Grade 3 lesion in which the joint has been violated, leading to septic arthritis and osteomyelitis. Further progression leads to a Grade 4 lesion or gangrene of the forefoot and to Grade 5, gangrene of the entire foot. Specific protocols have been developed for each grade of lesion.

As noted above, Grade 0 represents a foot at risk. Ordinarily, undue localized pressure can be relieved by custom inserts placed in shoes that comfortably accommodate both the foot and the insert. At times, this is not feasible and a prophylactic osteotomy is done to reduce or remove the offending bony prominence. Diligent foot care thereafter should prevent sores.

In Grades 1 and 2, provided that infection does not supervene, weight relief is necessary until the lesion is firmly healed. There are a number of non-weightbearing options. Using crutches or a walker is awkward at best, and these devices are frequently ignored by the patient because the ulcer causes no pain. They also make it difficult to carry objects and, therefore, are a nuisance. A wheelchair is sometimes useful for patients with lesions on both feet. Bed rest is to be condemned for its debilitating effect. Since their introduction by brand, healing casts have been used for the healing of insensate ulcers in patients with Hansen disease. They are extremely effective in distributing forces during weightbearing over the entire foot, thus reducing pressure over the prominent area. Recently, shoes have been introduced that bear major weight on the heel with little or none through the forefoot. These are excellent for forefoot lesions, but healing casts are still the best option for hindfoot lesions. Once healing has been achieved, protective shoes as described above should continue to be used.

Grade 3 and 4 lesions should be cultured aerobically and anaerobically. Coverage with broad spectrum antibiotics is given, pending the results of sensitivity testing, due to the polymicrobial nature of most diabetic food infections. Diabetic control should then be initiated. This may be difficult to accomplish in the presence of infection. Treating the infection with antibiotics, on the other hand, will be only partially effective because of the inhibitory effect of hyperglycemia on leukocyte functions. The interdependence of these factors reinforces the case for early excisional debridement of necrotic and infected tissue.

Determining the circulatory status of the affected limb will ensure surgery is performed at the appropriate level. Segmental systolic blood pressure measurement by Doppler is useful if peripheral vessels have not become overly stiffened from calcification secondary to diabetes. These values are compared to the systolic pressure in the brachial artery to obtain the ischemic index. This should be at least 0.45 to 0.5 in the affected area if reliable healing is to occur at that level. Pressures are recorded at the base of the toes with a cuff around the forefoot, as well as the ankle, with a supramalleolar cuff to provide information about the entire foot.

Grade 3 and 4 lesions will require excisional debridement of all infected and necrotic tissue. While the gangrenous tissue in Grade 4 lesions may be dry, more often it is wet due to infection. (Gangrenous changes occur due to thrombosis of local vessels surrounded by purulent material.) The patient must understand the procedure is somewhat exploratory in nature; and based on information acquired from the blood flow studies, the surgeon will be as conservative as possible in removing tissue.

However, the first priority is controlling the disease. Both the patient and surgeon must be willing to redebride the lesion as necessary, either at the bedside or more formally in the operating room if the patient's loss of sensitivity is not sufficient to permit this procedure without anesthesia. Following complete debridement, weight-bearing must be limited until the wound is fully healed, whether it has been closed primarily or allowed to heal by secondary intention.

In instances where the wound can be closed primarily, the procedure consists of two parts. These are debridement of all necrotic and infected tissue, including bone, followed by reconstruction of the foot using all viable remaining tissue (provided the wound can be closed primarily according to criteria discussed later in this section). It is common to fashion nonstandard flaps using any residual noninfected viable tissue. In the case of osteomyelitis of the distal phalanx of the great toe, if sufficient skin can be salvaged to cover the proximal phalanx, the patient's gait definitely will be enhanced, as opposed to removing the toe at the metatarsophalangeal joint. Infection of the distal phalanx of the lesser toes also can be treated by removing only that phalanx. Removing the entire great toe produces some disability that will require shoe corrections. Removing only the second toe removes the support needed by the first toe to prevent bunion formation. It is often better, therefore, to remove the entire second metatarsal down to its proximal metaphysis to allow the foot to narrow. If one of the lateral three toes is removed, the others tend to shift and fill in the gap.

As Grade 4 lesions are gangrene of part or all of the forefoot, they require a partial foot amputation or Syme ankle disarticulation, followed by a prosthetic fitting and lifelong follow-up. Here we need to consider the role of transverse versus longitudinal amputations. With a longitudinal amputation, such as a single lesser ray resection, only the width of the residual foot lever is affected. Rollover function and overall foot balance during terminal stance should be minimally affected.

Ray resections are excellent examples of conservative forefoot amputations. The best ray resections, from a functional point of view, are those of single lesser rays. With barefoot walking, there is never a good first ray amputation because an intact medial column in forward propulsion is important. If the first metatarsal is infected, the length of the shaft of the first metatarsal should be preserved as much as possible. If sufficient length has been saved, an adequate custom-molded insert can be made to support the medial arch of the foot in proper shoewear. Removing two or more central rays is not good functionally or cosmetically. If necessary, all lateral rays and portions of metatarsals can be removed in an oblique fashion and still provide a good functional result if the first ray remains intact.

Transmetatarsal Amputation

Transmetatarsal amputation can be performed when all of the distal forefoot is involved transversely, and the blood flow to the soft tissues is sufficient to support the flap fashioned from the distal plantar skin. This procedure provides a reasonably long foot lever that can be quite functional in a shoe with a stiff sole or sole plate and rocker. Some patients, who are not too concerned about cosmesis, will elect a short shoe.

The Lisfranc and Chopart levels have considerably less to recommend them. If these are attempted in infected cases and fail, it is very difficult to salvage a Syme level. Patients also tend to develop equinus deformity and foot imbalance since insertions of the foot's extrinsic muscles are disrupted. Therefore, percutaneous fractional heel cord lengthening and proper balancing of the foot by reinsertion of extrinsic foot muscles should be done at the time of amputation. A postoperative cast is also helpful in maintaining the proper plantigrade position. In fitting transmetatarsal, Lisfranc, and Chopart amputations, special care must be exercised to avoid excessive direct and shear forces at the interface of the prosthesis and residual foot.

Following excisional debridement, with or without partial foot amputation, a decision must be made regarding primary closure vs. open management of the wounds created. Prior to the pioneering work of Kritter, these wounds were invariably left open. His studies led to a revolution in the management of these problems.[3] By following his principles, primary healing can be achieved in three to four weeks in virtually all cases; this avoids lengthy healing by secondary intention that might take four to six months in many cases. It also avoids skin grafting, resulting in better cosmesis.

This method works well when certain criteria are met. Pus in the presenting wound must be either absent or minimal. When the debridement is complete, the wound should be clean with minimal inflammation of the remaining tissues. A 14- or 16-gauge polyethylene intravenous catheter, equipped with its own insertion needle, is passed through the skin into the depths of the wound. The needle is withdrawn and the catheter hub is sutured in place to the skin. A bag of normal saline is then attached to the catheter. Once the system has been noted to be running well, the skin is closed loosely with a few deep, widely spaced simple cutaneous sutures. Widely spaced sutures let the fluid escape from the wound to be absorbed in a soft dressing. The wound is irrigated in this flow-through manner for three days at a rate of one liter of normal saline every 24 hours. Intravenous antibiotics are given concomitantly. At the end of three days, if there is any evidence of purulence, the wound can simply be opened and packed at the bedside. This rarely occurs, however, if the criteria described are met.

Long-Term Management

Once healing has been achieved, it is essential patients become involved in an effective program for the long-term management of their insensate/dysvascular feet. In general, the problems related to diabetes have not been approached from a holistic point of view, but rather from a fragmented one related to the various organ systems affected. Therefore, it is important to take a more organized approach in foot management if true preventive rehabilitation is to be achieved. A team dedicated to the prevention of foot loss is ideal and must be both interdisciplinary and interactive.

In our institution [Patient-Family Education Clinic at the University of Miami School of Medicine], orthopaedics and diabetology work closely together to ensure the proper overall care of the patient. The vascular surgeon is ready for consultation, as necessary, in cases where reconstruction or recanalization of vessels might be indicated. The dietitian, physical therapist, psychologist, and social worker all have major roles to play. The pedorthist plays a special role in providing the proper shoewear and shoe inserts. The patient is probably the most important member of the team because without his or her compliance, little can be accomplished.

Specific instructions on shoewear include: avoiding tight, noncompliant materials, high heels, and inward-facing seams. Favored features include roominess for toes and a high, wide toe box, pliant leather rather than rigid plastics, and proper padding in the form of inserts depending on the individual conformation of the sole of the foot. We have found that well-fitted in-depth shoes with custom-molded inserts meet most patients' foot protection needs. Patients are encouraged to check their shoes, socks, and feet daily for problems and are warned to avoid barefoot walking.

Further preventive instructions include avoiding thermal injury, keratolytic callus removers, and "bathroom surgery." Rational walking programs are stressed to prevent excessive weightbearing trauma.

Psychological risk factors include denial, depression, and displacement of the locus of control. These all affect compliance with the foot care program and can be addressed by the social worker and the psychologist. This counseling can be done in individual and group sessions in both inpatient and outpatient phases of care.

Summary

Peripheral neuropathy complicating diabetes mellitus is the leading cause of insensate foot problems in the developed world. The risk factors associated with this problem have been discussed. A systematic approach to the management of insensate foot lesions, based on the work of Wagner and Meggitt, is described. Proper application of the principles noted by all members of the interdisciplinary team, including the patient, should lead to prevention of major limb loss.

—by John H. Bowker, MD

References

1.   Boulton, A.J.M., Kubrusly, D.B., Bowker, J.H., Gadia, M.T., Quintero, L., Becker, D.M., Skyler, J.S., Sosenko, J.M. Impaired vibratory perception and diabetic foot infection. *Diabetic Medicine* 1986; 3:335-337.

2.   Wagner, F.W., Jr. Orthopaedic rehabilitation of the dysvascular limb. *Orthopaedic Clinics of North America* 1978; 9:325-350.

3. Kritter, A.L. A technique for salvage of the infected diabetic foot. *Orthopaedic Clinics of North America* 1973; 4:21-30.

Section 40.4

Preventing Lower Extremity Amputations in Insensate Feet

"The LEAP Program," Bureau of Primary Health Care, Health Resources and Services Administration, 2001.

A comprehensive prevention program has been developed at the Bureau of Primary Health Care that can dramatically reduce lower extremity amputations in individuals with diabetes mellitus, Hansen disease, or any condition that results in loss of protective sensation in the feet.

The LEAP Program consists of five relatively simple activities:

• annual foot screening
• patient education
• daily self inspection of the foot
• appropriate footwear selection
• management of simple foot problems

Annual Foot Screening

The foundation of this prevention program is a foot screen that identifies those patients who have lost protective sensation. While it is well known that patients with diabetes frequently have vascular insufficiency in their extremities, the initial plantar ulcer usually results from an injury to a foot that has lost sensation. In the absence of protective sensation, even normal walking can result in such injuries.

The LEAP Diabetic Foot Screen uses a 5.07 monofilament, which delivers 10 grams of force, to identify patients with a foot at risk of developing problems. An initial foot screen should be performed on all patients with diabetes and at least annually thereafter. Patients who are at risk should be seen at least four times a year to check their feet and shoes to help prevent foot problems from occurring.

Patient Education

Teaching the patient self-management skills is the second component of the LEAP Program. Once taught simple self-management techniques, the patient assumes personal responsibility and becomes a full partner with the health care team in preventing foot problems.

Daily Self-Inspection

Daily self-inspection is an integral part of the self-management program. Every individual who has lost protective sensation must regularly and properly examine his/her feet on a daily basis. Studies have shown that daily self-inspection is the single most effective way to protect feet in the absence of the pain warning system.

Early detection of foot injuries (blister, redness, or swelling), callus, or toenail problems (thick, tender, long, or discolored) is necessary to prevent potentially more serious problems. Some problems should be reported immediately to a health care provider while the patient can manage others if he/she has been taught simple, basic self-management techniques.

Footwear Selection

Shoes, like feet, come in a variety of styles and shapes. A person with normal sensation in his/her feet can wear almost any shoe style with little risk of injury. But with diabetes, if the patient has lost protective sensation, poorly designed or improperly fitting shoes can seriously complicate the condition of the feet.

Once a patient has lost protective sensation, he/she should never walk barefoot, even around the house. The patient should never wear narrow toe shoes or boots, heeled shoes, shoes with vinyl tops, thongs, or any shoe that is too loose or too tight. This person will need special assistance in selecting the appropriate style and fit of shoes.

The shoe should fit the shape of the foot. There should be at least one-half inch between the longest toe and the end of the shoe. In a properly fitting shoe, a small amount of leather can be pinched up. The patient, the family, and the health care team need to recognize that wearing appropriately styled shoes that fit can prevent most foot problems.

Management of Simple Foot Problems

In addition to causing loss of protective sensation, diabetes can also affect the autonomic nerves in the foot and lead to dry, cracked skin, increasing the probability of foot injuries and wounds.

This prevention program emphasizes the importance of reporting all injuries to the health care provider. [For more information on the LEAP program go to their homepage at http://www.bphc.hrsa.gov/leap. For further contact information, see the resource directory at the end of this book.]

Section 40.5

Care of Skin and Nails of the Neuropathic Foot

The Skin

Healthy skin is soft and flexible and slightly moist and acidic. It is the largest organ of the body, covering 3,000 square inches on the average adult. It weighs approximately six pounds (almost twice the weight of the brain and liver). The skin receives about one-third of all circulating blood of the body. Its two main parts, the epidermis and the corneum (the dermis), serve as a protective barrier against microorganisms. It insulates against heat and cold, helps eliminate body wastes in the form of perspiration, and its sense receptors enable the body to feel pain, cold, heat, touch, and pressure. The epidermis is thickest on the palms and soles of the feet and becomes thinner over the surface of the trunk.

The Nail

Nails are composed of hard keratin, a modification of the horny epidermal cells of the skin. The white crescent shape of the lunula at the proximal end of each nail is caused by air mixed in the keratin matrix. The nail plate originates from the proximal nail fold and attaches to the nail bed. It grows about 1 mm per week unless inhibited by disease. Regeneration of a lost toenail occurs in six to eight months.

Facts about Nails[1]

- Nails grow approximately 0.1 mm per day or 3 mm per month.

- Nails grow faster in daytime and summer.

- Fever and serious illness slow growth rates.

- Pregnancy enhances growth.

- Nails grow more rapidly in men and younger people than in women and the elderly.

- Toenails grow 1/2 to 1/3 the rate of fingernails.

Skin and Nail Care

Before starting skin and nail care, thoroughly inspect feet and ankles for breaks in the skin. Have a mirror available to examine the heels. Look for ulcers, heel fissures, maceration between the toes, or embedded objects. When nails are neglected and grow too long, they can break the skin of the neighboring toe. Abnormal nails that are not given routine care can accumulate excess keratin and debris under the nails and in the nail folds, creating an ideal environment for bacteria to grow.[2] Poor hygiene necessitates routine foot care.

The procedure for basic foot care is as follows:

1. Wash hands.

2. Submerge patient's feet into warm water (not more than 95° F).

3. While wearing gloves, make a paste of baby shampoo (or any mild soap) and baking soda in the palm of your hand and gently massage over the entire foot. (You can also use water that

is three parts water and one part vinegar to clean the feet. Vinegar softens the skin and nails.[3])

4. Rinse and wrap feet individually.

5. Expose toes and apply cuticle remover.

6. Using a curette, gently remove dead skin and loose cuticle from the toes.

7. Rinse.

8. Using nail clippers, cut nail straight across. Don't cut what you can't see. Always have good lighting.

9. Thinner, more fragile nails can be cut using smaller cuticle nippers.

10. Ingrown toenails are a puncture wound. To prevent them, use an ingrown nail file to smooth sharp corners that can dig into the skin.

11. Smooth rough edges of nails with emery board. Patient may take the emery board home for self-care.

12. Massage emollient into feet but not between toes. Avoid lotions with fragrance because of drying, alcohol content. Vaseline, lanolin, or even Crisco may be used. Pat excess off with paper towel. Remind patient to use caution when using emollient to prevent slipping and falling. Removing excess and wearing socks help minimize the hazard.

13. Educate patient regarding appropriate footwear.

There are nails that are difficult to trim. The safest way to trim the pincer type nail is to file it straight across, rather than risk cutting the skin. Some nails have grown into a "tent" shape, usually formed by being squeezed into tight pointed shoes for years. When trimming this type nail be aware of the skin under the nail at the apex. A condition called onycholysis (separation of the nail plate from the nail bed) can be caused by nail traumas and disorders. If onycholysis has been present for a long time (six months or more) the structure of the nail bed can change and the nail plate will no longer attach to the nail bed. At this point, the condition becomes permanent. Keep the patient's nails short to prevent the nail from catching on something and tearing off.[4]

Helpful Foot Aids

- Tube foam is ideal for protecting bunion deformities, soft corns, and maceration between the toes.

- Lamb's wool aids in protection between the toes from maceration and provides cushioning.

- Toe socks help with overlapping toes and controlling maceration in interdigit spaces.

- Socks that are designed to wick moisture away from the skin are desirable, especially in a foot that sweats excessively. Avoid socks with tight elastic tops.

Care of the Hypertrophic Nail

A hypertrophic nail may be caused by damage to the matrix, fungal infection, age, or circulation problems.

Hypertrophic nails that have been neglected for a long period need to be thinned to make shoe fit possible and to help prevent secondary infection if the prominent nail is traumatized.

The most effective and expedient way to thin the nail is to use a cordless rotary Dremel tool with an abrasive disc. These discs are easily interchangeable and should be discarded between patients.

It is important to protect yourself and the patient from airborne dust by wearing a mask and, preferably, hair covering. Using a government-rated high efficiency particulate arrester (HEPA) air filter device would give added protection to limit the amount of dust in the air.

Procedure for Reducing Hypertrophic Nails

1. Begin by washing your hands and donning gloves.

2. Examine the skin around the nail for any damage.

3. If there are no signs of broken skin or infection, secure toe to be worked on with the thumb and index finger and move other toes out of the way.

4. Turn Dremel on and move sander in a proximal to distal direction in even strokes until nail is thinned. Caution must be exercised when thinning these nails because of unanticipated raised nail beds.

5. Wash and dry thinned nail with water or water/vinegar solution (three parts water/one part vinegar) and apply an antifungal cream such as Teniacide. Use of this, or a similar product, will allow consecutive nail care to be more effective by keeping the nail and surrounding skin conditioned.

—by Joan Conlan, LVN, CPed

References

1. Kechiijian, P. How do nails grow? *Nails*. May 1993:78–79.

2. O'Neal, L.W. Surgical pathways of the foot and clinical pathological conditions. In: Bowker, J.H., Pfeifer, M.A., eds. *The Diabetic Foot*, ed. 6. St. Louis: C.V. Mosby; 2000:501–506.

3. Ruscin, C., Cunningham, G., Blaylock, A. Foot care protocol for the older client. *Geriatric Nursing*. July/August 1993: 210–212.

4. Scher, R.K. The nail doctor. *Nails*. December 1997:93–95.

Chapter 41

Rheumatic Diseases

Chapter Contents

Section 41.1

Arthritis of the Foot and Ankle

Reproduced with permission from "Arthritis of the Foot and Ankle," in Johnson, TR, (ed): *Your Orthopaedic Connection,* Rosemont, IL, American Academy of Orthopaedic Surgeons. Available at http://orthoinfo.aaos.org. Co-developed by the American Orthopaedic Foot and Ankle Society. Published December 2001.

There are more than 100 different types of arthritis. But when most people talk about arthritis, they are usually referring to the most common form, osteoarthritis ("osteo" means bone). Osteoarthritis develops as we age and is often called "wear-and-tear" arthritis. Over the years, the thin covering (cartilage) on the ends of bones becomes worn and frayed. This results in inflammation, swelling, and pain in the joint.

An injury to a joint, even if treated properly, can cause osteoarthritis to develop in the future. This is often referred to as traumatic arthritis. It may develop months or years after a severe sprain, torn ligament, or broken bone.

Anatomy

There are 28 bones and over 30 joints in the foot. Tough bands of tissue, called ligaments, hold the bones and joints in place. If arthritis develops in one or more of these joints, your balance and walk may be affected. The foot joints most commonly affected by arthritis include:

- the ankle (tibiotalar joint), where the shinbone (tibia) rests on the uppermost bone of the foot (the talus);

- the three joints of the hindfoot: the subtalar or talocalcaneal joint, where the bottom of the talus connects to the heel bone (calcaneus); the talonavicular joint, where the talus connects to the inner midfoot bone (naviculus), and the calcaneocuboid joint, where the heel bone connects to the outer midfoot bone (cuboid);

- the midfoot (metatarsocuneiform joint), where one of the fore-foot bones (metatarsals) connects to the smaller midfoot bones (cuneiforms);

- the great toe (first metatarsophalangeal joint), where the first metatarsal connects to the toe bone (phalange); this is also where bunions usually develop.

Signs and Symptoms

Signs and symptoms of arthritis of the foot vary, depending on which joint is affected. Common symptoms include pain or tenderness, stiffness or reduced motion, and swelling. Walking may be difficult.

Diagnosing Arthritis of the Foot and Ankle

Your doctor will begin by getting your medical history and giving you a physical exam. The following are among the questions you may be asked:

- When did the pain start? Is it worse at night? Does it get worse when you walk or run? Is it continuous, or does it come and go?

- Have you ever had an injury to your foot or ankle? What kind of injury? When did it occur? How was it treated?

- Is the pain in both feet or just one? Where is the pain centered?

- What kinds of shoes do you normally wear? Are you taking any medications?

Your doctor may do a gait analysis. This shows how the bones in your leg and foot line up as you walk, measures your stride, and tests the strength of your ankles and feet. You may also need some diagnostic tests. X-rays can show changes in the spacing between bones or in the shape of the bones themselves. A bone scan, computed tomography (CT) scan, or magnetic resonance image (MRI) may also be used in the evaluation.

Treating Your Arthritis

Depending on the type, location, and severity of your arthritis, there are many types of treatment available. Nonsurgical treatment options include the following:

- taking pain relievers and anti-inflammatory medication to reduce swelling

- putting a pad, arch support, or other type of insert in your shoe

- wearing a custom-made shoe, such as a stiff-soled shoe with a rocker bottom

- using an ankle-foot orthosis (AFO)

- wearing a brace or using a cane

- participating in a program of physical therapy and exercises

- controlling your weight or taking nutritional supplements

- getting a dose of steroid medication injected into the joint

If your arthritis doesn't respond to such conservative treatments, surgical options are available. The type of surgery that's best for you will depend on the type of arthritis you have, the impact of the disease on your joints, and the location of the arthritis. Sometimes more than one type of surgery will be needed. The primary surgeries performed for arthritis of the foot and ankle are as follows:

- **Arthroscopic debridement:** Arthroscopic surgery may be helpful in the early stages of arthritis. A pencil-sized instrument (arthroscope) with a small lens, a miniature camera, and a lighting system is inserted into a joint. This projects three-dimensional images of the joint on a television monitor, enabling the surgeon to look directly inside the joint and identify the trouble. Tiny probes, forceps, knives, and shavers can then be used to clean the joint area by removing foreign tissue and bony outgrowths (spurs).

- **Arthrodesis, or fusion:** This surgery eliminates the joint completely by welding the bones together. Pins, plates, and screws or rods through the bone are used to hold the bones together until they heal. A bone graft is sometimes needed. Your doctor may be able to use a piece of your own bone, taken from one of the lower leg bones or the hip, for the graft. This surgery is normally quite successful. A very small percentage of patients have problems with wound healing. These complications can be addressed by bracing or additional surgery.

- **Arthroplasty, or joint replacement:** In rare cases, your doctor may recommend replacing the ankle joint with artificial implants. However, total ankle joint replacement is not as advanced or successful as total hip or knee joint replacement. The implant may loosen or fail, resulting in the need for additional surgery.

Outcomes and Rehabilitation

Initially, foot and ankle surgery can be quite painful, so you will be given pain relievers both in the hospital and after you are released. After surgery, you will have to restrict activities for a time. You may have to wear a cast and use crutches, a walker, or a wheelchair, depending on the type of surgery you had. Keeping your foot elevated above the level of your heart will be very important for the first week or so.

You will not be able to put any weight on your foot for at least four to six weeks, and full recovery takes four to nine months. You may also need to participate in a physical therapy program for several months to regain strength in the foot and restore range of motion. Usually, you can return to ordinary daily activities in three to four months, although you may have to wear special shoes or braces. In the vast majority of cases, surgery brings pain relief and makes it easier for you to do daily activities.

Section 41.2

Stiff Big Toe (Hallux Rigidus)

Reproduced with permission from "Stiff Big Toe," in Johnson, TR, (ed): *Your Orthopaedic Connection.* Rosemont, IL, American Academy of Orthopaedic Surgeons. Available at http://orthoinfo.aaos.org. Co-developed by the American Orthopaedic Foot and Ankle Society. Published May 1, 2002.

The most common site of arthritis in the foot is at the base of the big toe. This joint is called the metatarsophalangeal, or MTP joint. It's important because it has to bend every time you take a step. If the joint starts to stiffen, walking can become painful and difficult.

In the MTP joint, as in any joint, the ends of the bones are covered by a smooth articular cartilage. If wear-and-tear or injury damage the articular cartilage, the raw bone ends can rub together. A bone spur, or overgrowth, may develop on the top of the bone. This overgrowth can prevent the toe from bending as much as it needs to when you walk. The result is a stiff big toe, or hallux rigidus.

Hallux rigidus usually develops in adults between the ages of 30 and 60 years. No one knows why it appears in some people and not others. It may result from an injury to the toe that damages the articular cartilage or from differences in foot anatomy that increase stress on the joint.

Signs and Symptoms

- pain in the joint when you are active, especially as you push-off on the toes when you walk
- swelling around the joint
- a bump, like a bunion or callus, that develops on the top of the foot
- stiffness in the great toe and an inability to bend it up or down

Diagnosing the Problem

If you find it difficult to bend your toe up and down or find that you are walking on the outside of your foot because of pain in the toe, see your doctor right away. Hallux rigidus is easier to treat when the condition is caught early. If you wait until you see a bony bump on the top of your foot, the bone spurs will have already developed and the condition will be more difficult to treat.

Your physician will examine your foot and look for evidence of bone spurs. He or she may move the toe around to see how much motion is possible without pain. X-rays will show the location and size of any bone spurs, as well as the degree of degeneration in the joint space and cartilage.

Nonoperative Treatment Options

Pain relievers and anti-inflammatory medications such as ibuprofen may help reduce the swelling and ease the pain. Applying ice packs or taking contrast baths (described below) may also help reduce inflammation and control symptoms for a short period of time. But they aren't enough to stop the condition from progressing. Wearing a shoe with a large toe box will reduce the pressure on the toe, and you will probably have to give up wearing high heels. Your doctor may recommend that you get a stiff-soled shoe with a rocker or roller bottom design and possibly even a steel shank or metal brace in the sole. This type of shoe supports the foot when you walk and reduces the amount of bend in the big toe.

A contrast bath uses alternating cold and hot water to reduce inflammation. You'll need two buckets, one with water as cold as you can tolerate and the other with water as warm as you can tolerate. Immerse your foot in the cold water for 30 seconds, then immediately place it in the hot water for 30 seconds. Continue to alternate between cold and hot for five minutes, ending in the cold water. You can do contrast baths up to three times a day. However, be careful to avoid extreme temperatures in the water, especially if your feet aren't very sensitive to heat or cold.

Surgical Options

Cheilectomy (kI-lek'-toe-me)

This surgery is usually recommended when damage is mild or moderate. It involves removing the bone spurs as well as a portion of the foot bone, so the toe has more room to bend. The incision is made on the top of the foot. The toe and the operative site may remain swollen for several months after the operation, and you will have to wear

407

a wooden-soled sandal for at least two weeks after the surgery. But most patients do experience long-term relief.

Arthrodesis (are-throw-dee'-sis)

Fusing the bones together (arthrodesis) is often recommended when the damage to the cartilage is severe. The damaged cartilage is removed and pins, screws, or a plate are used to fix the joint in a permanent position. Gradually, the bones grow together. This type of surgery means that you will not be able to bend the toe at all. However, it is the most reliable way to reduce pain in these severe cases.

For the first six weeks after surgery, you will have to wear a cast and then use crutches for about another six weeks. You won't be able to wear high heels, and you may need to wear a shoe with a rocker-type sole.

Arthroplasty (are-throw-plas'-tee)

Older patients who place few functional demands on the feet may be candidates for joint replacement surgery. The joint surfaces are removed and an artificial joint is implanted. This procedure may relieve pain and preserve joint motion.

Section 41.3

Reactive Arthritis

"Questions and Answers about Reactive Arthritis," National Institute of Arthritis and Musculoskeletal and Skin Diseases, National Institutes of Health, NIH Publication No. 02-5039, August 2002.

This text contains general information about reactive arthritis. It describes what reactive arthritis is and how it develops. It also explains how reactive arthritis is diagnosed and treated. If you have further questions after reading this section, you may wish to discuss them with your doctor.

What is reactive arthritis?

Reactive arthritis is a form of arthritis, or joint inflammation, that occurs as a "reaction" to an infection elsewhere in the body. Inflammation is a characteristic reaction of tissues to injury or disease and is marked by swelling, redness, heat, and pain. Besides this joint inflammation, reactive arthritis is associated with two other symptoms: redness and inflammation of the eyes (conjunctivitis) and inflammation of the urinary tract (urethritis). These symptoms may occur alone, together, or not at all.

Reactive arthritis is also known as Reiter syndrome, and your doctor may refer to it by yet another term, as a seronegative spondyloarthropathy. The seronegative spondyloarthropathy are a group of disorders that can cause inflammation throughout the body, especially in the spine. (Examples of other disorders in this group include psoriatic arthritis, ankylosing spondylitis, and the kind of arthritis that sometimes accompanies inflammatory bowel disease.)

In many patients, reactive arthritis is triggered by a venereal infection in the bladder, the urethra, or, in women, the vagina (the urogenital tract) that is often transmitted through sexual contact. This form of the disorder is sometimes called genitourinary or urogenital reactive arthritis. Another form of reactive arthritis is caused by an infection in the intestinal tract from eating food or handling substances that are contaminated with bacteria. This form of arthritis is sometimes called enteric or gastrointestinal reactive arthritis.

The symptoms of reactive arthritis usually last three to twelve months, although symptoms can return or develop into a long-term disease in a small percentage of people.

What causes reactive arthritis?

Reactive arthritis typically begins about one to three weeks after infection. The bacterium most often associated with reactive arthritis is *Chlamydia trachomatis*, commonly known as chlamydia (pronounced "kla-MID-e-a"). It is usually acquired through sexual contact. Some evidence also shows that respiratory infections with *Chlamydia pneumoniae* may trigger reactive arthritis.

Infections in the digestive tract that may trigger reactive arthritis include Salmonella, Shigella, Yersinia, and Campylobacter. People may become infected with these bacteria after eating or handling improperly prepared food, such as meats that are not stored at the proper temperature.

Doctors do not know exactly why some people exposed to these bacteria develop reactive arthritis and others do not, but they have identified a genetic factor, human leukocyte antigen (HLA) *B27*, that increases a person's chance of developing reactive arthritis. Approximately 80 percent of people with reactive arthritis test positive for *HLA-B27*. However, inheriting the *HLA-B27* gene does not necessarily mean you will get reactive arthritis. Eight percent of healthy people have the *HLA-B27* gene, and only about one-fifth of them will develop reactive arthritis if they contract the triggering infections.

Is reactive arthritis contagious?

Reactive arthritis is not contagious; that is, a person with the disorder cannot pass the arthritis on to someone else. However, the bacteria that can trigger reactive arthritis can be passed from person to person.

Who gets reactive arthritis?

Overall, men between the ages of 20 and 40 are most likely to develop reactive arthritis. However, evidence shows that although men are nine times more likely than women to develop reactive arthritis due to venereally acquired infections, women and men are equally likely to develop reactive arthritis as a result of food-borne infections. Women with reactive arthritis often have milder symptoms than men.

What are the symptoms of reactive arthritis?

Reactive arthritis most typically results in inflammation of the urogenital tract, the joints, and the eyes. Less common symptoms are mouth ulcers and skin rashes. Any of these symptoms may be so mild that patients do not notice them. They usually come and go over a period of several weeks to several months.

Urogenital Tract Symptoms: Reactive arthritis often affects the urogenital tract, including the prostate or urethra in men and the urethra, uterus, or vagina in women. Men may notice an increased need to urinate, a burning sensation when urinating, and a fluid discharge from the penis. Some men with reactive arthritis develop prostatitis (inflammation of the prostate gland). Symptoms of prostatitis can include fever and chills, as well as an increased need to urinate and a burning sensation when urinating.

Women with reactive arthritis may develop problems in the urogenital tract, such as cervicitis (inflammation of the cervix) or urethritis (inflammation of the urethra), which can cause a burning sensation during urination. In addition, some women also develop salpingitis (inflammation of the fallopian tubes) or vulvovaginitis (inflammation of the vulva and vagina). These conditions may or may not cause any arthritic symptoms.

Joint Symptoms: The arthritis associated with reactive arthritis typically involves pain and swelling in the knees, ankles, and feet. Wrists, fingers, and other joints are affected less often. People with reactive arthritis commonly develop inflammation of the tendons (tendonitis) or at places where tendons attach to the bone (enthesitis). In many people with reactive arthritis, this results in heel pain or irritation of the Achilles tendon at the back of the ankle. Some people with reactive arthritis also develop heel spurs, which are bony growths in the heel that may cause chronic (long-lasting) foot pain. Approximately half of people with reactive arthritis report low-back and buttock pain.

Reactive arthritis also can cause spondylitis (inflammation of the vertebrae in the spinal column) or sacroiliitis (inflammation of the joints in the lower back that connect the spine to the pelvis). People with reactive arthritis who have the *HLA-B27* gene are even more likely to develop spondylitis and/or sacroiliitis.

Eye Involvement: Conjunctivitis, an inflammation of the mucous membrane that covers the eyeball and eyelid, develops in approximately

411

half of people with reactive arthritis. Some people may develop uveitis, which is an inflammation of the inner eye. Conjunctivitis and uveitis can cause redness of the eyes, eye pain and irritation, and blurred vision. Eye involvement typically occurs early in the course of reactive arthritis, and symptoms may come and go.

Other Symptoms: Between 20 and 40 percent of men with reactive arthritis develop small, shallow, painless sores (ulcers) on the end of the penis. A small percentage of men and women develop rashes or small, hard nodules on the soles of the feet and, less often, on the palms of their hands or elsewhere. In addition, some people with reactive arthritis develop mouth ulcers that come and go. In some cases, these ulcers are painless and go unnoticed.

How is reactive arthritis diagnosed?

Doctors sometimes find it difficult to diagnose reactive arthritis because there is no specific laboratory test to confirm that a person has it. A doctor may order a blood test to detect the genetic factor *HLA-B27*, but even if the result is positive, the presence of *HLA-B27* does not always mean that a person has the disorder.

At the beginning of an examination, the doctor will probably take a complete medical history and note current symptoms as well as any previous medical problems or infections. Before and after seeing the doctor, it is sometimes useful for the patient to keep a record of the symptoms that occur, when they occur, and how long they last. It is especially important to report any flu-like symptoms, such as fever, vomiting, or diarrhea, because they may be evidence of a bacterial infection.

The doctor may use various blood tests besides the *HLA-B27* test to help rule out other conditions and confirm a suspected diagnosis of reactive arthritis. For example, the doctor may order rheumatoid factor or antinuclear antibody tests to rule out reactive arthritis. Most people who have reactive arthritis will have negative results on these tests. If a patient's test results are positive, he or she may have some other form of arthritis, such as rheumatoid arthritis or lupus. Doctors also may order a blood test to determine the erythrocyte sedimentation rate (sed rate), which is the rate at which red blood cells settle to the bottom of a test tube of blood. A high sed rate often indicates inflammation somewhere in the body. Typically, people with rheumatic diseases, including reactive arthritis, have an elevated sed rate.

The doctor also is likely to perform tests for infections that might be associated with reactive arthritis. Patients generally are tested for a *Chlamydia* infection because recent studies have shown that early treatment of *Chlamydia*-induced reactive arthritis may reduce the progression of the disease. The doctor may look for bacterial infections by testing cell samples taken from the patient's throat as well as the urethra in men or cervix in women. Urine and stool samples also may be tested. A sample of synovial fluid (the fluid that lubricates the joints) may be removed from the arthritic joint. Studies of synovial fluid can help the doctor rule out infection in the joint.

Doctors sometimes use x-rays to help diagnose reactive arthritis and to rule out other causes of arthritis. X-rays can detect some of the symptoms of reactive arthritis, including spondylitis, sacroiliitis, swelling of soft tissues, damage to cartilage or bone margins of the joint, and calcium deposits where the tendon attaches to the bone.

What type of doctor treats reactive arthritis?

A person with reactive arthritis probably will need to see several different types of doctors because reactive arthritis affects different parts of the body. However, it may be helpful to the doctors and the patient for one doctor, usually a rheumatologist (a doctor specializing in arthritis), to manage the complete treatment plan. This doctor can coordinate treatments and monitor the side effects from the various medicines the patient may take. The following specialists treat other features that affect different parts of the body.

- A ophthalmologist treats eye disease.
- A gynecologist treats genital symptoms in women.
- A urologist treats genital symptoms in men and women.
- A dermatologist treats skin symptoms.
- An orthopaedist performs surgery on severely damaged joints.
- A physiatrist supervises exercise regimens.

How is reactive arthritis treated?

Although there is no cure for reactive arthritis, some treatments relieve symptoms of the disorder. The doctor is likely to use one or more of the following treatments:

- **Nonsteroidal anti-inflammatory drugs (NSAIDs):** NSAIDs reduce joint inflammation and are commonly used to treat patients with reactive arthritis. Some traditional NSAIDs, such as

413

aspirin and ibuprofen, are available without a prescription, but others that are more effective for reactive arthritis, such as indomethacin and tolmetin, must be prescribed by a doctor. Less is known about whether a new class of NSAIDs, called COX-2 inhibitors, is effective for reactive arthritis, but they may reduce the risk of gastrointestinal complications associated with traditional NSAIDs.

- **Corticosteroid injections:** For people with severe joint inflammation, injections of corticosteroids directly into the affected joint may reduce inflammation. Doctors usually prescribe these injections only after trying unsuccessfully to control arthritis with NSAIDs.

- **Topical corticosteroids:** These corticosteroids come in a cream or lotion and can be applied directly on the skin lesions, such as ulcers, associated with reactive arthritis. Topical corticosteroids reduce inflammation and promote healing.

- **Antibiotics:** The doctor may prescribe antibiotics to eliminate the bacterial infection that triggered reactive arthritis. The specific antibiotic prescribed depends on the type of bacterial infection present. It is important to follow instructions about how much medicine to take and for how long; otherwise the infection may persist. Typically, an antibiotic is taken for seven to ten days or longer. Some doctors may recommend a person with reactive arthritis take antibiotics for a long period of time (up to three months). Current research shows that in most cases, this practice is necessary.

- **Immunosuppressive medicines:** A small percentage of patients with reactive arthritis have severe symptoms that cannot be controlled with any of the above treatments. For these people, medicine that suppresses the immune system, such as sulfasalazine or methotrexate, may be effective.

- **TNF inhibitors:** Several relatively new treatments that suppress tumor necrosis factor (TNF), a protein involved in the body's inflammatory response, may be effective for reactive arthritis and other spondyloarthropathies. They include etanercept and infliximab. These treatments were first used to treat rheumatoid arthritis.

- **Exercise:** Exercise, when introduced gradually, may help improve joint function. In particular, strengthening and range-of-motion exercises will maintain or improve joint function. Strengthening exercises builds up the muscles around the joint to better support it. Muscle-tightening exercises that do not move any joints can be done even when a person has inflammation and pain. Range-of-motion exercises improve movement and flexibility and reduce stiffness in the affected joint. For patients with spine pain or inflammation, exercises to stretch and extend the back can be particularly helpful in preventing long-term disability. Aquatic exercise also may be helpful. Before beginning an exercise program, patients should talk to a health professional who can recommend appropriate exercises.

What is the prognosis for people who have reactive arthritis?

Most people with reactive arthritis recover fully from the initial flare of symptoms and are able to return to regular activities two to six months after the first symptoms appear. In such cases, the symptoms of arthritis may last up to 12 months, although these are usually very mild and do not interfere with daily activities. Approximately 20 percent of people with reactive arthritis will have chronic (long-term) arthritis, which usually is mild. Studies show that between 15 and 50 percent of patients will develop symptoms again sometime after the initial flare has disappeared. It is possible that such relapses may be due to reinfection. Back pain and arthritis are the symptoms that most commonly reappear. A small percentage of patients will have chronic, severe arthritis that is difficult to control with treatment and may cause joint deformity.

What are researchers learning about reactive arthritis?

Researchers continue to investigate the causes of reactive arthritis and study treatments for the condition. The following are examples:

- Researchers are trying to better understand the relationship between infection and reactive arthritis. In particular, they are trying to determine why an infection triggers arthritis and why some people who develop infections get reactive arthritis while others do not. Scientists also are studying why people with the genetic factor *HLA-B27* are more at risk than others.

- Researchers are developing methods to detect the location of the triggering bacteria in the body. Some scientists suspect that after the bacteria enter the body, they are transported to the joints, where they can remain in small amounts indefinitely.

- Researchers are testing combination treatments for reactive arthritis. In particular, they are testing the use of antibiotics in combination with TNF inhibitors and with other immunosuppressant medicines, such as methotrexate and sulfasalazine.

Section 41.4

Ankle Sprains Can Lead to Arthritis

"Reoccurring Ankle Sprains Can Lead to Loss of Ankle Mobility,"
© 2006 American Orthopaedic Foot and Ankle Society.
Reprinted with permission.

Repeated ankle sprains and other ankle injuries can lead to severe ankle arthritis, sometimes the inability to walk (end-stage arthritis), and should be treated aggressively, according to a study presented at the American Orthopaedic Foot and Ankle Society's Annual Winter Meeting [March 13, 2004].

The goal of this study was to uncover the causes of ankle arthritis, severe discomfort, and loss of mobility. Ankle arthritis is a common ailment that can result in the need for total ankle replacement surgery. Misalignment, ankle instability, and flat foot can also contribute to arthritis.

Ankle arthritis differs from hip or knee arthritis in that it usually results from trauma rather than the everyday wear and tear associated with old age. "Post traumatic arthritis was seen in 58 percent of the examined patients and is the leading cause for end stage ankle arthritis" said Matthew Roberts, MD, New York, NY, the primary author of this study.

The study showed that 18 percent of the patients suffering from end-stage ankle arthritis have a history of chronic instability, and repeated ankle sprains. "This is a very significant percentage. People are suffering from end-stage ankle arthritis as a result of reoccurring ankle sprains," said Dr. Roberts. "It's as simple as twisting your ankle as you walk down the street."

He noted that most people don't realize that little reoccurring ankle sprains can lead to such severe pain and an inability to walk. "If something as simple as reoccurring ankle sprains can have this effect, do we need to be more proactive in treating these patients from their first ankle sprain?" said Dr. Roberts. "I say the answer is 'yes!'"

The results of this study point to a need for doctors to search the underlying causes behind the arthritis, instead of looking at the ankle alone. Learning about a patient's history will help in the diagnosis of problems and in deciding on the most effective treatment. "In asking why, we'll know how to better administer effective treatment," said Dr. Roberts. This retrospective study shows that taking better care of everyday injuries can have a valuable long-term effect, and prevent end-stage ankle arthritis.

The study was conducted on 455 ankles, from 435 patients with an average age of 55. All suffered from end-stage arthritis. In 58 percent of the patients, this resulted from post-traumatic arthritis, 29 percent from secondary arthritis, which includes instability, 13 percent from complication of swelling and infection, and less than 1 percent was attributed to primary osteoarthritis.

Section 41.5

Psoriatic Arthritis

Psoriatic arthritis is an inflammatory arthritis associated with psoriasis, a chronic skin and nail disease. There are five types of this disease:

- arthritis involving primarily the small joints of fingers or toes

- asymmetrical arthritis, which involves joints of the extremities

- symmetrical polyarthritis, which resembles rheumatoid arthritis

- arthritis mutilans, which is rare but very deforming and destructive

- arthritis of the sacroiliac joints and spine (psoriatic spondylitis)

The exact prevalence of each of these forms of arthritis is difficult to establish. Patterns may themselves change with time in individual patients, and some patients may show overlapping features or more than one type. Sometimes arthritis is associated with inflammation of the eyes, or inflammation at the bony sites of attachment of ligaments and tendons, causing local pain, for example at the heels.

Cause

The exact cause is unknown, but an interplay of immune, genetic, and environmental factors are suspected. Up to 40 percent of patients with psoriatic arthritis may have a history of psoriasis or arthritis in family members. Both psoriasis and psoriatic arthritis flare up in the presence of immunodeficiency due to HIV infection (AIDS).

Health Impact

- Psoriatic arthritis affects at least 10 percent of the 3 million people with psoriasis in the United States.

- It affects men and women equally and usually begins between 30–50 years of age, but can begin in childhood.

- Psoriatic arthritis may precede the onset or the diagnosis of psoriasis in up to 15 percent of patients.

Diagnosis

Skin and nail changes characteristic of psoriasis must be demonstrated before a diagnosis can be made with certainty. Elevated erythrocyte sedimentation rate (ESR), mild anemia, and elevated levels of blood uric acid can be seen in some patients. Gout must be excluded.

Treatment

Initial treatment of psoriatic arthritis consists of the use of non-steroidal anti-inflammatory drugs (NSAIDs), but methotrexate may be needed for arthritis that doesn't respond. An antimalarial drug, hydroxychloroquine, may be effective, but some patients experience a flare of their psoriasis. Sulfasalazine has been found to be very beneficial for some psoriatic arthritis patients. Azathioprine may be used in severe cases of the disease.

Corticosteroid injections directly into the joints can be useful. Cyclosporin has been used recently with some good results, but because of kidney side effects, it should be reserved for patients with progressive disease unresponsive to other measures. Proper exercise is very important. Surgery can be helpful in patients who develop joint destruction.

The Rheumatologist's Role in Treating Psoriatic Arthritis

Rheumatologists have great experience and are more likely to make the proper diagnosis of the disease in its various forms which may be easily confused with other diseases. Rheumatologists also have unique experience in determining the optimal therapy for the patient's psoriatic arthritis.

For More Information

If you want to find a rheumatologist in your area, check the American College of Rheumatology membership directory. If you want more information on this or any other form of arthritis, contact the Arthritis Foundation. [Contact information for both organizations can be found in Chapter 48, A Directory of Foot and Ankle Health Resources.]

Section 41.6

Gout

"Fast Facts about Gout," National Institute of Arthritis and Musculoskeletal and Skin Diseases, National Institutes of Health, March 2005. Brand names included in this text are provided as examples only, and their inclusion does not mean that these products are endorsed by the National Institutes of Health or any other government agency. Also, if a particular brand name is not mentioned, this does not mean or imply that the product is unsatisfactory.

What is gout?

Gout is one of the most painful forms of arthritis. It occurs when too much uric acid builds up in the body. The buildup of uric acid can lead to the following conditions:

- sharp uric acid crystal deposits in joints, often in the big toe
- deposits of uric acid (called tophi) that look like lumps under the skin
- kidney stones from uric acid crystals in the kidneys

For many people, the first attack of gout occurs in the big toe. Often, the attack wakes a person from sleep. The toe is very sore, red, warm, and swollen.

Gout can cause the following:

- pain
- swelling
- redness
- heat
- stiffness in joints

In addition to the big toe, gout can affect the following parts of the body:

- instep
- ankles
- heels
- knees
- wrists
- fingers
- elbows

A gout attack can be brought on by stressful events, alcohol or drugs, or another illness. Early attacks usually get better within three to ten days, even without treatment. The next attack may not occur for months or even years.

What causes gout?

Gout is caused by the buildup of too much uric acid in the body. Uric acid comes from the breakdown of substances called purines. Purines are found in all of your body's tissues. They are also in many foods, such as liver, dried beans and peas, and anchovies.

Normally, uric acid dissolves in the blood. It passes through the kidneys and out of the body in urine. But uric acid can build up in the blood when the following occur:

- the body increases the amount of uric acid it makes
- the kidneys do not get rid of enough uric acid
- a person eats too many foods high in purines

When uric acid levels in the blood are high, it is called hyperuricemia. Most people with hyperuricemia do not develop gout. But if excess uric acid crystals form in the body, gout can develop.

You are more likely to have gout if you:

- have family members with the disease;
- are a man;
- are overweight;
- drink too much alcohol;
- eat too many foods rich in purines;
- have an enzyme defect that makes it hard for the body to break down purines;
- are exposed to lead in the environment;

- have had an organ transplant;
- use some medicines such as diuretics, aspirin, cyclosporine, or levodopa;
- take the vitamin niacin.

How is gout diagnosed?

Your doctor will ask about your symptoms, medical history, and family history of gout. Signs and symptoms of gout include the following:

- hyperuricemia (high level of uric acid in the blood)
- uric acid crystals in joint fluid
- more than one attack of acute arthritis
- arthritis that develops in one day, producing a swollen, red, and warm joint
- attack of arthritis in only one joint, usually the toe, ankle, or knee

To confirm a diagnosis of gout, your doctor may draw a sample of fluid from an inflamed joint to look for crystals associated with gout.

How is gout treated?

Doctors use medicines to treat an acute attack of gout, including the following:

- nonsteroidal anti-inflammatory drugs (NSAIDs), such as Motrin
- corticosteroids, such as prednisone
- colchicine, which works best when taken within the first 12 hours of an acute attack

Sometimes doctors prescribe NSAIDs or colchicine in small daily doses to prevent future attacks. There are also medicines that lower the level of uric acid in the blood.

What can people with gout do to stay healthy?

Some things that you can do to stay healthy are as follows:

- Take the medicines your doctor prescribes as directed.
- Tell your doctor about all the medicines and vitamins you take.
- Plan follow-up visits with your doctor.
- Maintain a healthy, balanced diet. Avoid foods that are high in purines, and drink plenty of water.
- Exercise regularly and maintain a healthy body weight. Ask your doctor about how to lose weight safely. Fast or extreme weight loss can increase uric acid levels in the blood.

What research is being done on gout?

Scientists are studying: which NSAIDs are the most effective treatments for gout; new medicines that safely lower uric acid in the blood and reduce symptoms; and enzymes that break down purines in the body. Scientists are also studying the role of genetics and environmental factors in hyperuricemia and gout.

Chapter 42

Lupus and the Feet

Does lupus cause foot problems?

The foot is a complex structure and foot problems are very common in the general population especially amongst older people. Lupus, however, can cause specific joint and muscle pains in the feet; joints may ache even though there are no obvious signs of inflammation or swelling. Even a stiff hip or back can affect the way we walk, perhaps by causing us to favor one leg, and so cause trouble elsewhere. Abnormal walking patterns can lead to misshapen feet with toe deformities such as bunions and hammer toes. Toe deformities can then increase the risk of friction and pressure inside the shoes causing calluses and corns. Foot complaints tend to be underreported amongst lupus patients, perhaps because other problems are more obvious and more important.

Can skin problems affect the feet?

Corns and callus occur frequently in older patients, those with problems walking, or those who wear badly fitting shoes. Lupus and the drugs used to treat lupus can aggravate the problem of this hard skin. Specific skin problems associated with lupus can occur on the feet but these are rare. Verrucae [warts] can sometimes be a nuisance to people who are taking immunosuppressants. But, contrary to popular belief, verrucae are not often very painful and although they are caused by a virus and can be spread they are not highly contagious. They tend to occur only where the skin is damaged. However, they can linger when the immune system is compromised and may need specialized treatment if they are troublesome.

Does lupus affect toenails?

Twenty-five percent (25%) of people with lupus have some sort of nail problem. In some patients nail growth can be slow, leading to weak, thin nails sometimes with pitting in the nail plate and the nail may become loose. In others, inflammation around the nail or Raynaud phenomenon can lead to thickened or ridged nails. Black or brown marks in the nail are sometimes seen due to tiny bleeding points in the nail bed. Nail problems are generally cosmetic although involuted (curved) or ingrown toenails are common. These can be very sensitive and it is important to get professional help to prevent ingrown toenails from becoming infected.

So what are the risks to the foot in lupus?

Serious foot problems are rare, but any condition that can reduce the amount of blood reaching the toes can lead to ulceration and infection. This can be prevented with effective care. About 20–30 percent of lupus patients develop Raynaud phenomenon (spasms in the blood vessels causing cold or white fingers or toes). Chilblains (small, red, itchy swellings) are also common, often in association with Raynaud. They can become painful and are an abnormal reaction to cold, usually on toes and fingers. They can dry out leaving cracks in the skin, which expose it to infection. It is important to keep the feet warm but not to warm them up too quickly if they are cold.

Vasculitis occasionally causes very painful toes and feet and can lead to infections. It may cause small red lines in the cuticle or nail fold, or little red bumps on the legs; sometimes painful red nodules can form on the legs. Occasionally these red bumps can ulcerate. Steroids can make the skin thinner and more prone to damage and infection. So it is especially important to look after the feet, which are prone to pressure, rubbing, and damage from shoes.

How can I help myself?

Generally, lupus does not cause major foot problems, but no feet will stand up to too much abuse or neglect. Nails must be cut carefully—it is often easier and safer to file them rather than cut them, particularly if they are thick or uneven. The feet should be washed and examined daily for any damage or problems. Any dry skin should be kept moist with a good moisturizing cream to prevent cracks from occurring.

It is vital to wear well-fitting, supportive footwear. Ideally, shoes should have a soft cushioned sole, a pliable yielding upper, and fasten firmly round the instep, preferably with laces. There should be no high-pressure areas on the feet which rub the skin. Feet must be kept warm. Two thin pairs of socks are warmer than one thick pair, and in cold weather thermal insoles should be put in shoes and bed socks worn at night.

Lupus patients should attend a chiropodist (now often called a podiatrist) on at least one occasion for foot care advice. Sometimes the chiropodist will recommend regular checkups even if there are no current problems.

Chapter 43

Raynaud Phenomenon

What is Raynaud phenomenon?

Raynaud phenomenon is a condition that affects the blood vessels in the extremities—generally, the fingers and toes. It is characterized by episodic attacks, called vasospastic attacks, in which the blood vessels in the digits (fingers and toes) constrict (narrow), usually in response to cold temperatures and/or emotional stress. When this condition occurs on its own, it is called primary Raynaud phenomenon. When it occurs with another condition such as scleroderma or lupus, it is called secondary Raynaud phenomenon.

Who gets Raynaud phenomenon?

Although people of any age can have Raynaud phenomenon, the primary form typically begins between the ages of 15 and 25. Women are more likely than men to have Raynaud phenomenon. It appears to be more common in people who live in colder climates. This is likely

"Questions and Answers about Raynaud's Phenomenon," National Institute of Arthritis and Musculoskeletal and Skin Diseases (NIAMS), National Institutes of Health (NIH), NIH Publication No. 06-4911, Publication Date May 2001, Revised June 2006. Brand names included in this fact sheet are provided as examples only, and their inclusion does not mean that these products are endorsed by the National Institutes of Health or any other government agency. Also, if a particular brand name is not mentioned, this does not mean or imply that the product is unsatisfactory.

true because people with the disorder have more Raynaud attacks during periods of colder weather.

Although estimates vary, most studies show that Raynaud phenomenon affects about 3 percent of the general population. For most, the symptoms are mild and not associated with any blood vessel or tissue damage.

Most people with Raynaud phenomenon have the primary form, which is not associated with any underlying disease. In fact, in these individuals it is thought to be an exaggeration of normal responses to cold temperature and/or stress.

When Raynaud phenomenon is caused by or associated with an underlying disease, it is referred to as secondary Raynaud phenomenon. Secondary Raynaud phenomenon tends to begin later in life than the primary form, typically after 35 to 40 years of age.

It is common for patients with a connective tissue disease to have Raynaud phenomenon. It occurs in more than 90 percent of patients with scleroderma, and in about 30 percent of patients with systemic lupus erythematosus and with Sjögren syndrome. Secondary Raynaud phenomenon may also be associated with exposure to vibrating tools such as jackhammers, which cause trauma to the hands and wrists. And it may be linked to certain drugs, such as chemotherapy agents, or to chemicals such as vinyl chloride.

What happens during an attack?

Attacks of Raynaud phenomenon are caused by an intensification of the body's natural response to cold. When a person is exposed to cold, the body's normal response is to slow the loss of heat and preserve its core temperature. Blood vessels in the surface of the skin are called thermoregulatory vessels because they react to changes in the ambient temperature. To maintain normal core temperature, these specialized blood vessels in the skin surface constrict and move blood from arteries near the surface to veins deeper in the body. But for people who have Raynaud phenomenon, the thermoregulatory vessels overreact to cold exposure with sudden and intense spasmodic contractions of these small blood vessels that supply blood to the skin of the fingers, toes, ears, face, and other body areas.

Once an attack begins, a person may experience three phases (though not all people have all three) of skin color changes—typically from white to blue to red—in the fingers or toes. Whiteness (called pallor) may occur in response to spasms of the arterioles (small branches of an artery) and the resulting collapse of the arteries supplying the fingers and toes. Blueness (cyanosis) may appear because the fingers or toes are not getting enough oxygen-rich blood. Finally, as the arterioles dilate (relax) and blood returns to the digits, redness (rubor) may occur.

During the attack, the fingers or toes may feel cold and numb as blood flow to them is interrupted. As the attack ends and blood flow returns, fingers or toes may throb and tingle. Typically, the blood flow to the skin will remain low until the skin is rewarmed. After warming, it usually takes 15 minutes to recover normal blood flow to the skin.

What is the difference between primary and secondary Raynaud phenomenon?

In medical literature, primary Raynaud phenomenon may also be called idiopathic Raynaud phenomenon, primary Raynaud syndrome, or Raynaud disease. There is no known cause for primary Raynaud phenomenon. It is more common than the secondary form and often is so mild the patient never seeks medical attention. It generally is an annoyance that causes little disability. Secondary Raynaud phenomenon is a more complex and serious disorder.

The most common cause of secondary Raynaud phenomenon is connective tissue disease. The condition most commonly occurs with scleroderma or lupus, but is also associated with Sjögren syndrome, dermatomyositis, and polymyositis. Some of these diseases reduce blood flow to the fingers and toes by causing blood vessel walls to thicken and the vessels to constrict too easily.

Other possible causes of secondary Raynaud phenomenon are carpal tunnel syndrome and obstructive arterial disease (blood vessel disease). Some drugs are also linked to Raynaud phenomenon. They include beta-blockers, such as Lopressor or Cartrol, used to treat high blood pressure; ergotamine preparations, such as Cafergot or Wigraine, used for migraine headaches; certain agents used in cancer chemotherapy; and drugs, such as over-the-counter cold medication and narcotics, that cause vasoconstriction.

People in certain occupations may be more vulnerable to secondary Raynaud phenomenon. Some workers in the plastics industry who are exposed to vinyl chloride, for example, develop a scleroderma-like illness, of which Raynaud phenomenon can be a part. Workers who operate vibrating tools can develop a type of Raynaud phenomenon called vibration-induced white finger.

Severe cases of Raynaud phenomenon—usually of the secondary form—can lead to problems such as skin ulcers (sores) or gangrene (tissue death) in the fingers and toes, which can be painful and difficult to treat.

How does a doctor diagnose Raynaud phenomenon?

Most doctors find it fairly easy to diagnose Raynaud phenomenon but find it more difficult to identify the form of the disorder.

Physicians can now distinguish primary from secondary Raynaud phenomenon with a complete history and physical examination. Sometimes, special blood testing is needed. If the evaluation and special testing studies are normal, then the diagnosis of primary Raynaud phenomenon can be made and it is unlikely to change into a secondary form. Interestingly, about 30 percent of first-degree relatives of patients with primary Raynaud phenomenon also have the condition. This finding suggests that primary Raynaud phenomenon is determined by some yet-to-be discovered genetic trait.

A few tests can help the doctor distinguish between primary and secondary Raynaud phenomenon. They are as follows:

Nail fold capillaroscopy—During this test, the doctor puts a drop of oil on the patient's nail folds, the skin at the base of the fingernail. The doctor then examines the nail folds under a microscope to look for problems in the tiny blood vessels called capillaries. If the capillaries are enlarged or malformed, the patient may have a connective tissue disease.

Antinuclear antibody (ANA) test—In this blood test, the doctor determines whether the body is producing special proteins called antibodies that are directed against the nuclei of the body's cells. These abnormal antibodies are often found in people who have connective tissue diseases or other autoimmune disorders.

Erythrocyte sedimentation rate (ESR or sed rate)—This is a laboratory test for inflammation that measures how quickly red blood cells fall to the bottom of a test tube of unclotted blood. Rapidly descending cells (an elevated sed rate) indicate inflammation in the body.

What is the treatment for Raynaud phenomenon?

The aims of treatment are to reduce the number and severity of attacks and to prevent tissue damage and loss of tissue in the fingers and toes. Most doctors are conservative in treating patients with primary Raynaud phenomenon because they do not get tissue damage. For these patients, doctors tend to recommend nondrug treatments before moving onto medications. For patients with secondary Raynaud phenomenon, medications are more often prescribed, because severe attacks with ulcers or tissue damage are more likely.

In the most severe cases, Raynaud causes ulcers and serious tissue damage that does not respond to medications. Doctors may use a surgical procedure called a digital sympathectomy with adventitial stripping (which involves removing the tissue and nerves around the blood vessels supplying the affected digits). While this procedure may result in reducing symptoms and healing tissue, it only helps temporarily and therefore is reserved for difficult cases.

The most common treatments and self-help measures are described below.

Nondrug Treatments and Self-Help Measures

The following nondrug treatments and self-help measures can decrease the severity of Raynaud attacks and promote overall well-being.

Take action during an attack. You can decrease both its length and severity by a few simple actions. The first and most important one is avoid the cold. Warming the body and the hands or feet is also helpful. If you're outside and the weather is cold, go indoors. Run warm water over your fingers or toes or soak them in a bowl of warm water to warm them. If a stressful situation triggers the attack, get out of the stressful situation, if possible, and relax. While biofeedback and similar nondrug methods are used, formal studies have suggested they are not helpful.

Keep warm. It is important not only to keep the extremities warm but also to avoid chilling any part of the body. Remember, a drop in the body's core temperature triggers the attack. Shifting temperature (for example, rapidly moving from 90 degrees outside to a 70 degree air-conditioned room) and damp rainy weather are to be avoided. In cold weather, pay particular attention to dressing. Several layers of loose clothing, socks, hats, and gloves or mittens are recommended. A hat is important because a great deal of body heat is lost through the scalp. Keep feet warm and dry. Some people find it helpful to wear mittens and socks to bed during the winter. Chemical warmers, such as small heating pouches that can be placed in pockets, mittens, boots, or shoes, can give added protection during long periods outdoors.

People who have secondary Raynaud phenomenon should talk to their doctors before exercising outdoors in cold weather.

In warm weather, be aware that air conditioning also can trigger attacks. Setting the thermostat for a higher temperature or wearing a sweater indoors can help prevent an attack. Some people find it helpful to use insulated drinking glasses and to put on gloves before handling frozen or refrigerated foods.

Do not smoke. The nicotine in cigarettes causes the skin temperature to drop, which may lead to an attack.

Avoid aggravating medications such as vasoconstrictors, which cause the blood vessels to narrow. Vasoconstrictors include beta-blockers, many cold preparations, caffeine, narcotics, some migraine headache medications, some chemotherapeutic drugs, and clonidine, a blood pressure medication. Some studies also associate the use of estrogen with Raynaud phenomenon.

Control stress. Because stress and emotional upsets may trigger an attack, particularly for people who have primary Raynaud phenomenon, learning to recognize and avoid stressful situations may help control the number of attacks. Many people have found that relaxation can help decrease the number and severity of attacks. Local hospitals and other community organizations, such as schools, often offer programs in stress management.

Exercise regularly. Many doctors encourage patients who have Raynaud phenomenon—particularly the primary form—to exercise regularly. Most people find that exercise promotes overall well-being, increases energy level, helps control weight, and promotes cardiovascular fitness and restful sleep. Patients with Raynaud phenomenon should talk to their doctors before starting an exercise program.

See a doctor. People with Raynaud phenomenon should see their doctors if they are worried or frightened about attacks or if they have questions about caring for themselves. They should always see their doctors if episodes occur only on one side of the body (one hand or one foot) and any time one results in sores or ulcers on the fingers or toes.

Treatment with Medications

People with secondary Raynaud phenomenon are more likely than those with the primary form to be treated with medications. Many doctors believe that the most effective and safest drugs for Raynaud phenomenon are calcium channel blockers such as nifedipine (Procardia) or amlodipine (Norvasc). These drugs, which are used to treat high blood pressure, work by relaxing the smooth muscle and dilating the small blood vessels. This decreases the frequency and severity of Raynaud attacks. These drugs can also help heal skin ulcers on the fingers or toes.

Some patients have found relief with alpha receptor blockers, which are high blood pressure medications such as prazosin (Minipress) or doxazosin (Cardura). These medications counteract the actions of norepinephrine, a hormone that constricts blood vessels. Effects are reported to be modest and side effects are associated with long-term use. However, preliminary research has found that a more highly targeted blocker for a specific alpha receptor shows promise. This receptor blocker is under investigation.

To help heal skin ulcers, some doctors prescribe a nonspecific vasodilator (drug that relaxes blood vessels) such as nitroglycerin paste, which is applied to the fingers. Many new agents that vasodilate are being used in cases that do not respond. These include the antidepressant fluoxetine (Prozac); phosphodiesterase inhibitors such as cilostazol (Pletal), pentoxifylline (Trental), and sildenafil (Viagra); and an angiotensin II receptor antagonist (used for blood pressure control), losartan (Cozaar). Patients should keep in mind that the treatment for Raynaud phenomenon is not always successful. Often, patients with the secondary form will not respond as well to treatment as those with the primary form of the disorder. In cases of critical digital ischemia (where the blood flow will not return and finger loss may result), intravenous vasodilator therapy is used with prostaglandins such as epoprostenol (Flolan).

Patients may find that one drug works better than another. Some people may experience side effects that require stopping the medication. For other people, a drug may become less effective over time. Women of childbearing age should know that the medications used to treat Raynaud phenomenon may affect the growing fetus. Therefore, women who are pregnant or who might become pregnant should avoid taking these medications if possible. Interestingly, Raynaud phenomenon gets better or goes away during pregnancy.

Self-Help Reminders

- Take action during an attack.
- Keep warm.
- Don't smoke.

- Avoid aggravating medications.
- Control stress.
- Exercise regularly.
- See a doctor if questions or concerns develop.

What research is being conducted to help people who have Raynaud phenomenon?

Researchers are studying techniques such as laser Doppler imaging to better diagnose Raynaud phenomenon and to predict and monitor its course and responsiveness to treatment.

They are also evaluating the use of new treatments to improve blood flow for those who have Raynaud phenomenon. These include the high blood pressure drug losartan (Cozaar); prostaglandins such as iloprost and alprostadil (Caverject, Edex); the male erectile dysfunction drug sildenafil (Viagra); the blood-clot-preventing drug ticlopidine (Ticlid); and the herbal remedy gingko biloba.

Treatments such as L-arginine, taken orally, have been studied as a way to reverse Raynaud-related damage to tissue in the toes and fingers, but they have been found ineffective in most studies.

Basic investigators are studying the molecular mechanisms behind Raynaud phenomenon, the anatomy of blood vessels, and possible genetic associations. Researchers in scleroderma and other connective tissue diseases are also investigating Raynaud phenomenon in relation to these diseases.

For Your Information

This publication contains information about medications used to treat the health condition discussed here. When this book was printed, the most up-to-date (accurate) information available was included. Occasionally, new information on medication is released.

For updates and for any questions about any medications you are taking, please contact the U.S. Food and Drug Administration at 888-INFO-FDA (888-463-6332, a toll-free call) or visit their website at http://www.fda.gov.

Chapter 44

Hansen Disease
(Leprosy)

What is Hansen disease?

Hansen disease (HD), erroneously associated with biblical leprosy, is a complex infectious disease. Although recognized for more than two thousand years and found over a century ago to be caused by a bacterium, the disease is still not completely understood. Dr. Gerhard Armauer Hansen, a Norwegian scientist, first discovered the HD bacillus in 1873. Considerable progress has been made over the last 40 years so that today we can treat the majority of cases without undue difficulty and counteract most of the fears generated by the folklore surrounding this disease.

HD is in the same bacterial family as *Mycobacterium tuberculosis,* but is uniquely a disease of the peripheral nerves. It also affects the skin and sometimes other tissues, notably the eye, the mucosa of the upper respiratory tract, muscles, bone, and testes.

There are both localized and disseminated forms of HD. If left untreated, HD causes nerve damage, which can result in loss of muscle control and crippling of hands and feet. Eye involvement can result in blindness.

"Frequently Asked Questions," U.S. Department of Health and Human Services, Health Resources and Services Administration, Bureau of Primary Health Care, National Hansen's Disease Programs, May 2005.

Where is Hansen disease found?

In 1994 the World Health Organization estimated that there were 2.4 million cases of HD worldwide with 1.7 million cases registered on treatment. The estimates for 1985 were 10–12 million and 5.4 million respectively. According to these estimates, in 1994, 70 percent of those who should be on treatment are now being treated. In 1992 there were 690,000 new cases reported and in 1993, 591,000 cases. There are also an estimated 2–3 million cases who have completed treatment but still have residual disabilities. These cases are not included in the 1994 totals. The largest numbers of Hansen disease patients continue to be in Southeast Asia and Central Africa with smaller numbers in South and Central America. The largest number of patients in the Western Hemisphere are in Brazil.

In the United States there are approximately 6,500 cases on the registry which includes all cases reported since the registry began and still living. The number of cases with active disease and requiring drug treatment is approximately 600. There are 200–250 new cases reported to the registry annually with about 175 of these being new cases diagnosed for the first time. The largest number of cases in the United States (U.S.) are in California, Texas, Hawaii, Louisiana, Florida, New York, and Puerto Rico.

The National Hansen's Disease Programs (NHDP) in Baton Rouge, Louisiana, is the only institution in the United States (U.S.) exclusively devoted to Hansen disease. The center functions as a referral and consulting center with related research and training activities. Most patients in the U.S. are treated under U.S. Public Health Service grants at clinics in major cities or by private physicians.

How does HD spread?

The most commonly accepted theory is that it is transmitted by way of the respiratory tract since large numbers of bacteria can be found in the nose of some untreated patients. The degree of susceptibility of the person, the extent of exposure, and environmental conditions are among factors probably of great importance in transmission.

Is Hansen disease contagious?

Yes, but far less so than other infectious diseases. Most specialists agree that more than 95 percent of the world's population has a natural immunity to the disease. Health care workers rarely contract the disease. Cases of HD which respond satisfactorily to treatment become noninfectious within a short time.

Is there effective treatment?

Although the sulfone drugs, introduced at Carville in 1941, continue to be an important weapon against the Hansen bacillus [*Mycobacterium leprae*], the rising incidence of sulfone resistant disease necessitates treating all patients with more than one drug. There is very effective treatment for Hansen disease in the form of antibiotics. The three most commonly used are Dapsone, Rifampin, and Clofazimine. Other antibiotics such as Clarithromycin, Ofloxacin, Levofloxacin, and Minocycline also have excellent antibacterial activity against *M. leprae*. Treatment rapidly renders the disease noncommunicable by killing nearly all the bacilli. These dead bacilli are then cleared from the body within a variable number of years. Treatment regimens differ depending upon the form of the disease. Information on treatment can be obtained by contacting National Hansen's Disease Programs (NHDP).

Are there different forms of Hansen disease?

Yes. There is a limited form of the disease called tuberculoid or paucibacillary (few bacilli) and a more generalized form called lepromatous or multibacillary (many bacilli).

Are both forms of Hansen disease contagious?

No. The tuberculoid or paucibacillary form is not contagious.

How do I know if I have Hansen disease?

Pale or slightly red areas on the skin which have lost feeling, or loss of feeling of the hands or feet may be the first signs of HD. Your doctor can make the diagnosis by doing a test called a skin biopsy.

Who is at greatest risk of contacting the disease?

Those at greatest risk are the household contacts of the untreated case possibly because of genetic factors relating to susceptibility and/ or the prolonged intimate contact. The spouse is the least at risk familial member. The greatest risk is for the children, brothers or sisters, or parents of someone with HD.

Must a patient be treated for life for Hansen disease?

No. Clinicians now use fixed duration treatment. Treatment will generally continue for one year for tuberculoid or paucibacillary disease and two years for lepromatous or multibacillary disease.

Is it passed on during pregnancy or through sex?

HD is not passed on from a mother to her unborn baby. You also do not get it through sexual contact.

What effects does it have on the body?

Because the bacteria like the cooler parts of the body, the skin and its nerves are affected. This can cause dryness and stiffness of the skin. In some cases affected nerves can swell, causing pain, loss of feeling, and weakness in the muscles of the hands or feet.

Are all patients disfigured with loss of fingers and toes?

No. Early diagnosis and treatment is very important and can prevent many of the complications associated with the disease. Many patients with tuberculoid or paucibacillary disease can even self heal without benefit of treatment, but it is the standard of care to treat all patients identified with the disease. Problems with fingers or toes can be prevented by avoiding injury and infections to these areas, and by taking the HD medicines.

Some patients report that they get worse after treatment has begun. How can that happen?

Some patients experience what is called reaction after treatment has begun. This is a response of the immune system to dead or dying bacteria and can cause worsening of the rash or a painful neuritis which can affect sensation and/or strength.

Is reaction harmful?

Reaction can be mild or severe. If mild, no treatment or only over-the-counter anti-inflammatory medication may be sufficient. More severe reaction can be harmful to nerves and should be promptly treated by a physician. If you think you are having a reaction of any type, it is best to notify your physician so that he can decide on appropriate treatment.

Why is diagnosis difficult and often delayed?

Unfortunately, the rash caused by Hansen disease often resembles other skin diseases. Lack of experience with this disease, because of its infrequent occurrence in our population, occasionally leads to lack of recognition and delay in diagnosis. Further complicating diagnosis is the inability to grow or culture this bacterium in the laboratory as we would do with other infections such as pneumonia or pharyngitis.

How does Hansen disease present itself?

Hansen disease mainly presents as a rash on the trunk or extremities. Frequently there is an associated decrease in light touch sensation in the area of the rash but not always. This change in sensation can be a valuable clue to diagnosis. Nasal congestion may be a sign of infection, but infection is usually associated with changes of the skin on the face, and perhaps thinning of the eyebrows or eyelashes.

How is diagnosis made?

The diagnosis is made by a combination of the characteristic clinical picture of rash with change in sensation plus a skin biopsy which reveals a particular pathologic pattern and demonstrates the specific "red" staining bacteria. By far the most important diagnostic tool is the biopsy of the rash.

Is there any medicine that I should take if I think I have been exposed to the disease?

No! Household contacts of patients with HD need only a good examination by a physician. These examinations should be repeated annually for five years. The degree of natural immunity is very high and there is no need for prophylaxis. Household contacts who have a questionable skin rash should have a skin biopsy to determine whether or not Hansen disease is present.

Is there any test that will tell if I have been exposed or if I have early disease?

No. Unfortunately there is no blood or skin test that will tell if you have been exposed or if you have pre-clinical disease.

Is there any way to prevent the disease such as a vaccine that would protect against exposure?

No. We do not as yet have a suitable vaccine to prevent Hansen disease, but it is an area of very active research.

Can I continue to work?

A person with HD can continue to work and lead an active life.

Where is treatment available?

Medicine for HD can be provided at no cost to patients by their family doctor or through the Hansen's Disease Clinic closest to them. [For information on Hansen's Disease Clinics or to contact the National Hansen's Disease Program, see the contact information under Lower Extremity Amputation Prevention Program (LEAP) in Chapter 48, "A Directory of Foot and Ankle Health Resources," at the end of this book.]

Part Six

Additional Help and Information

Chapter 45

Glossary of Podiatric Terms

abduction: Movement of the digits away from the median plane (of the foot).

ablation: Removal of a body part or the destruction of its function, as by a surgical procedure, morbid process, or noxious substance.

ambulatory: Walking about or able to walk about.

ankylosis: Stiffening or fixation of a joint as the result of a disease process, with fibrous or bony union across the joint.

apophysis: An outgrowth or projection, especially one from a bone. A bony process or outgrowth that lacks an independent center of ossification.

arthroplasty: (1) Creation of an artificial joint to correct advanced degenerative arthritis, (2) An operation to restore as far as possible the integrity and functional power of a joint.

avulsion: A tearing away or forcible separation.

bunion: A localized swelling at either the medial or dorsal aspect of the first metatarsophalangeal joint, caused by an inflammatory bursa; a medial bunion is usually associated with hallux valgus.

---

bursitis: Inflammation of a bursa (a closed sac containing fluid).

calcaneal: Relating to the calcaneus or heel bone.

carpopedal: Relating to the wrist and the foot, or the hands and feet; denoting especially carpopedal spasm.

cheilectomy: Chiseling away bony irregularities at osteochondral margin of a joint cavity that interfere with movements of the joint.

claudication: Limping, usually referring to intermittent claudication.

clawfoot: A condition of the foot characterized by hyperextension at the metatarsophalangeal joint and flexion at the interphalangeal joints, as a fixed contracture.

cosmesis: A concern in therapeutics for the appearance of the patient; i.e., an operation that improves appearance.

dermatophyte: A fungus that causes superficial infections of the skin, hair, and/or nails, i.e., keratinized tissues. Species of *Epidermophyton*, *Microsporum*, and *Trichophyton* are regarded as dermatophytes, but causative agents of tinea versicolor, tinea nigra, and cutaneous candidiasis are not so classified.

digits of foot (dactyl, dactylus, digitus): Toe.

dorsiflexion: Upward movement (extension) of the foot or toes.

ecchymosis: A purplish patch caused by extravasation of blood into the skin, differing from petechiae only in size (larger than 3 mm diameter).

edema: An accumulation of an excessive amount of watery fluid in cells or intercellular tissues.

epiphyseal plate (growth plate): The disc of cartilage between the metaphysis and the epiphysis of an immature long bone permitting growth in length.

erythema: Redness due to capillary dilation.

eversion: A turning outward, as of the foot.

fascia: A sheet of fibrous tissue that envelops the body beneath the skin; it also encloses muscles and groups of muscles, and separates their several layers or groups.

fasciotomy: Incision through a fascia; used in the treatment of certain disorders and injuries when marked swelling is present or anticipated which could compromise blood flow.

flexion: Bending the foot or toes toward the plantar surface.

gait: Manner of walking.

hallux (big toe): Great toe I, the first digit of the foot.

hallux rigidus (stiff toe): A condition in which stiffness appears in the first metatarsophalangeal joint; usually associated with the development of bone spurs on the dorsal surface.

hallux valgus: A deviation of the tip of the great toe, or main axis of the toe, toward the outer or lateral side of the foot.

hyperkeratosis: Thickening of the horny layer of the epidermis.

interossei (dorsal interossei, interosseous muscles): Muscles which arise from and run between the long (metacarpal and metatarsal) bones of the hand and foot, extending to and producing movement of the digits.

lesion: A wound or injury.

malleolus: A rounded bony prominence such as those on either side of the ankle joint. Plural: malleoli.

metatarsal bones (long bones): The five long bones numbered I to V beginning with the bone on the medial side forming the skeleton of the anterior portion of the foot, articulating posteriorly with the three cuneiform and the cuboid bones, anteriorly with the five proximal phalanges.

metatarsalgia: Pain in the forefoot in the region of the heads of the metatarsals.

neuritis (neuropathy): Inflammation of a nerve.

onychomycosis (ringworm of nails): Very common fungus infections of the nails, causing thickening, roughness, and splitting, often caused by *Trichophyton rubrum* or *T. mentagrophytes*, *Candida*, and occasionally molds.

orthosis: An external orthopaedic appliance, as a brace or splint, that prevents or assists movement of the spine or the limbs.

orthotics: The science concerned with the making and fitting of orthopaedic appliances.

osteotomy: Cutting a bone, usually by means of a saw or osteotome.

pes cavus, talipes cavus: An exaggeration of the normal arch of the foot.

pes planus, talipes planus (flat foot): A condition in which the longitudinal arch is broken down, the entire sole touching the ground.

phalanx: One of the long bones of the digits, 14 in number for each hand or foot, two for the thumb or great toe, and three each for the other four digits; designated as proximal, middle, and distal, beginning from the metacarpus. Plural: phalanges.

plantar: Relating to the sole of the foot.

plantar fascia: Deep fascia of the sole of the foot; includes thick central part, the plantar aponeurosis, covering the central compartment of the sole of the foot, and thinner medial and lateral parts covering the hallucis and digit minimi muscles (compartments), respectively.

plantar wart: See verruca plantaris.

pronation: The condition of being prone; the act of assuming or of being placed in a prone position; a specific rotational motion of the foot in which the plantar surface is rotated outward.

prophylaxis: Prevention of disease or of a process that can lead to disease.

sesamoid bone: A bone formed after birth in a tendon where it passes over a joint.

supination of the foot: Inversion and abduction of the foot, causing an elevation of the medial edge.

talipes: Any deformity of the foot involving the talus.

talonavicular: Relating to the talus and the navicular bone.

talus (ankle): The bone of the foot that articulates with the tibia and fibula to form the ankle joint.

tarsal bones: The seven bones of the instep: talus, calcaneus, navicular, three cuneiform (wedge), and cuboid bones.

tinea pedis (athlete's foot): Dermatophytosis of the feet, especially of the skin between the toes, caused by one of the dermatophytes, usually a species of *Trichophyton* or *Epidermophyton;* the disease consists of small vesicles, fissures, scaling, maceration, and eroded areas between the toes and on the plantar surface of the foot; other skin areas may be involved.

valgus: Bent or twisted outward away from the midline or body; modern accepted usage, particularly in orthopedics, erroneously transposes the meaning of varus to valgus, as in genu valgum (knock-knee).

varus: Bent or twisted inward toward the midline of the limb or body; modern accepted usage, particularly in orthopedics, erroneously transposes the meaning of valgus to varus, as in genu varum (bow-leg).

vasculitis (angiitis): Inflammation of a blood vessel (arteritis, phlebitis) or lymphatic vessel (lymphangitis).

verruca plantaris (plantar wart): An often painful wart on the sole, usually caused by human papillomavirus type 1.

Chapter 46

Podiatric Patients
and Financial Concerns

Chapter Contents

Section 46.1

Medicare Coverage for Therapeutic Footwear

"Medicare Coverage of Therapeutic Footwear for People with Diabetes" excerpted from *Feet Can Last a Lifetime: A Health Care Provider's Guide to Preventing Diabetes Foot Problems*, National Diabetes Education Program, a joint initiative of the National Institutes of Health and the Centers for Disease Control and Prevention, National Institute of Diabetes and Digestive and Kidney Diseases, November 2000. Contact information verified in July 2006.

Medicare provides coverage for depth-inlay shoes, custom-molded shoes, and shoe inserts for people with diabetes who qualify under Medicare Part B. Designed to prevent lower-limb ulcers and amputations in people who have diabetes, this Medicare benefit can prevent suffering and save money.

How Individuals Qualify

The MD or DO treating the patient for diabetes must certify that the individual meets the following requirements:

1. has diabetes

2. has one or more of the following conditions in one or both feet:

    *   history of partial or complete foot amputation

    *   history of previous foot ulceration

    *   history of pre-ulcerative callus

    *   peripheral neuropathy with evidence of callus formation

    *   poor circulation

    *   foot deformity

3. is being treated under a comprehensive diabetes care plan and needs therapeutic shoes and/or inserts because of diabetes

Type of Footwear Covered

If an individual qualifies, he/she is limited to one of the following footwear categories within each calendar year:

1. one pair of depth shoes and three pairs of inserts

2. one pair of custom-molded shoes (including inserts) and two additional pairs of inserts

Separate inserts may be covered under certain criteria. Shoe modification is covered as a substitute for an insert, and a custom-molded shoe is covered when the individual has a foot deformity that cannot be accommodated by a depth shoe.

What the Physician Needs to Do

1. The certifying physician (the MD or DO) overseeing the diabetes treatment must review and sign a "Statement of Certifying Physician for Therapeutic Shoes" (see form online at http://www.ndep.nih.gov/diabetes/pubs/Feet_HCGuide.pdf).

2. The prescribing physician (the DPM, DO, or MD) must complete a footwear prescription (see form online at http://www.ndep.nih.gov/diabetes/pubs/Feet_HCGuide.pdf). Once the patient has the signed statement and the prescription, he/she can see a podiatrist, orthotist, prosthetist, or pedorthist to have the prescription filled. The supplier will then submit the Medicare claim form (Form HCFA 1500) to the appropriate Durable Medical Equipment Regional Carrier (DMERC), keeping copies of the claim form and the original statement and prescription.

Note: In most cases, the certifying physician and the prescribing physician will be two different individuals.

Patient Responsibility for Payment

Medicare will pay for 80 percent of the payment amount allowed. The patient is responsible for a minimum of 20 percent of the total payment amount and possibly more if the dispenser does not accept Medicare assignment and the dispenser's usual fee is higher than the payment amount. The maximum payment amounts per pair as of 2000 can be found in Table 46.1.

453

Table 46.1. Maximum payment amounts.

	Total Amount Allowed	Amount Covered by Medicare
Depth shoes	$126.00	$100.80
Custom-molded shoes	$378.00	$302.40
Inserts or modifications	$64.00	$51.20

ICD-9 Codes

Because this benefit is available only to people with diabetes, an appropriate ICD-9 code (250.00-250.93) is required when completing the Statement of Certifying Physician.

Section 46.2

Financial Assistance for Amputees

"In Search of Funding," by Bill Dupes, Amputee Coalition of America Information Specialist. Reprinted with permission from *First Step: A Guide for Adapting to Limb Loss*, Volume 3. © 2003 Amputee Coalition of America. All rights reserved. Contact information verified July 2006.

With the constant development of new technology, more and more options exist to enable people with disabilities to work, achieve higher levels of education, and live independently.

It is easy to become frustrated as these individuals seek access to assistive technology; financial aid for their education, home, school, and office modifications; adaptive driving equipment; and funding for a variety of needs.

Fortunately, funding is available for those who qualify and who know how to find it. This section provides a basic overview of the types of assistance that amputees might be able to obtain.

Child Assistance

St. Jude Children's Research Hospital: Acceptance for treatment is based solely on a patient's eligibility for an ongoing clinical trial. (Birth–18)

St. Jude Children's Research Hospital
332 North Lauderdale
Memphis, TN 38105
Toll-Free: 866-2STJUDE
Phone: 901-495-3300
Website: http://www.stjude.org

Medicaid: Individuals get Medicaid services automatically if they receive Supplemental Security Income (SSI) or Aid to Families with Dependent Children (AFDC). If they're ineligible for either of these programs, however, they might still qualify for Medicaid.

Medicaid
7500 Security Boulevard
Baltimore, MD 21244
Toll-Free: 877-267-2323
Website: http://www.cms.hhs.gov/medicaid/stateplans/map.asp

Early and Periodic Screening, Diagnosis, and Treatment (EPSDT): This Medicaid program provides a wide range of healthcare coverage to low-income children. (Birth–21)

EPSDT
Phone: 410-786-5916
Website: http://www.cms.hhs.gov/MedicaidEarlyPeriodicScrn

Blue Cross Blue Shield: Some Blue Cross Blue Shield companies have established "Caring for Children Foundations" that provide free or low-cost coverage to children who are not insurable through Medicaid or private insurance. Services and eligibility requirements vary. Website: http://www.bcbs.com

Variety Clubs International: The organization's purpose is to improve the quality of life of children who are sick, disabled, or disadvantaged by social circumstances. Website: http://www.usvariety.org. (Birth–21)

Lions Clubs International: Lions clubs provide a variety of services, including senior citizen programs and medical care for those in need.

Lions Clubs International
300 West 22nd Street
Oak Brook, IL 60523-8842
Phone: 630-571-5466
Website: http://www.lionsclubs.org

Rotary International: This worldwide organization of business leaders provides humanitarian service through more than 30,000 Rotary Clubs. (Birth-21)

Rotary International
One Rotary Center
1560 Sherman Avenue
Evanston, IL 60201
Phone: 847-866-3000
Website: http://www.rotary.org/index.html

The Benevolent and Protective Order of Elks: Services and opportunities vary from one community to another and include summer camps, educational grants and scholarships, healthcare, and home modification assistance. (Birth-21)

The Benevolent and Protective Order of Elks
2750 North Lakeview Avenue
Chicago, IL 60614-1889
Phone: 773-755-4700
Website: http://www.elks.org

Shriners: All children under 18 are eligible for prostheses. If a child has insurance, the insurance is billed first and Shriners pays the rest. If there is no insurance, Shriners pays the entire bill, including travel expenses. They will even transport patients to their facility by van or plane. (Birth-21)

Shriners
Toll-Free: 800-237-5055
Website: http://www.shrinershq.org/hospit.html

Transportation Resources

If individuals can't afford the travel expenses to see their prosthe-tist, most major airlines have programs to which people can donate their frequent-flier miles for charitable or medical use. In addition, there are several networks of volunteer pilots willing to provide trans-portation for those with medical and financial need.

National Patient Air Transport Helpline
Toll-Free: 800-296-1217
Website: http://www.npath.org

AirLifeLine
Toll-Free: 877-247-5433
Website: http://www.airlifeline.org/a1/servlet/visit

Angel Flights
Toll-Free: 877-858-7788
Website: http://www.angelflightamerica.org

Nonprofit Organizations

The following organizations help those who can't afford assistive technology or related services and have exhausted the usual funding methods.

Amputee Resource Foundation of America
Phone: 612-812-7875
Website: http://www.amputeeresource.org

Barr/United Amputee Assistance Fund
Phone: 407-359-5500
Website: http://www.oandp.com/organiza/barr/index2.htm
E-mail:barr@oandp.com

Limbs for Life Foundation
5929 North May, Suite 511
Oklahoma City, OK 73112
Toll-Free: 888-235-5462
Phone: 405-843-5174
Website: http://www.limbsforlife.org
E-mail:admin@limbsforlife.org

New Beginnings Prosthetic Ministries
Website: http://www.newbeginnings2000.org

Prosthetics for Diabetics Foundation
Website: http://www.expage.com/page/pfdfoundation

Vocational Rehabilitation (VR): Individuals who are unemployed and don't have Medicare, Medicaid, or private insurance should check with their state VR office to see what funding programs are available. VR may pay for assistive technology or offer other services, including counseling, referrals to other funding sources, independent living training, or advocacy. Many states also provide the equivalent of VR for children. Anyone applying for funds, however, is expected to demonstrate that the service or assistive technology will enhance their employability. If employment isn't an option, they must show that it will enable them to function independently. Toll-Free: 800-772-1213.

Technical Assistance Project (TAP): TAP is funded to help reduce barriers and increase access to assistive technology and services.

TAP
1700 North Moore Street, Suite 1540
Arlington, VA 22209
Phone: 703-524-6686
Website: http://www.resna.org/taproject/at/statecontacts.html

Special Education: School systems may provide a range of assistive technology and services. A child must receive any assistive technology or services needed to transport him or her to school. In addition, training may also be provided to parents if it will benefit their children who receive special education services. (Ages 3-21)

U.S. Department of Education
Office for Civil Rights—Customer Service Team
550 12th Street, SW
Washington, DC 20202-1100
Phone: 800-421-3481
Fax: 202-245-6840
TDD: 877-521-2172
Website: http://www.ed.gov/about/offices/list/ocr/504faq.html
E-mail: OCR@ed.gov

Student Aid Resources

Students with disabilities may apply for a variety of scholarships offered by various organizations. Information on special student aid is also available through state VR offices. (Ages 18+)

Higher Education and Adult Training for People with Handicaps
Toll-Free: 800-544-3284
Website: http://www.heath-resource-center.org

International Center for Disability Resources on the Internet
5212 Covington Bend Drive
Raleigh, NC 27613
Phone: 919-349-6661
Website: http://www.icdri.org

FinAid
Website: http://www.finaid.org/otheraid/disabled.phtml

American Association of People with Disabilities
Website: http://www.aapd.com

Organizations for Disabled Athletes

Challenged Athletes Foundation (CAF)
Phone: 858-866-0959
Website: http://www.challengedathletes.org

National Sports Center for the Disabled (NSCD)
Phone: 303-293-5711
Website: http://www.nscd.org

Home Modification Resources

How accessible a home is depends on the nature of the individual's disability. Without the appropriate assistive technology, people with disabilities can feel as if they are trapped in their own home. The solution might be as simple as adding grab bars and a tub seat in the bathroom, or, for wheelchair users, adding ramps, widening doors, and lowering counters. Fortunately, assistance is available.

Fair Housing Act (FHA): The FHA requires landlords to allow renters to make their residence accessible. Though renters must agree to return the interior of the residence to its original condition when they leave, they don't have to remove exterior modifications such as ramps.

FHA
Phone: 202-708-1112
Website: http://www.hud.gov/offices/fheo/FHLaws/index.cfm

Departments of Energy/Health and Human Services: The Low Income Home Energy Assistance Program (LIHEAP) and the Weatherization Assistance Program (WAP) provide funds to weatherize the homes of lower income individuals. You may want to contact the National Energy Assistance Referral (NEAR) project. NEAR is a free service for persons who want information on where to apply for LIHEAP help.

LIHEAP/NEAR
Toll-Free: 866-674-6327
Website: http://www.acf.hhs.gov/programs/liheap
E-mail: energyassistance@neat.org (please include your city, county, and state along with your e-mail message)

WAP
Toll-Free: 877-337-3463
Website: http://www.eren.doe.gov/buildings/weatherization_assistance/contacts.html
E-mail: eereic@ee.doe.gov

Community Development: Many cities and towns use CD Block Grants to help low-income citizens upgrade their homes.

Community Development
Phone: 202-708-1112
Website: http://www.hud.gov/offices/cpd/communitydevelopment/programs/contacts/index.cfm

Social Security Administration (SSA): Under the SSA's work incentive programs, the amount individuals pay for home modifications is deducted from their earned income, allowing them to receive the applicable amount of benefits. They must prove, however, that these modifications will enable them to go to work. Toll-Free: 800-772-1213.

Habitat for Humanity: Habitat for Humanity may provide volunteer labor to construct a ramp if materials are provided.

Habitat for Humanity
Phone: 229-924-6935, ext. 2552
Website: http://www.habitat.org/local

Independent Living: Independent Living Centers (ILCs) are nonresidential, community-based organizations providing services and advocacy for all people with disabilities. Their purpose is to help individuals achieve their maximum potential within their families and communities.

ILC
Phone: 703-525-3406
Website: http://www.virtualcil.net/cils

Veterans Administration (VA): The VA offers income, medical, educational, and vocational rehabilitation assistance to qualified veterans. Veterans with certain mobility impairments can also receive funds for home modifications. The VA may also help them buy, adapt, or repair a vehicle.

Veterans Administration
Toll-Free: 800-827-1000
Website: http://www.va.gov

Vehicle Modification Resources

Nearly 383,000 modified vehicles are currently on the road. A new vehicle with modifications can range from $20,000 to $80,000. Still, no matter what modifications a person needs, there's probably more than one way to soften the blow. Here's a list of opportunities potential buyers might want to explore.

Manufacturer rebates: Most major automobile manufacturers offer rebates of up to $1,000 toward the cost of aftermarket modifications on new vehicles. Website: http://www.nhtsa.dot.gov/cars/rules/adaptive/brochure/index.html.

Used model: Buying a used vehicle for modification can save a person a lot of money, both in retail price and insurance costs. Those

461

who want a new vehicle, on the other hand, should consider waiting until the end of the model year. At this time, dealers are motivated to move their inventory to make room for new models, which gives the buyer a bargaining edge.

Sales tax exemption: Many states will waive the sales tax on adaptive equipment if the buyer has a doctor's prescription for it. The dealer can provide more details.

Tax deductions: Buyers may be able to claim their vehicle modification as a medical expense on their income tax return. A tax consultant can help them determine whether their expenses qualify.

Long-term versus short-term financing: Some dealers will roll the cost of the vehicle and the modifications into a single package that can be financed over a period up to ten years. The good news: lower monthly payments. The bad news: higher interest.

Additional information: The following organizations can provide additional information or help buyers locate companies that adhere to industry standards.

National Highway Traffic Safety Administration (NHTSA)
400 Seventh Street, SW
Washington, DC 20590
Toll-Free: 888-327-4236
Website: http://www.nhtsa.dot.gov

National Mobility Equipment Dealers Association (NMEDA)
3327 West Bears Avenue
Tampa, FL 33618
Toll-Free: 800-833-0427
Fax: 813-962-8970
Website: http://www.nmeda.org
E-mail: nmeda@aol.com

Adaptive Driving Alliance
Phone: 623-434-0722
Website: http://www.adamobility.com

Association for Driver Rehabilitation Specialists
711 South Vienna Street
Ruston, LA 71270
Toll-Free: 800-290-2344
Website: http://www.driver-ed.org

Senior Assistance

Department of Agriculture: The Rural Development program offers 1 percent interest repair loans (up to $15,000) or grants (up to $5,000) to low-income and elderly homeowners. (Ages 62+)

Department of Agriculture—Rural Development Program
Phone: 859-224-7322
Website: http://www.rurdev.usda.gov/recd_map.html

Medicare: Medicare is a health insurance program for people who receive Social Security Administration (SSA) benefits. Most people don't have to apply for Medicare benefits; SSA notifies them when they become eligible. Medicare provides two kinds of coverage. Part A covers inpatient hospital services, nursing facility and home health services, and hospice care. Part B is medical insurance. Individuals pay premiums through an automatic deduction from their SSA check or they get a quarterly bill. Part B covers durable medical equipment (DME), ambulance or doctor's fees, and rehabilitation services. Both Part A and Part B services cover assistive technology. If a person is also eligible for Medicaid, it will cover some or all of the costs not covered by Medicare. (Ages 65+)

Medicare
Toll-Free: 800-633-4227
Website: http://www.medicare.gov/Contacts/Home.asp

Special Purchasing Assistance and Techniques

Medical Discount Programs: Companies that offer medical discount programs negotiate with healthcare providers for discounts on medical goods and services. While such companies stress that they are not a replacement for health insurance, individuals with a preexisting condition or those who cannot afford insurance coverage may find these programs an option worth investigating. Even if a person has insurance, these programs may provide savings on services not covered by insurance. Examples of medical discount programs currently available are as follows:

HealthCove
8016 Buckdale
Indio, CA 92201
Toll-Free: 800-796-5558
Website: http://www.healthcove.com

Care Entrée
Phone: 972-522-2000
Website: http://www.careentree.com

Pharmacy Assistance Programs: Thirty-four states have established or authorized some type of program to provide pharmaceutical coverage or assistance to low-income elderly or disabled individuals who don't qualify for Medicaid.

Pharmacy Assistance Programs
7500 Security Boulevard
Baltimore, MD 21244-1850
Toll-Free: 800-633-4227
Website: http://www.medicare.gov/Prescription/Home.asp

Patient Assistance Programs: These programs are offered by many drug manufacturers to help those who can't afford their medicines obtain them at no cost or low cost. Individuals may call or write the companies to determine if their medication is covered and request the necessary information and paperwork. If a medication isn't covered, there may be an alternative drug available that might qualify. After the paperwork is submitted and approved, the company will ship the medication to the individual through his or her physician. A list of participating companies may be found at http://www.seniorliving .about.com/gi/dynamic/offsite.htm?site=http://needymeds.com.

Making Payments: If asked, prosthetists will occasionally make special payment arrangements for those who simply can't pay for prostheses in any other way.

"One Step at a Time": A common misconception is that if there is a problem with a prosthesis, getting a new one is the only way to go, since insurers often won't cover repairs. If possible, however, individuals can save their money and get one thing done at a time, repairing or replacing components as needed.

Used Equipment: Individuals seeking used DME may advertise in support group newsletters for the components they need, asking readers with unused parts to donate or sell them. A local prosthetist might be willing to install them at low or no cost. Although liability issues can complicate this, individuals can make a "hold-harmless" agreement with those willing to help. They should, however, discuss this with their attorney first.

Several organizations, such as Easter Seals and TAP, accept donated equipment to loan or sell at discount prices. Others serve as a "classifieds" forum where individuals can buy, trade, and sell their equipment.

Easter Seals
Toll-Free: 800-221-6827
Website: http://www.easter-seals.org/site/PageServer

Disabled Dealer Magazine
Toll-Free: 888-521-8778
Website: http://www.disableddealer.com

Worldwide Wheelchairs and Used Medical Equipment
Toll-Free: 800-786-8231
Website: http://www.usedwheelchairs.com

Advocacy

Sometimes, no matter how hard individuals try, or how well they prepare, it may take a third party to overcome obstacles that block the way to the assistance they need. Advocate organizations serve as mediators between them and their insurer, employer, or creditors to resolve insurance, employment, or financial problems related to their medical condition. The following organizations or directories may be able to help:

Patient Advocate Foundation
700 Thimble Shoals Boulevard, Suite 200
Newport News, VA 23606
Toll-Free: 800-532-5274
Website: http://www.patientadvocate.org

National Patient Advocate Foundation

725 15th Street NW, 10th Floor
Washington, DC 20005
Phone: 757-873-0438
Website: http://www.npaf.org

American Bar Association

Toll-Free: 800-285-2221
Website: http://www.abanet.org/disability

Neighborhood Legal Services

Phone: 716-847-0650
Website: http://www.nls.org

National ADA Attorney List

2641-C Chateau Lane
Tallahassee, FL 32311-9453
Phone: 850-942-5505
Website: http://www.istal.com/smoke/smoke4.htm

Chapter 47

Further Reading on Disorders, Diseases, and Injuries of the Foot

Databases

Ankle Injuries and Disorders
http://www.health.nih.gov/result.asp/973

Foot Health
http://www.nlm.nih.gov/medlineplus/foothealth.html

Foot Injuries and Disorders
http://www.nlm.nih.gov/medlineplus/footinjuriesanddisorders.html

Information Websites

PodiatryChannel
http://www.podiatrychannel.com
A medical information website of Healthcommunities.com, Inc., PodiatryChannel is developed and monitored by board-certified physicians and provides comprehensive, trustworthy information about conditions that affect the legs and feet, such as diabetes, osteoarthritis, and heel pain and about treatments, including orthotics.

Resources listed in this chapter were compiled from a variety of sources. Inclusion does not constitute endorsement. This list is not considered complete; it is merely intended to serve as a starting point for readers interested in pursuing additional information. Websites were all verified and accessed in July 2006.

PodiatryNetwork
http://www.podiatrynetwork.com
PodiatryNetwork.com is a comprehensive health information website designed to provide the general public with health information relating to the lower extremities.

Cold Weather Injuries of the Feet

Cold Hurts: Frostbite, Frostnip, and Immersion Foot
http://www.uaf.edu/seagrant/bookstore/pubs/SG-ED-27.pdf

Cold Weather Injuries and Treatment
http://afsafety.af.mil/SEG/crossfeed/documents/coldwet.doc

Environmental Health: Cold Weather
http://www.detrick.army.mil/tenants/ih/ehcold.cfm

Fighting Jack Frost
http://www.narmc.amedd.army.mil/kacc/Pat_Ed/fighting_JF.htm

Outdoor Action Guide to Hypothermia and Cold Weather Injuries
http://www.princeton.edu/~oa/safety/hypocold.shtml

Diagnostic and Treatment Options

Bunion Removal
http://www.nlm.nih.gov/medlineplus/ency/article/002962.htm

Foot Fitness, Health, and Safety

Feet, Legs, and Hips: Maintaining Movement and Independence
http://fcs.tamu.edu/health/Health_Education_Rural_Outreach/Health_Hints/1999/June/Foot.php

Foot Care Library (North Shore Podiatry)
http://www.bunionbusters.com

Foot Fitness for Life: The AOFAS Guide to Keeping Your Feet Young and Healthy
http://www.orthoassociates.com/feet1.htm

Foot Health Conditions and Concerns (APMA pamphlet series)
http://www.foothealthfdn.org

Foot Health Guide (Dr. Scholl's)
http://www.drscholls.com

Pedicure Protection Program
http://www.pedicureprotection.com

Pedicures: Protecting Yourself at the Nail Salon
http://www.mass.gov/dpl/current/tip2004/tip0799.htm

Stepping Up: Foot Care in Later Life
http://extension.oregonstate.edu/fcd/vprograms/fcelessons/fcepdffiles/
footcareparticipant.pdf

Taking Care of Your Feet in **FDA Consumer Magazine March-April 2006**
http://www.fda.gov/fdac/features/2006/206_feet.html

Foot and Leg Problems

Common Foot Disorders
http://www.pubmedcentral.nih.gov/articlerender.fcgi?artid=1183444

Foot Pain: Half of Americans Suffer from Foot Pain
http://www.apma.org/s_apma/doc.asp?CID&DID=19437

Foot Pain
http://adam.about.com/reports/000061_2htm.fullarticle=000061.htm

Leg Problems (Flow Chart to Use to Find Information about Pain, Swelling, or Lumps in the Lower Leg)
http://www.familydoctor.org/x2564.xml

Other Medical Conditions and Their Effect on the Feet

Feet Are a Common Spot for Skin Cancer
http://www.seniorhealthweek.org/NewsStories/skincancer-story
-n2.htm

Diabetes-Related Foot Problems

Feet Can Last a Lifetime: A Health Care Provider's Guide to Preventing Diabetes Foot Problems
http://www.ndep.nih.gov/diabetes/pubs/Feet_HCGuide.pdf

Take Care of Your Feet for a Lifetime
http://ndep.nih.gov/diabetes/pubs/Feet_broch_Eng.pdf
Easy-to read, illustrated patient booklet; provides step-by-step instructions for proper foot care.

Muscular Dystrophy: Putting Your Best Foot Forward in Quest *(Muscular Dystrophy Association)*

http://www.mdausa.org/publications/quest/q125feet.aspx

Stroke: Foot Care after Stroke *(Heart and Stroke Foundation)*

http://ww2.heartandstroke.ca/Page.asp?PageID=33&ArticleID=456&Src=stroke&From=SubCategory

Information about Shoes and Socks

Protective Footwear *(The American National Standards Institute Standard)*

http://www.apparelandfootwear.org/pressreleases/21605PR.pdf

Shoe List *(AAPSM)*

http://www.aapsm.org
The Association of Podiatric Sports Medicine maintains an updated list of recommended shoes for various foot types and activities.

The Ten Points of Proper Shoe Fit

http://www.aofas.org/i4a/pages/index.cfm?pageid=3300

Women's Shoes and Foot Problems *(AOFAS Position Statement)*

http://www.aofas.org/i4a/pages/index.cfm?pageid=3681

Footwear Tips: Toe, Foot, and Ankle Problems, etc. *(Yale New Haven Health—Health Library)*

http://www.ynhh.org/healthlink/womens/womens_6_01.html

Socks and Your Feet

http://www.aapsm.org/socknov97.html

Sports-Related Issues Concerning the Feet

Best Foot Forward Campaign (Road Runners Club of America)
http://www.rrca.org/news/index.php?article=1861

Sports Health and Safety
http://www.pueblo.gsa.gov/cfocus/cfsports05/focus.htm

How Running Impacts the Foot
http://www.feetforlife.org/cgi-bin/item.cgi?ap=1&id=1233&d=pnd& dateformat=%250-%25B

Running and Your Feet
http://www.aapsm.org/running.html

Sports Injuries (NIH Publication No. 04-5278)
http://www.niams.nih.gov/hi/topics/sports_injuries/SportsInjuries.htm

Turf Toe
http://www.ubsportsmed.buffalo.edu/education/turf.html

Chapter 48

A Directory of Foot and Ankle Health Resources

American Academy of Dermatology (AAD)
P.O. Box 4014
Schaumburg, IL 60618-4014
Toll-Free: 866-503-SKIN (7546)
Phone: 847-330-0230
Fax: 847-240-1859
Website: http://www.aad.org
E-mail: MRC@aad.org

The American Academy of Dermatology (AAD) was founded in 1938 to encourage and provide continuing education in dermatology. The Academy sponsors a number of educational events for its membership throughout the year. Educational materials are available for dermatologists, physicians, medical students, allied health professionals, schools, and the public.

American Academy of Family Physicians (AAFP)
11400 Tomahawk Creek Parkway
Leawood, KS 66211-2672
Toll-Free: 800-274-2237
Phone: 913-906-6000

Information on organizations listed in this chapter was compiled from a variety of sources. All contact information was verified in July 2006. Inclusion does not constitute endorsement.

Website: http://www.aafp.org
E-mail: fp@aafp.org

The American Academy of Family Physicians (AAFP) was founded in 1947 to represent the interests of family physicians, provide opportunities for continuing education, and maintain high standards of family practice care. AAFP requires continuing education from its members and promotes the development of family practice medical education. A public education program is conducted to inform the public about family practice.

American Academy of Orthopaedic Surgeons (AAOS)
P.O. Box 2058
Des Plaines, IL 60017
Toll-Free: 800-824-BONE (2663)
Website: http://www.aaos.org

The American Academy of Orthopaedic Surgeons (AAOS) provides education and practice management services for orthopedic surgeons and allied health professionals. It also serves as an advocate for improved patient care and informs the public about the science of orthopedics. The orthopedist's scope of practice includes disorders of the body's bones, joints, ligaments, muscles, and tendons.

American Academy of Orthotists and Prosthetists (AAOP)
526 King Street, Suite 201
Alexandria, VA 22314
Phone: 703-836-0788
Fax: 703-836-0737
Website: http://www.oandp.org

The American Academy of Orthotists and Prosthetists (AAOP) is dedicated to promoting professionalism and advancing the standards of patient care through education, literature, research, advocacy, and collaboration.

American Academy of Pediatrics (AAP)
141 Northwest Point Boulevard
Elk Grove Village, IL 60007
Phone: 847-434-4000
Fax: 847-434-8000
Website: http://www.aap.org

The American Academy of Pediatrics (AAP) and its member pediatricians dedicate their efforts and resources to the health, safety, and well-being of infants, children, adolescents, and young adults. Activities of the AAP include advocacy for children and youth, public education, research, professional education, and membership service and advocacy for pediatricians.

American Academy of Podiatric Sports Medicine (AAPSM)
109 Greenwich Drive
Walkersville, MD 21793-9121
Toll-Free: 888-854-FEET (3338)
Fax: 301-962-3850
Website: http://www.aapsm.org
E-mail: info@aapsm.org

A professional, member organization, AAPSM was founded in 1970 by a group of podiatric sports physicians who saw the need for a podiatric sports medicine association devoted to the treatment of athletic injuries. The major objectives of the AAPSM are: to provide and stimulate programs for research and education; to promote and encourage publication of research findings and other literature pertaining to podiatric sports medicine; to provide a consultative service for those persons engaged in sports medicine; to increase awareness of the medical profession, sports population, and general public to the profession of podiatric sports medicine and modalities available to those who participate in sports; to coordinate student chapters; and to acquaint the podiatric medical student with the needs and demands placed upon athletes.

American Association of Colleges of Podiatric Medicine (AACPM)
15850 Crabbs Branch Way, Suite 320
Rockville, MD 20855
Toll-Free: 800-922-9266
Website: http://www.aacpm.org
E-mail: info@aacpm.org

Doctors of Podiatric Medicine (DPMs) strive to improve the overall health of their patients by focusing on preventing, diagnosing, and treating conditions associated with the foot and ankle. They treat a variety of conditions and employ innovative treatments to improve the well-being of their patients. The American Association of Colleges of Podiatric Medicine's (AACPM) mission is to enhance academic podiatric medicine. AACPM's membership consists of eight colleges and more than 200 hospitals and institutions that offer postdoctoral training in podiatric medicine. The Association serves as a national forum for the exchange of ideas, issues formation and concerns relating to podiatric medical education.

American College of Foot and Ankle Orthopedics and Medicine (ACFAOM)

5272 River Road, Suite 630
Bethesda, MD 20816
Toll-Free: 800-265-8263
Phone: 301-718-6505
Fax: 301-656-0989
Website: http://www.acfaom.org

ACFAOM was founded in 1949 and incorporated in 1951 as the American College of Foot Orthopedists (ACFO). The name was changed in the early 1990's to better reflect the scope of interest of the membership. ACFAOM's purpose is to support scientific study and research to enhance the field of foot orthopedics and related matters in podiatric medicine.

American College of Foot and Ankle Surgeons (ACFAS)

8725 West Higgins Road, Suite 555
Chicago, IL 60631-2724
Toll-Free: 800-421-2237
Phone: 773-693-9300
Fax: 773-693-9304
Website: http://www.acfas.org; Patient Information: http://www.foot physicians.com
E-mail: info@acfas.org

The American College of Foot and Ankle Surgeons is a medical specialty society comprised of more than 6,000 physician members. The mission of the College is to advance the competency of foot and ankle surgeons and the care of their patients by providing continuing education, publishing research, and serving as a source of information to the public.

American College of Rheumatology

1800 Century Place, Suite 250
Atlanta, GA 30345

Phone: 404-633-3777
Fax: 404-633-1870
Website: http://www.rheumatology.org
E-mail: acr@rheumatology.org

The American College of Rheumatology/Association of Rheumatology Health Professionals provides referrals to rheumatologists and physical and occupational therapists who have experience working with people who have a rheumatic disease. The organization also provides educational materials and guidelines about many different rheumatic diseases.

American College of Sports Medicine (ACSM)
401 West Michigan Street
Indianapolis, IN 46202-3233
P.O. Box 1440
Indianapolis, IN 46206-1440
Phone: 317-637-9200 (National Center)
Fax: 317-634-7817
Website: http://www.acsm.org/index.asp

The American College of Sports Medicine (ACSM) is a nonprofit, multi-disciplinary professional membership organization which is dedicated to generating and disseminating knowledge concerning the motivation, responses, adaptations, and health aspects of persons engaged in sport and exercise. ACSM sponsors an annual meeting, a team physician's conference, a variety of workshops and lecture tours; provides continuing medical education; certifies program directors, exercise specialists, exercise test technologists, health/fitness directors, instructors, and aerobic exercise leaders.

American Diabetes Association (ADA)
National Service Center
1701 North Beauregard Street
Alexandria, VA 22311
Toll-Free: 800-DIABETES (342-2383)
Fax: 703-549-6995
Website: http://www.diabetes.org
E-mail: customerservice@diabetes.org

The American Diabetes Association (ADA), formed in 1940, was created to fight diabetes through education and research. Local chapters and affiliates use volunteers to organize educational and screening programs and to conduct fundraising activities to support research aimed at care, control, and cure of diabetes. The Association supports research into the nature and cause of diabetes, more effective means of treatment, factors leading to complications, and prevention and cure of diabetes. Five professional journals keep the medical and scientific communities up to date in their respective fields. Patient educational programs are conducted by the State and metropolitan affiliates.

American Medical Society for Sports Medicine (AMSSM)
11639 Earnshaw
Overland Park, KS 66210
Phone: 913-327-1415
Fax: 913-327-1491
Website: http://www.amssm.org
E-mail: office@amssm.org

The American Medical Society for Sports Medicine (AMSSM) is a multi-disciplinary organization of physicians whose members are dedicated to education, research, collaboration, and fellowship within the field of Sports Medicine. Founded in 1991, the AMSSM is now comprised of over 900 Sports Medicine Physicians whose goal is to provide a link between the rapidly expanding core of knowledge related to sports medicine and its application to patients in a clinical setting.

American Orthopaedic Foot and Ankle Society (AOFAS)
6300 North River Road, Suite 510
Rosemont, IL 60018
Toll-Free: 800-235-4855
Phone: 847-698-4654
Fax: 847-692-3315
Website: http://www.aofas.org
E-mail: aofasinfo@aofas.org

The American Orthopaedic Foot and Ankle Society (AOFAS) is the leading professional organization for orthopedic surgeons specializing in disorder of the foot and ankle. Orthopedic surgeons are medical doctors with extensive training in the diagnosis and treatment of the musculoskeletal system that includes bones, joints, ligaments, tendons, muscles, and nerves.

American Orthopaedic Society for Sports Medicine (AOSSM)
6300 North River Road, Suite 500
Rosemont, IL 60018
Phone: 847-292-4900
Fax: 847-292-4905
Website: http://www.aossm.org
E-mail: aossm@aossm.org

The American Orthopaedic Society for Sports Medicine (AOSSM) is an organization of orthopedic surgeons and allied health professionals dedicated to educating health care professionals and the general public about sports medicine. It promotes and supports educational and research programs in sports medicine, including those concerned with fitness, as well as programs designed to advance knowledge of the recognition, treatment, rehabilitation, and prevention of athletic injuries.

American Physical Therapy Association (APTA)
1111 North Fairfax Street
Alexandria, VA 22314-1488
Toll-Free: 800-999-2782, ext. 3395
Phone: 703-684-2782
Fax: 703-684-7343
Website: http://www.apta.org

The American Physical Therapy Association (APTA) is a national professional organization of physical therapists, physical therapist assistants, and physical therapy students. APTA's objectives are to improve physical therapy practice, research, and education to promote, restore, and maintain optimal physical function, wellness, fitness, and quality of life, especially as they relate to movement and health.

American Podiatric Medical Association (APMA)
9312 Old Georgetown Road
Bethesda, MD 20814-1698
Toll-Free: 800-ASK-APMA
Phone: 301-571-9200
Fax: 301-530-2752
Website: http://www.apma.org
E-mail: askapma@apma.org

The American Podiatric Medical Association (APMA), formerly the American Podiatry Association, was founded in 1912 to improve the quality of foot care in the United States, to attract young people to the profession, and to increase understanding of the profession. It publishes a monthly scientific journal, a monthly magazine, as well as informative brochures. APMA encourages continuing education. It participates in national and community health medicine.

Amputee Coalition of America (ACA)
900 East Hill Avenue, Suite 285
Knoxville, TN 37915-2568
Toll-Free: 888-AMP-KNOW (267-5669)
Phone: 865-524-8772
Fax: 865-525-7917
TTY: 865-525-4512
Website: http://www.amputee-coalition.org

The mission of the Amputee Coalition of America (ACA) is to reach out to people with limb loss and to empower them through education, support and advocacy. The ACA operates the National Limb Loss Information Center (NLLIC), the nation's most comprehensive source of information for people with limb differences.

Arthritis Foundation
1330 West Peachtree Street
Atlanta, GA 30309
Toll-Free: 800-283-7800
Phone: 404-872-7100
Website: http://www.arthritis.org

The Arthritis Foundation is the main voluntary organization devoted to arthritis. The foundation publishes a monthly magazine for members that provides up-to-date information on arthritis. The foundation can also provide physician and clinical referrals.

Charcot-Marie-Tooth Association (CMTA)
2700 Chestnut Street
Chester, PA 19013-4867
Toll-Free: 800-606-2682
Phone: 610-499-9264
Fax: 610-499-9267
Website: http://www.charcot-marie-tooth.org
E-mail: CMTAssoc@aol.com

Provides education and support to persons with Charcot-Marie-Tooth disorders, their families, and the health professionals who treat them.

Lower Extremity Amputation Prevention Program (LEAP)
National Hansen's Disease Programs (NHDP)
1770 Physicians Park Drive
Baton Rouge, Louisiana 70816
Toll-Free: 800-642-2477
Fax: 225-756-3806
Website: http://www.bphc.hrsa.gov

A comprehensive prevention program has been developed at the Bureau of Primary Health Care that can dramatically reduce lower extremity amputations in individuals with diabetes mellitus, Hansen disease, or any condition that results in loss of protective sensation in the feet. The LEAP Program consists of five relatively simple activities: annual foot screening, patient education, daily self inspection of the foot, appropriate footwear selection, and management of simple foot problems

Lupus Foundation of America, Inc. (LFA)
2000 L Street, Northwest, Suite 710
Washington, DC 20036
Toll-Free: 800-558-0121
Phone: 202-349-1155
Fax: 202-349-1156
Website: http://www.lupus.org
E-mail: info@lupus.org

The Lupus Foundation of America, Inc. (LFA) is the main voluntary organization devoted to lupus. The LFA offers information and referral services, health fairs, newsletters, publications, seminars, support group meetings, hospital visits, and telephone help lines.

March of Dimes Birth Defects Foundation
1275 Mamaroneck Avenue
White Plains, NY 10605
Toll-Free: 888-663-4637 (English); 800-925-1855 (Spanish)
Phone: 914-428-7100
Fax: 914-997-4763
Website: http://www.marchofdimes.com

The March of Dimes Birth Defects Foundation was established in 1938. Its mission is to improve the health of babies by preventing birth defects and infant mortality. The mission is carried out through research, community services, education, and advocacy. The March of Dimes public health education materials are targeted to students, school personnel, parents, health professionals, adults of childbearing age, pregnant women, and people in the workplace, to give them information about and help them understand perinatal health, birth defects and related newborn health problems. The Pregnancy and Newborn Health Education Center provides information and referral on pregnancy, pre-pregnancy, birth defects, genetics, drugs, and environmental hazards during pregnancy and related topics.

Muscular Dystrophy Association (MDA)
3300 East Sunrise Drive
Tucson, AZ 85718-3208
Toll-Free: 800-344-4863
Phone: 520-529-2000
Fax: 520-529-5300
Website: http://www.mdausa.org
E-mail: mda@mdausa.org

The Muscular Dystrophy Association, (MDA), is a voluntary health agency aimed at conquering more than 40 neuromuscular diseases that affect more than a million Americans. The diseases in MDA's program include nine forms of muscular dystrophy, amyotrophic lateral sclerosis (Lou Gehrig disease), spinal muscular atrophy, Charcot-Marie-Tooth disease, and other neuromuscular conditions. It conducts programs of worldwide research, comprehensive medical and community services, and far-reaching professional and public education. Services include medical examinations at a network of some 235 hospital-affiliated MDA clinics, support groups, MDA summer camps for youngsters, and assistance with wheelchair purchase and communication devices.

National Diabetes Education Program (NDEP)
1 Diabetes Way
Bethesda, MD 20892-3600
Toll-Free: 800-438-5383
Website: http://ndep.nih.gov

The National Diabetes Education Program (NDEP) is a federally sponsored initiative, involving public and private partners. NDEP's goal is to reduce the morbidity and mortality associated with diabetes and its complications by improving the treatment and outcomes for people with diabetes, promoting early diagnosis, and ultimately, preventing the onset of diabetes. The National Institute of Diabetes and Digestive and Kidney Diseases (NIDDK) of the National Institutes of Health (NIH) and the Centers for Disease Control and Prevention (CDC) are jointly sponsoring the development of the program.

National Diabetes Information Clearinghouse (NDIC)
1 Information Way
Bethesda, MD 20892-3560
Phone: 301-654-3327
Website: http://www.niddk.nih.gov/health/diabetes/ndic

The National Digestive Diseases Information Clearinghouse (NDDIC) is an information and referral service of the NIDDK, one of the National Institutes of Health. A central information resource on the prevention and management of digestive diseases, the Clearinghouse responds to written inquiries, develops and distributes publications about digestive diseases, and provides referrals to digestive disease organizations. Publications distributed by the Clearinghouse are indexed on the Combined Health Information Database (CHID), available on the web at the internet address http://chid.nih.gov. Access is free of charge.

National Institute on Aging
Information Center
P.O. Box 8057
Gaithersburg, MD 20898-8057
Toll-Free: 800-222-2225
TTY: 800-222-4225
Website: http://www.nih.gov/nia

The National Institute on Aging (NIA) was established in 1974 to conduct and support biomedical, social, and behavioral research and training relating to the aging process, and the diseases and other special problems and needs of the aged. The Institute provides for the study of biomedical, psychological, social, educational, and economic aspects of aging through in-house research conducted at its Gerontology Research Center in Baltimore, MD, and through grant support of extramural and collaborative research programs at universities, hospitals, medical centers, and nonprofit institutions throughout the country.

National Institute of Arthritis and Musculoskeletal and Skin Diseases (NIAMS)

National Institutes of Health
1 AMS Circle
Bethesda, MD 20892-3675
Toll-Free: 877-22-NIAMS (266-4267)
Phone: 301-495-4484
Fax: 301-718-6366
TTY: 301-565-2966
Website: http://www.niams.nih.gov

The National Institute of Arthritis and Musculoskeletal and Skin Diseases Information Clearinghouse (NIAMS) provides information about various forms of arthritis and rheumatic disease and bone, muscle, and skin diseases. It distributes patient and professional education materials and refers people to other sources of information.

National Institute of Neurological Disorders and Stroke (NINDS)

P.O. Box 5801
Bethesda, MD 20824
Toll-Free: 800-352-9424
Website: http://www.ninds.nih.gov

The National Institute of Neurological Disorders and Stroke (NINDS) was originally established in 1950. The NINDS conducts and supports research and research training on the causes, prevention, diagnosis, and treatment of neurological disorders and stroke. The Institute awards grants for research projects, program projects, and center grants; provides training support to institutions and fellowships to individuals in the fields of neurological disorders and stroke; conducts intramural and collaborative research; and collects and disseminates research information.

National Parkinson Foundation (NPF)

1501 Northwest Ninth Avenue
Bob Hope Road
Miami, FL 33136
Toll-Free: 800-327-4545
Phone: 305-243-6666; 305-547-6666
Fax: 305-243-5595
Website: http://www.parkinson.org

The National Parkinson Foundation (NPF), founded in 1957, provides answers to patients and their families on problems relating to Parkinson disease and maintains the Bob Hope National Parkinson Research and Rehabilitation Institute, devoted to the diagnosis, treatment, and rehabilitation of Parkinsonism. Physical, speech, and occupational therapies are available at the Institute on an outpatient basis. NPF also conducts research in the cause and possible cure of the disease. NPF sponsors a variety of educational programs, including a national awareness program designed to explain the workings of the Institute and to help the public understand the nature of Parkinson disease. Its toll-free number is for information on the disease, publications, and physician referrals.

Neuropathy Association
P.O. Box 26226
New York, NY 10165-0999
Phone: 212-692-0662
Fax: 212-692-0668
Website: http://www.ncuropathy.org
E-mail: info@neuropathy.org

The mission of this nonprofit organization is to: support research into the causes and treatment of peripheral neuropathies; provide support through education and sharing information and experiences related to peripheral neuropathy; increase public awareness of the nature and extent of peripheral neuropathy and the need for early intervention and research; encourage pharmaceutical and biotechnology companies to develop new therapies and devices for treatment of neuropathy; encourage government support for research into the causes and treatments of neuropathy, and the need for special accommodations and facilities for people with neuropathy; encourage medical providers, including hospitals, HMOs and insurance companies, to provide coverage, proper care and treatment; and participate in national and international awareness, research and information exchange.

Nicholas Institute for Sports Medicine and Athletic Trauma
130 East 77th Street, 10th Floor
New York, NY 10021
Phone: 212-434-2700
Website: http://www.nismat.org

The Nicholas Institute of Sports Medicine and Athletic Trauma (NISMAT)—the first hospital-based facility dedicated to the study of sports medicine in the country—was established at Lenox Hill Hospital in 1973. Since its founding as a research, teaching and clinical center, NISMAT's approach to the treatment of athletic injuries has brought a new perspective to the relationship between exercise and fitness in all age groups. Its ongoing work provides information relevant to everyone who participates in exercise or sports, whether it is a child at play or an elderly person exercising to keep fit, a weekend athlete or a marathon runner.

Pedorthic Footwear Association
7150 Columbia Gateway Drive, Suite G
Columbia, MD 21046-1151
Toll-Free: 800-673-8447 Phone: 410-381-7278
Fax: 410-381-1167
Website: http://www.pedorthics.org

The Pedorthic Footwear Association (PFA), founded in 1958, is the not-for-profit professional association which represents the interests of the certified and/or licensed pedorthist and supports the pedorthic profession at large. Through the efforts of PFA, pedorthics—the design, manufacture, modification and fit of shoes and foot orthoses to alleviate problems caused by disease, congenital condition, overuse or injury—is a well-established allied health profession which makes an invaluable contribution to public health.

St. Jude Children's Research Hospital
332 North Lauderdale
Memphis, TN 38105
Toll-Free: 866-278-5833, ext. 3621
Phone: 901-495-3300
Website: http://www.stjude.org

St. Jude Children's Research Hospital, located in Memphis, TN, is one of the world's premier centers for research and treatment of catastrophic diseases in children, primarily pediatric cancers. The mission of St. Jude Children's Research Hospital is to find cures for children with catastrophic diseases through research and treatment. Patients at St. Jude are accepted by physician referral when the children or adolescents are newly diagnosed or have a disease under research and treatment by the St. Jude staff. St. Jude is the only pediatric research center where families never pay for treatment not covered by insurance, and families without insurance are never asked to pay.

Scleroderma Foundation

300 Rosewood Drive
Suite 105
Danvers, MA 01923
Toll-Free: 800-722-HOPE (4673)
Fax: 978-463-5809
Website: http://www.scleroderma.org
E-mail: sfinfo@scleroderma.org

The Scleroderma Foundation is a voluntary organization which publishes information on scleroderma and funds research. It also offers patient education seminars, support groups, physician referrals, and information hotlines.

Shriners International Headquarters

2900 Rocky Point Drive
Tampa, FL 33607-1460
Toll-Free: 813-281-0300
Website: http://www.shrinershq.org

Shriners Hospitals is a network of 22 pediatric specialty hospitals that provide free orthopedic and burn care to children under the age of 18. There are 18 orthopedic Shriners Hospitals, three Shriners Hospitals dedicated to treating children with burns, and one Shriners Hospital that provides burn and spinal cord injury care. The Hospitals accept neither government funds nor insurance moneys; all care is paid for entirely by Shriners Hospitals. Shriners hospitals serve as a valuable resource for families whose children need specialized expert care but who cannot afford it.

Spondylitis Association of America

P.O. Box 5872
Sherman Oaks, CA 91413
Toll-Free: 800-777-8189
Phone: 818-981-1616
Website: http://www.spondylitis.org
E-mail: info@spondylitis.org

The Spondylitis Association of America is the main voluntary organization devoted to all forms of spondylitis, including reactive arthritis. The association publishes patient and professional materials and a newsletter for members.

Schools of Podiatry

Barry University—School of Graduate Medical Sciences
Podiatric Medicine and Surgery Program
11300 Northeast 2nd Avenue
Miami Shores, FL 33161-6695
Toll-Free: 800-756-6000, ext. 3249
Phone: 305-899-3249
Website: http://www.barry.edu/podiatry/default.asp
E-mail: mweiner@mail.barry.edu

*Arizona Podiatric Medicine Program (AZPod)
at Midwestern University*
19555 North 59th Avenue
Glendale AZ 85308
Toll-Free: 888-247-9277
Phone: 623-572-3275
Website: http://www.midwestern.edu/azpod
E-mail: admissaz@midwestern.edu

*California School of Podiatric Medicine
at Samuel Merritt College*
370 Hawthorne Avenue
Oakland, CA 94609
Toll-Free: 800-607-6377
Phone: 510-869-6727
Fax: 510-869-6525
Website: http://www.samuelmerritt.edu/default.cfm
E-mail: information@samuelmerritt.edu

*College of Podiatric Medicine and Surgery
at Des Moines University*
3200 Grand Avenue
Des Moines, IA 50312
Phone: 515-271-7497
Fax: 515-271-7075
Website: http://www.dmu.edu/cpms
E-mail: cpmsadmit@dmu.edu

New York College of Podiatric Medicine
1800 Park Avenue
New York, NY 10035
Toll-Free: 800-526-6966
Phone: 212-410-8053
Fax: 212-722-4918
Website: http://www.nycpm.edu
E-mail: admissions@nycpm.edu

Ohio College of Podiatric Medicine
10515 Carnegie Avenue
Cleveland, OH 44106-9990
Toll-Free: 800-238-7903
Phone: 216-231-3300
Fax: 216-231-6537
Website: http://www.ocpm.edu

Scholl College of Podiatric Medicine
at Rosalind Franklin University of Medicine and Science
3333 Green Bay Road
North Chicago, IL 60064
Toll-Free: 800-843-3059
Phone: 847-578-8400
Website: http://www.rosalindfranklin.edu/scpm
E-mal: scholl.admission@rosalindfranklin.edu

Temple University School of Podiatric Medicine
Eighth at Race Street
Philadelphia, PA 19107
Toll-Free: 800-220-FEET
Phone: 215-625-5448
Fax: 215-627-2815
Website: http://podiatry.temple.edu

Index

Index

Page numbers followed by 'n' indicate a footnote. Page numbers in *italics* indicate a table or illustration.

A

AACPM *see* American Association of Colleges of Podiatric Medicine
AAD *see* American Academy of Dermatology
AAFP *see* American Academy of Family Physicians
AAOP *see* American Academy of Orthotists and Prosthetists
AAOS *see* American Academy of Orthopaedic Surgeons
AAP *see* American Academy of Pediatrics
AAPSM *see* American Academy of Podiatric Sports Medicine
abduction, defined 445
ablation, defined 445
ACA *see* Amputee Coalition of America
accessory navicular 302–4
acetaminophen 346
ACFAOM *see* American College of Foot and Ankle Orthopedics and Medicine

ACFAS *see* American College of Foot and Ankle Surgeons
Achilles tendon
    calcaneovalgus 35
    clubfoot 35
    described 7, 31
    diabetic foot ulcers 368–69
    flat feet 178
Achilles tendonitis
    described 7, 42
    heel pain 170
    overview 257–61
Achilles tendon rupture 258
ACSM *see* American College of Sports Medicine
acute injury, *versus* chronic injury 84–85
acute strain, described 224
ADA *see* American Diabetes Association
A.D.A.M., Inc., publications
    ankle replacement 139n
    foot spasms 197n
    hammer toe 319n
    hand spasms 197n
    peripheral swelling 329n
    pes planus 299n
Adaptive Driving Alliance, contact information 462

Health Reference Series

COMPLETE CATALOG

List price $87 per volume. **School and library price $78 per volume.**

Adolescent Health Sourcebook, 2nd Edition

Basic Consumer Health Information about the Physical, Mental, and Emotional Growth and Development of Adolescents, Including Medical Care, Nutritional and Physical Activity Requirements, Puberty, Sexual Activity, Acne, Tanning, Body Piercing, Common Physical Illnesses and Disorders, Eating Disorders, Attention Deficit Hyperactivity Disorder, Depression, Bullying, Hazing, and Adolescent Injuries Related to Sports, Driving, and Work

Along with Substance Abuse Information about Nicotine, Alcohol, and Drug Use, a Glossary, and Directory of Additional Resources

Edited by Joyce Brennfleck Shannon. 683 pages. 2006. 978-0-7808-0943-7.

"It is written in clear, nontechnical language aimed at general readers. . . . Recommended for public libraries, community colleges, and other agencies serving health care consumers."
— *American Reference Books Annual, 2003*

"Recommended for school and public libraries. Parents and professionals dealing with teens will appreciate the easy-to-follow format and the clearly written text. This could become a 'must have' for every high school teacher." — *E-Streams, Jan '03*

"A good starting point for information related to common medical, mental, and emotional concerns of adolescents." — *School Library Journal, Nov '02*

"This book provides accurate information in an easy to access format. It addresses topics that parents and caregivers might not be aware of and provides practical, useable information."
— *Doody's Health Sciences Book Review Journal, Sep-Oct '02*

"Recommended reference source."
— *Booklist, American Library Association, Sep '02*

AIDS Sourcebook, 3rd Edition

Basic Consumer Health Information about Acquired Immune Deficiency Syndrome (AIDS) and Human Immunodeficiency Virus (HIV) Infection, Including Facts about Transmission, Prevention, Diagnosis, Treatment, Opportunistic Infections, and Other Complications, with a Section for Women and Children, Including Details about Associated Gynecological Concerns, Pregnancy, and Pediatric Care

Along with Updated Statistical Information, Reports on Current Research Initiatives, a Glossary, and Directories of Internet, Hotline, and Other Resources

Edited by Dawn D. Matthews. 664 pages. 2003. 978-0-7808-0631-3.

"The 3rd edition of the *AIDS Sourcebook*, part of Omnigraphics' *Health Reference Series*, is a welcome update. . . . This resource is highly recommended for academic and public libraries."
— *American Reference Books Annual, 2004*

"Excellent sourcebook. This continues to be a highly recommended book. There is no other book that provides as much information as this book provides."
— *AIDS Book Review Journal, Dec-Jan '00*

"Recommended reference source."
— *Booklist, American Library Association, Dec '99*

Alcoholism Sourcebook, 2nd Edition

Basic Consumer Health Information about Alcohol Use, Abuse, and Dependence, Featuring Facts about the Physical, Mental, and Social Health Effects of Alcohol Addiction, Including Alcoholic Liver Disease, Pancreatic Disease, Cardiovascular Disease, Neurological Disorders, and the Effects of Drinking during Pregnancy

Along with Information about Alcohol Treatment, Medications, and Recovery Programs, in Addition to Tips for Reducing the Prevalence of Underage Drinking, Statistics about Alcohol Use, a Glossary of Related Terms, and Directories of Resources for More Help and Information

Edited by Amy L. Sutton. 653 pages. 2006. 978-0-7808-0942-0.

"This title is one of the few reference works on alcoholism for general readers. For some readers this will be a welcome complement to the many self-help books on the market. Recommended for collections serving general readers and consumer health collections."
— *E-Streams, Mar '01*

"This book is an excellent choice for public and academic libraries."
— *American Reference Books Annual, 2001*

"Recommended reference source."
— *Booklist, American Library Association, Dec '00*

"Presents a wealth of information on alcohol use and abuse and its effects on the body and mind, treatment, and prevention." — *SciTech Book News, Dec '00*

"Important new health guide which packs in the latest consumer information about the problems of alcoholism." — *Reviewer's Bookwatch, Nov '00*

SEE ALSO Drug Abuse Sourcebook,

517

Allergies Sourcebook, 2nd Edition

Basic Consumer Health Information about Allergic Disorders, Triggers, Reactions, and Related Symptoms, Including Anaphylaxis, Rhinitis, Sinusitis, Asthma, Dermatitis, Conjunctivitis, and Multiple Chemical Sensitivity

Along with Tips on Diagnosis, Prevention, and Treatment, Statistical Data, a Glossary, and a Directory of Sources for Further Help and Information

Edited by Annemarie S. Muth. 598 pages. 2002. 978-0-7808-0376-3.

"This book brings a great deal of useful material together. . . . This is an excellent addition to public and consumer health library collections."
— *American Reference Books Annual, 2003*

"This second edition would be useful to laypersons with little or advanced knowledge of the subject matter. This book would also serve as a resource for nursing and other health care professions students. It would be useful in public, academic, and hospital libraries with consumer health collections." — *E-Streams, Jul '02*

Alternative Medicine Sourcebook

SEE *Complementary & Alternative Medicine Sourcebook, 3rd Edition*

Alzheimer's Disease Sourcebook, 3rd Edition

Basic Consumer Health Information about Alzheimer's Disease, Other Dementias, and Related Disorders, Including Multi-Infarct Dementia, AIDS Dementia Complex, Dementia with Lewy Bodies, Huntington's Disease, Wernicke-Korsakoff Syndrome (Alcohol-Related Dementia), Delirium, and Confusional States

Along with Information for People Newly Diagnosed with Alzheimer's Disease and Caregivers, Reports Detailing Current Research Efforts in Prevention, Diagnosis, and Treatment, Facts about Long-Term Care Issues, and Listings of Sources for Additional Information

Edited by Karen Bellenir. 645 pages. 2003. 978-0-7808-0666-5.

"This very informative and valuable tool will be a great addition to any library serving consumers, students and health care workers."
— *American Reference Books Annual, 2004*

"This is a valuable resource for people affected by dementias such as Alzheimer's. It is easy to navigate and includes important information and resources."
— *Doody's Review Service, Feb '04*

"Recommended reference source."
— *Booklist, American Library Association, Oct '99*

SEE ALSO *Brain Disorders Sourcebook*

Arthritis Sourcebook, 2nd Edition

Basic Consumer Health Information about Osteoarthritis, Rheumatoid Arthritis, Other Rheumatic Disorders, Infectious Forms of Arthritis, and Diseases with Symptoms Linked to Arthritis, Featuring Facts about Diagnosis, Pain Management, and Surgical Therapies

Along with Coping Strategies, Research Updates, a Glossary, and Resources for Additional Help and Information

Edited by Amy L. Sutton. 593 pages. 2004. 978-0-7808-0667-2.

"This easy-to-read volume is recommended for consumer health collections within public or academic libraries." — *E-Streams, May '05*

"As expected, this updated edition continues the excellent reputation of this series in providing sound, usable health information. . . . Highly recommended."
— *American Reference Books Annual, 2005*

"Excellent reference." — *The Bookwatch, Jan '05*

Asthma Sourcebook, 2nd Edition

Basic Consumer Health Information about the Causes, Symptoms, Diagnosis, and Treatment of Asthma in Infants, Children, Teenagers, and Adults, Including Facts about Different Types of Asthma, Common Co-Occurring Conditions, Asthma Management Plans, Triggers, Medications, and Medication Delivery Devices

Along with Asthma Statistics, Research Updates, a Glossary, a Directory of Asthma-Related Resources, and More

Edited by Karen Bellenir. 609 pages. 2006. 978-0-7808-0866-9.

"A worthwhile reference acquisition for public libraries and academic medical libraries whose readers desire a quick introduction to the wide range of asthma information." — *Choice, Association of College & Research Libraries, Jun '01*

"Recommended reference source."
— *Booklist, American Library Association, Feb '01*

"Highly recommended." — *The Bookwatch, Jan '01*

"There is much good information for patients and their families who deal with asthma daily."
— *American Medical Writers Association Journal, Winter '01*

"This informative text is recommended for consumer health collections in public, secondary school, and community college libraries and the libraries of universities with a large undergraduate population."
— *American Reference Books Annual, 2001*

Attention Deficit Disorder Sourcebook

Basic Consumer Health Information about Attention Deficit/Hyperactivity Disorder in Children and Adults,

Including Facts about Causes, Symptoms, Diagnostic Criteria, and Treatment Options Such as Medications, Behavior Therapy, Coaching, and Homeopathy

Along with Reports on Current Research Initiatives, Legal Issues, and Government Regulations, and Featuring a Glossary of Related Terms, Internet Resources, and a List of Additional Reading Material

Edited by Dawn D. Matthews. 470 pages. 2002. 978-0-7808-0624-5.

"Recommended reference source."
—Booklist, American Library Association, Jan '03

"This book is recommended for all school libraries and the reference or consumer health sections of public libraries." —American Reference Books Annual, 2003

Back & Neck Sourcebook, 2nd Edition

Basic Consumer Health Information about Spinal Pain, Spinal Cord Injuries, and Related Disorders, Such as Degenerative Disk Disease, Osteoarthritis, Scoliosis, Sciatica, Spina Bifida, and Spinal Stenosis, and Featuring Facts about Maintaining Spinal Health, Self-Care, Pain Management, Rehabilitative Care, Chiropractic Care, Spinal Surgeries, and Complementary Therapies

Along with Suggestions for Preventing Back and Neck Pain, a Glossary of Related Terms, and a Directory of Resources

Edited by Amy L. Sutton. 633 pages. 2004. 978-0-7808-0738-9.

"Recommended . . . an easy to use, comprehensive medical reference book." —E-Streams, Sep '05

"The strength of this work is its basic, easy-to-read format. Recommended." —Reference and User Services Quarterly, American Library Association, Winter '97

Blood & Circulatory Disorders Sourcebook, 2nd Edition

Basic Consumer Health Information about the Blood and Circulatory System and Related Disorders, Such as Anemia and Other Hemoglobin Diseases, Cancer of the Blood and Associated Bone Marrow Disorders, Clotting and Bleeding Problems, and Conditions That Affect the Veins, Blood Vessels, and Arteries, Including Facts about the Donation and Transplantation of Bone Marrow, Stem Cells, and Blood and Tips for Keeping the Blood and Circulatory System Healthy

Along with a Glossary of Related Terms and Resources for Additional Help and Information

Edited by Amy L. Sutton. 659 pages. 2005. 978-0-7808-0746-4.

"Highly recommended pick for basic consumer health reference holdings at all levels."
—The Bookwatch, Aug '05

"Recommended reference source."
—Booklist, American Library Association, Feb '99

"An important reference sourcebook written in simple language for everyday, non-technical users. "
—Reviewer's Bookwatch, Jan '99

Brain Disorders Sourcebook, 2nd Edition

Basic Consumer Health Information about Acquired and Traumatic Brain Injuries, Infections of the Brain, Epilepsy and Seizure Disorders, Cerebral Palsy, and Degenerative Neurological Disorders, Including Amyotrophic Lateral Sclerosis (ALS), Dementias, Multiple Sclerosis, and More

Along with Information on the Brain's Structure and Function, Treatment and Rehabilitation Options, Reports on Current Research Initiatives, a Glossary of Terms Related to Brain Disorders and Injuries, and a Directory of Sources for Further Help and Information

Edited by Sandra J. Judd. 625 pages. 2005. 978-0-7808-0744-0.

"Highly recommended pick for basic consumer health reference holdings at all levels."
—The Bookwatch, Aug '05

"Belongs on the shelves of any library with a consumer health collection." —E-Streams, Mar '00

"Recommended reference source."
—Booklist, American Library Association, Oct '99

SEE ALSO Alzheimer's Disease Sourcebook

Breast Cancer Sourcebook, 2nd Edition

Basic Consumer Health Information about Breast Cancer, Including Facts about Risk Factors, Prevention, Screening and Diagnostic Methods, Treatment Options, Complementary and Alternative Therapies, Post-Treatment Concerns, Clinical Trials, Special Risk Populations, and New Developments in Breast Cancer Research

Along with Breast Cancer Statistics, a Glossary of Related Terms, and a Directory of Resources for Additional Help and Information

Edited by Sandra J. Judd. 595 pages. 2004. 978-0-7808-0668-9.

"This book will be an excellent addition to public, community college, medical, and academic libraries."
—American Reference Books Annual, 2006

"It would be a useful reference book in a library or on loan to women in a support group."
—Cancer Forum, Mar '03

"Recommended reference source."
—Booklist, American Library Association, Jan '02

"This reference source is highly recommended. It is quite informative, comprehensive and detailed in nature, and yet it offers practical advice in easy-to-read language. It could be thought of as the 'bible' of breast cancer for the consumer." — *E-Streams, Jan '02*

"From the pros and cons of different screening methods and results to treatment options, *Breast Cancer Sourcebook* provides the latest information on the subject."
— *Library Bookwatch, Dec '01*

"This thoroughgoing, very readable reference covers all aspects of breast health and cancer. . . . Readers will find much to consider here. Recommended for all public and patient health collections."
— *Library Journal, Sep '01*

SEE ALSO *Cancer Sourcebook for Women, Women's Health Concerns Sourcebook*

■

Breastfeeding Sourcebook

Basic Consumer Health Information about the Benefits of Breastmilk, Preparing to Breastfeed, Breastfeeding as a Baby Grows, Nutrition, and More, Including Information on Special Situations and Concerns Such as Mastitis, Illness, Medications, Allergies, Multiple Births, Prematurity, Special Needs, and Adoption

Along with a Glossary and Resources for Additional Help and Information

Edited by Jenni Lynn Colson. 388 pages. 2002. 978-0-7808-0332-9.

"Particularly useful is the information about professional lactation services and chapters on breastfeeding when returning to work. . . . *Breastfeeding Sourcebook* will be useful for public libraries, consumer health libraries, and technical schools offering nurse assistant training, especially in areas where Internet access is problematic."
— *American Reference Books Annual, 2003*

SEE ALSO *Pregnancy & Birth Sourcebook*

■

Burns Sourcebook

Basic Consumer Health Information about Various Types of Burns and Scalds, Including Flame, Heat, Cold, Electrical, Chemical, and Sun Burns

Along with Information on Short-Term and Long-Term Treatments, Tissue Reconstruction, Plastic Surgery, Prevention Suggestions, and First Aid

Edited by Allan R. Cook. 604 pages. 1999. 978-0-7808-0204-9.

"This is an exceptional addition to the series and is highly recommended for all consumer health collections, hospital libraries, and academic medical centers."
— *E-Streams, Mar '00*

"This key reference guide is an invaluable addition to all health care and public libraries in confronting this ongoing health issue."
— *American Reference Books Annual, 2000*

"Recommended reference source."
— *Booklist, American Library Association, Dec '99*

SEE ALSO *Dermatological Disorders Sourcebook*

Cancer Sourcebook, 4th Edition

Basic Consumer Health Information about Major Forms and Stages of Cancer, Featuring Facts about Head and Neck Cancers, Lung Cancers, Gastrointestinal Cancers, Genitourinary Cancers, Lymphomas, Blood Cell Cancers, Endocrine Cancers, Skin Cancers, Bone Cancers, Sarcomas, and Others, and Including Information about Cancer Treatments and Therapies, Identifying and Reducing Cancer Risks, and Strategies for Coping with Cancer and the Side Effects of Treatment

Along with a Cancer Glossary, Statistical and Demographic Data, and a Directory of Sources for Additional Help and Information

Edited by Karen Bellenir. 1,119 pages. 2003. 978-0-7808-0633-7.

"With cancer being the second leading cause of death for Americans, a prodigious work such as this one, which locates centrally so much cancer-related information, is clearly an asset to this nation's citizens and others."
— *Journal of the National Medical Association, 2004*

"This title is recommended for health sciences and public libraries with consumer health collections."
— *E-Streams, Feb '01*

". . . can be effectively used by cancer patients and their families who are looking for answers in a language they can understand. Public and hospital libraries should have it on their shelves."
— *American Reference Books Annual, 2001*

"Recommended reference source."
— *Booklist, American Library Association, Dec '00*

SEE ALSO *Breast Cancer Sourcebook, Cancer Sourcebook for Women, Pediatric Cancer Sourcebook, Prostate Cancer Sourcebook*

■

Cancer Sourcebook for Women, 3rd Edition

Basic Consumer Health Information about Leading Causes of Cancer in Women, Featuring Facts about Gynecologic Cancers and Related Concerns, Such as Breast Cancer, Cervical Cancer, Endometrial Cancer, Uterine Sarcoma, Vaginal Cancer, Vulvar Cancer, and Common Non-Cancerous Gynecologic Conditions, in Addition to Facts about Lung Cancer, Colorectal Cancer, and Thyroid Cancer in Women

Along with Information about Cancer Risk Factors, Screening and Prevention, Treatment Options, and Tips on Coping with Life after Cancer Treatment, a Glossary of Cancer Terms, and a Directory of Resources for Additional Help and Information

Edited by Amy L. Sutton. 715 pages. 2006. 978-0-7808-0867-6.

"An excellent addition to collections in public, consumer health, and women's health libraries."
— *American Reference Books Annual, 2003*

"Overall, the information is excellent, and complex topics are clearly explained. As a reference book for the consumer it is a valuable resource to assist them to make informed decisions about cancer and its treatments." — *Cancer Forum, Nov '02*

"Highly recommended for academic and medical reference collections." — *Library Bookwatch, Sep '02*

"This is a highly recommended book for any public or consumer library, being reader friendly and containing accurate and helpful information." — *E-Streams, Aug '02*

"Recommended reference source." — *Booklist, American Library Association, Jul '02*

SEE ALSO *Breast Cancer Sourcebook, Women's Health Concerns Sourcebook*

■

Cardiovascular Diseases & Disorders Sourcebook, 3rd Edition

Basic Consumer Health Information about Heart and Vascular Diseases and Disorders, Such as Angina, Heart Attacks, Arrhythmias, Cardiomyopathy, Valve Disease, Atherosclerosis, and Aneurysms, with Information about Managing Cardiovascular Risk Factors and Maintaining Heart Health, Medications and Procedures Used to Treat Cardiovascular Disorders, and Concerns of Special Significance to Women

Along with Reports on Current Research Initiatives, a Glossary of Related Medical Terms, and a Directory of Sources for Further Help and Information

Edited by Sandra J. Judd. 713 pages. 2005. 978-0-7808-0739-6.

"This updated sourcebook is still the best first stop for comprehensive introductory information on cardiovascular diseases." — *American Reference Books Annual, 2006*

"Recommended for public libraries and libraries supporting health care professionals." — *E-Streams, Sep '05*

"This should be a standard health library reference." — *The Bookwatch, Jun '05*

"Recommended reference source." — *Booklist, American Library Association, Dec '00*

". . . comprehensive format provides an extensive overview on this subject." — *Choice, Association of College & Research Libraries*

■

Caregiving Sourcebook

Basic Consumer Health Information for Caregivers, Including a Profile of Caregivers, Caregiving Responsibilities and Concerns, Tips for Specific Conditions, Care Environments, and the Effects of Caregiving

Along with Facts about Legal Issues, Financial Information, and Future Planning, a Glossary, and a Listing of Additional Resources

Edited by Joyce Brennfleck Shannon. 600 pages. 2001. 978-0-7808-0331-2.

"Essential for most collections." — *Library Journal, Apr 1, 2002*

"An ideal addition to the reference collection of any public library. Health sciences information professionals may also want to acquire the *Caregiving Sourcebook* for their hospital or academic library for use as a ready reference tool by health care workers interested in aging and caregiving." — *E-Streams, Jan '02*

"Recommended reference source." — *Booklist, American Library Association, Oct '01*

■

Child Abuse Sourcebook

Basic Consumer Health Information about the Physical, Sexual, and Emotional Abuse of Children, with Additional Facts about Neglect, Munchausen Syndrome by Proxy (MSBP), Shaken Baby Syndrome, and Controversial Issues Related to Child Abuse, Such as Withholding Medical Care, Corporal Punishment, and Child Maltreatment in Youth Sports, and Featuring Facts about Child Protective Services, Foster Care, Adoption, Parenting Challenges, and Other Abuse Prevention Efforts

Along with a Glossary of Related Terms and Resources for Additional Help and Information

Edited by Dawn D. Matthews. 620 pages. 2004. 978-0-7808-0705-1.

"A valuable and highly recommended resource for school, academic and public libraries whether used on its own or as a starting point for more in-depth research." — *E-Streams, Apr '05*

"Every week the news brings cases of child abuse or neglect, so it is useful to have a source that supplies so much helpful information. . . . Recommended. Public and academic libraries, and child welfare offices." — *Choice, Association of College & Research Libraries, Mar '05*

"Packed with insights on all kinds of issues, from foster care and adoption to parenting and abuse prevention." — *The Bookwatch, Nov '04*

SEE ALSO: *Domestic Violence Sourcebook, 2nd Edition*

■

Childhood Diseases & Disorders Sourcebook

Basic Consumer Health Information about Medical Problems Often Encountered in Pre-Adolescent Children, Including Respiratory Tract Ailments, Ear Infections, Sore Throats, Disorders of the Skin and Scalp, Digestive and Genitourinary Diseases, Infectious Diseases, Inflammatory Disorders, Chronic Physical and Developmental Disorders, Allergies, and More

Along with Information about Diagnostic Tests, Common Childhood Surgeries, and Frequently Used Medications, with a Glossary of Important Terms and Resource Directory

Edited by Chad T. Kimball. 662 pages. 2003. 978-0-7808-0458-6.

"This is an excellent book for new parents and should be included in all health care and public libraries." — *American Reference Books Annual, 2004*

SEE ALSO: *Healthy Children Sourcebook*

Colds, Flu & Other Common Ailments Sourcebook

Basic Consumer Health Information about Common Ailments and Injuries, Including Colds, Coughs, the Flu, Sinus Problems, Headaches, Fever, Nausea and Vomiting, Menstrual Cramps, Diarrhea, Constipation, Hemorrhoids, Back Pain, Dandruff, Dry and Itchy Skin, Cuts, Scrapes, Sprains, Bruises, and More

Along with Information about Prevention, Self-Care, Choosing a Doctor, Over-the-Counter Medications, Folk Remedies, and Alternative Therapies, and Including a Glossary of Important Terms and a Directory of Resources for Further Help and Information

Edited by Chad T. Kimball. 638 pages. 2001. 978-0-7808-0435-7.

"A good starting point for research on common illnesses. It will be a useful addition to public and consumer health library collections."
— *American Reference Books Annual, 2002*

"Will prove valuable to any library seeking to maintain a current, comprehensive reference collection of health resources. . . . Excellent reference."
— *The Bookwatch, Aug '01*

"Recommended reference source."
— *Booklist, American Library Association, Jul '01*

Communication Disorders Sourcebook

Basic Information about Deafness and Hearing Loss, Speech and Language Disorders, Voice Disorders, Balance and Vestibular Disorders, and Disorders of Smell, Taste, and Touch

Edited by Linda M. Ross. 533 pages. 1996. 978-0-7808-0077-9.

"This is skillfully edited and is a welcome resource for the layperson. It should be found in every public and medical library." — *Booklist Health Sciences Supplement, American Library Association, Oct '97*

Complementary & Alternative Medicine Sourcebook, 3rd Edition

Basic Consumer Health Information about Complementary and Alternative Medical Therapies, Including Acupuncture, Ayurveda, Traditional Chinese Medicine, Herbal Medicine, Homeopathy, Naturopathy, Biofeedback, Hypnotherapy, Yoga, Art Therapy, Aromatherapy, Clinical Nutrition, Vitamin and Mineral Supplements, Chiropractic, Massage, Reflexology, Crystal Therapy, Therapeutic Touch, and More

Along with Facts about Alternative and Complementary Treatments for Specific Conditions Such as Cancer, Diabetes, Osteoarthritis, Chronic Pain, Menopause,

Gastrointestinal Disorders, Headaches, and Mental Illness, a Glossary, and a Resource List for Additional Help and Information

Edited by Sandra J. Judd. 657 pages. 2006. 978-0-7808-0864-5.

"Recommended for public, high school, and academic libraries that have consumer health collections. Hospital libraries that also serve the public will find this to be a useful resource." — *E-Streams, Feb '03*

"Recommended reference source."
— *Booklist, American Library Association, Jan '03*

"An important alternate health reference."
— *MBR Bookwatch, Oct '02*

"A great addition to the reference collection of every type of library." — *American Reference Books Annual, 2000*

Congenital Disorders Sourcebook, 2nd Edition

Basic Consumer Health Information about Nonhereditary Birth Defects and Disorders Related to Prematurity, Gestational Injuries, Congenital Infections, and Birth Complications, Including Heart Defects, Hydrocephalus, Spina Bifida, Cleft Lip and Palate, Cerebral Palsy, and More

Along with Facts about the Prevention of Birth Defects, Fetal Surgery and Other Treatment Options, Research Initiatives, a Glossary of Related Terms, and Resources for Additional Information and Support

Edited by Sandra J. Judd. 647 pages. 2006. 978-978-0-7808-0945-1.

"Recommended reference source."
— *Booklist, American Library Association, Oct '97*

SEE ALSO *Pregnancy & Birth Sourcebook*

Contagious Diseases Sourcebook

Basic Consumer Health Information about Infectious Diseases Spread by Person-to-Person Contact through Direct Touch, Airborne Transmission, Sexual Contact, or Contact with Blood or Other Body Fluids, Including Hepatitis, Herpes, Influenza, Lice, Measles, Mumps, Pinworm, Ringworm, Severe Acute Respiratory Syndrome (SARS), Streptococcal Infections, Tuberculosis, and Others

Along with Facts about Disease Transmission, Antimicrobial Resistance, and Vaccines, with a Glossary and Directories of Resources for More Information

Edited by Karen Bellenir. 643 pages. 2004. 978-0-7808-0736-5.

"This easy-to-read volume is recommended for consumer health collections within public or academic libraries." — *E-Streams, May '05*

"This informative book is highly recommended for public libraries, consumer health collections, and secondary schools and undergraduate libraries."
— *American Reference Books Annual, 2005*

"Excellent reference." — *The Bookwatch, Jan '05*

Death & Dying Sourcebook, 2nd Edition

Basic Consumer Health Information about End-of-Life Care and Related Perspectives and Ethical Issues, Including End-of-Life Symptoms and Treatments, Pain Management, Quality-of-Life Concerns, the Use of Life Support, Patients' Rights and Privacy Issues, Advance Directives, Physician-Assisted Suicide, Caregiving, Organ and Tissue Donation, Autopsies, Funeral Arrangements, and Grief

Along with Statistical Data, Information about the Leading Causes of Death, a Glossary, and Directories of Support Groups and Other Resources

Edited by Joyce Brennfleck Shannon. 653 pages. 2006. 978-0-7808-0871-3.

"Public libraries, medical libraries, and academic libraries will all find this sourcebook a useful addition to their collections."
— *American Reference Books Annual, 2001*

"An extremely useful resource for those concerned with death and dying in the United States."
— *Respiratory Care, Nov '00*

"Recommended reference source."
—*Booklist, American Library Association, Aug '00*

"This book is a definite must for all those involved in end-of-life care." — *Doody's Review Service, 2000*

Dental Care & Oral Health Sourcebook, 2nd Edition

Basic Consumer Health Information about Dental Care, Including Oral Hygiene, Dental Visits, Pain Management, Cavities, Crowns, Bridges, Dental Implants, and Fillings, and Other Oral Health Concerns, Such as Gum Disease, Bad Breath, Dry Mouth, Genetic and Developmental Abnormalities, Oral Cancers, Orthodontics, and Temporomandibular Disorders

Along with Updates on Current Research in Oral Health, a Glossary, a Directory of Dental and Oral Health Organizations, and Resources for People with Dental and Oral Health Disorders

Edited by Amy L. Sutton. 609 pages. 2003. 978-0-7808-0634-4.

"This book could serve as a turning point in the battle to educate consumers in issues concerning oral health."
— *American Reference Books Annual, 2004*

"Unique source which will fill a gap in dental sources for patients and the lay public. A valuable reference tool even in a library with thousands of books on dentistry. Comprehensive, clear, inexpensive, and easy to read and use. It fills an enormous gap in the health care literature." — *Reference & User Services Quarterly, American Library Association, Summer '98*

"Recommended reference source."
—*Booklist, American Library Association, Dec '97*

Depression Sourcebook

Basic Consumer Health Information about Unipolar Depression, Bipolar Disorder, Postpartum Depression, Seasonal Affective Disorder, and Other Types of Depression in Children, Adolescents, Women, Men, the Elderly, and Other Selected Populations

Along with Facts about Causes, Risk Factors, Diagnostic Criteria, Treatment Options, Coping Strategies, Suicide Prevention, a Glossary, and a Directory of Sources for Additional Help and Information

Edited by Karen Belleni. 602 pages. 2002. 978-0-7808-0611-5.

"*Depression Sourcebook* is of a very high standard. Its purpose, which is to serve as a reference source to the lay reader, is very well served."
— *Journal of the National Medical Association, 2004*

"Invaluable reference for public and school library collections alike." — *Library Bookwatch, Apr '03*

"Recommended for purchase."
— *American Reference Books Annual, 2003*

Dermatological Disorders Sourcebook, 2nd Edition

Basic Consumer Health Information about Conditions and Disorders Affecting the Skin, Hair, and Nails, Such as Acne, Rosacea, Rashes, Dermatitis, Pigmentation Disorders, Birthmarks, Skin Cancer, Skin Injuries, Psoriasis, Scleroderma, and Hair Loss, Including Facts about Medications and Treatments for Dermatological Disorders and Tips for Maintaining Healthy Skin, Hair, and Nails

Along with Information about How Aging Affects the Skin, a Glossary of Related Terms, and a Directory of Resources for Additional Help and Information

Edited by Amy L. Sutton. 645 pages. 2005. 978-0-7808-0795-2.

". . . comprehensive, easily read reference book."
—*Doody's Health Sciences Book Reviews, Oct '97*

SEE ALSO Burns Sourcebook

Diabetes Sourcebook, 3rd Edition

Basic Consumer Health Information about Type 1 Diabetes (Insulin-Dependent or Juvenile-Onset Diabetes), Type 2 Diabetes (Noninsulin-Dependent or Adult-Onset Diabetes), Gestational Diabetes, Impaired Glucose Tolerance (IGT), and Related Complications, Such as Amputation, Eye Disease, Gum Disease, Nerve Damage, and End-Stage Renal Disease, Including Facts about Insulin, Oral Diabetes Medications, Blood Sugar Testing, and the Role of Exercise and Nutrition in the Control of Diabetes

Along with a Glossary and Resources for Further Help and Information

Edited by Dawn D. Matthews. 622 pages. 2003. 978-0-7808-0629-0.

"This edition is even more helpful than earlier versions. . . . It is a truly valuable tool for anyone seeking readable and authoritative information on diabetes."
— *American Reference Books Annual, 2004*

"An invaluable reference." — *Library Journal, May '00*

Selected as one of the 250 "Best Health Sciences Books of 1999." — *Doody's Rating Service, Mar-Apr '00*

"Provides useful information for the general public."
— *Healthlines, University of Michigan Health Management Research Center, Sep/Oct '99*

". . . provides reliable mainstream medical information . . . belongs on the shelves of any library with a consumer health collection." — *E-Streams, Sep '99*

"Recommended reference source."
— *Booklist, American Library Association, Feb '99*

Diet & Nutrition Sourcebook, 3rd Edition

Basic Consumer Health Information about Dietary Guidelines and the Food Guidance System, Recommended Daily Nutrient Intakes, Serving Proportions, Weight Control, Vitamins and Supplements, Nutrition Issues for Different Life Stages and Lifestyles, and the Needs of People with Specific Medical Concerns, Including Cancer, Celiac Disease, Diabetes, Eating Disorders, Food Allergies, and Cardiovascular Disease

Along with Facts about Federal Nutrition Support Programs, a Glossary of Nutrition and Dietary Terms, and Directories of Additional Resources for More Information about Nutrition

Edited by Joyce Brennfleck Shannon. 633 pages. 2006. 978-0-7808-0800-3.

"This book is an excellent source of basic diet and nutrition information." — *Booklist Health Sciences Supplement, American Library Association, Dec '00*

"This reference document should be in any public library, but it would be a very good guide for beginning students in the health sciences. If the other books in this publisher's series are as good as this, they should all be in the health sciences collections."
— *American Reference Books Annual, 2000*

"This book is an excellent general nutrition reference for consumers who desire to take an active role in their health care for prevention. Consumers of all ages who select this book can feel confident they are receiving current and accurate information." — *Journal of Nutrition for the Elderly, Vol. 19, No. 4, 2000*

SEE ALSO *Digestive Diseases & Disorders Sourcebook, Eating Disorders Sourcebook, Gastrointestinal Diseases & Disorders Sourcebook, Vegetarian Sourcebook*

Digestive Diseases & Disorders Sourcebook

Basic Consumer Health Information about Diseases and Disorders that Impact the Upper and Lower Digestive System, Including Celiac Disease, Constipation, Crohn's Disease, Cyclic Vomiting Syndrome, Diarrhea, Diverticulosis and Diverticulitis, Gallstones, Heartburn, Hemorrhoids, Hernias, Indigestion (Dyspepsia), Irritable Bowel Syndrome, Lactose Intolerance, Ulcers, and More

Along with Information about Medications and Other Treatments, Tips for Maintaining a Healthy Digestive Tract, a Glossary, and Directory of Digestive Diseases Organizations

Edited by Karen Bellenir. 335 pages. 2000. 978-0-7808-0327-5.

"This title would be an excellent addition to all public or patient-research libraries."
— *American Reference Books Annual, 2001*

"This title is recommended for public, hospital, and health sciences libraries with consumer health collections." — *E-Streams, Jul-Aug '00*

"Recommended reference source."
— *Booklist, American Library Association, May '00*

SEE ALSO *Eating Disorders Sourcebook, Gastrointestinal Diseases & Disorders Sourcebook*

Disabilities Sourcebook

Basic Consumer Health Information about Physical and Psychiatric Disabilities, Including Descriptions of Major Causes of Disability, Assistive and Adaptive Aids, Workplace Issues, and Accessibility Concerns

Along with Information about the Americans with Disabilities Act, a Glossary, and Resources for Additional Help and Information

Edited by Dawn D. Matthews. 616 pages. 2000. 978-0-7808-0389-3.

"It is a must for libraries with a consumer health section." — *American Reference Books Annual, 2002*

"A much needed addition to the Omnigraphics Health Reference Series. A current reference work to provide people with disabilities, their families, caregivers or those who work with them, a broad range of information in one volume, has not been available until now. . . . It is recommended for all public and academic library reference collections." — *E-Streams, May '01*

"An excellent source book in easy-to-read format covering many current topics; highly recommended for all libraries." — *Choice, Association of College & Research Libraries, Jan '01*

"Recommended reference source."
— *Booklist, American Library Association, Jul '00*

Domestic Violence Sourcebook, 2nd Edition

Basic Consumer Health Information about the Causes and Consequences of Abusive Relationships, Including Physical Violence, Sexual Assault, Battery, Stalking, and Emotional Abuse, and Facts about the Effects of Violence on Women, Men, Young Adults, and the Elderly, with Reports about Domestic Violence in Selected Populations, and Featuring Facts about Medical Care, Victim Assistance and Protection, Prevention Strategies, Mental Health Services, and Legal Issues

Along with a Glossary of Related Terms and Resources for Additional Help and Information

Edited by Dawn D. Matthews. 628 pages. 2004. 978-0-7808-0669-6.

"Educators, clergy, medical professionals, police, and victims and their families will benefit from this realistic and easy-to-understand resource."
— American Reference Books Annual, 2005

"Recommended for all collections supporting consumer health information. It should also be considered for any collection needing general, readable information on domestic violence." — E-Streams, Jan '05

"This sourcebook complements other books in its field, providing a one-stop resource . . . Recommended."
— Choice, Association of College & Research Libraries, Jan '05

"Interested lay persons should find the book extremely beneficial. . . . A copy of Domestic Violence and Child Abuse Sourcebook should be in every public library in the United States."
— Social Science & Medicine, No. 56, 2003

"This is important information. The Web has many resources but this sourcebook fills an important societal need. I am not aware of any other resources of this type." — Doody's Review Service, Sep '01

"Recommended reference source."
— Booklist, American Library Association, Apr '01

"Important pick for college-level health reference libraries." — The Bookwatch, Mar '01

"Because this problem is so widespread and because this book includes a lot of issues within one volume, this work is recommended for all public libraries."
— American Reference Books Annual, 2001

SEE ALSO Child Abuse Sourcebook

Drug Abuse Sourcebook, 2nd Edition

Basic Consumer Health Information about Illicit Substances of Abuse and the Misuse of Prescription and Over-the-Counter Medications, Including Depressants, Hallucinogens, Inhalants, Marijuana, Stimulants, and Anabolic Steroids

Along with Facts about Related Health Risks, Treatment Programs, Prevention Programs, a Glossary of Abuse and Addiction Terms, a Glossary of Drug-Related Street Terms, and a Directory of Resources for More Information

Edited by Catherine Ginther. 607 pages. 2004. 978-0-7808-0740-2.

"Commendable for organizing useful, normally scattered government and association-produced data into a logical sequence."
— American Reference Books Annual, 2006

"This easy-to-read volume is recommended for consumer health collections within public or academic libraries." — E-Streams, Sep '05

"An excellent library reference."
— The Bookwatch, May '05

"Containing a wealth of information, this book will be useful to the college student just beginning to explore the topic of substance abuse. This resource belongs in libraries that serve a lower-division undergraduate or community college clientele as well as the general public." — Choice, Association of College & Research Libraries, Jun '01

"Recommended reference source."
— Booklist, American Library Association, Feb '01

SEE ALSO Alcoholism Sourcebook

Ear, Nose & Throat Disorders Sourcebook, 2nd Edition

Basic Consumer Health Information about Disorders of the Ears, Hearing Loss, Vestibular Disorders, Nasal and Sinus Problems, Throat and Vocal Cord Disorders, and Otolaryngologic Cancers, Including Facts about Ear Infections and Injuries, Genetic and Congenital Deafness, Sensorineural Hearing Disorders, Tinnitus, Vertigo, Ménière Disease, Rhinitis, Sinusitis, Snoring, Sore Throats, Hoarseness, and More

Along with Reports on Current Research Initiatives, a Glossary of Related Medical Terms, and a Directory of Sources for Further Help and Information

Edited by Sandra J. Judd. 659 pages. 2006. 978-0-7808-0872-0.

"Overall, this sourcebook is helpful for the consumer seeking information on ENT issues. It is recommended for public libraries."
— American Reference Books Annual, 1999

"Recommended reference source."
— Booklist, American Library Association, Dec '98

Eating Disorders Sourcebook, 2nd Edition

Basic Consumer Health Information about Anorexia Nervosa, Bulimia Nervosa, Binge Eating, Compulsive Exercise, Female Athlete Triad, and Other Eating Disorders, Including Facts about Body Image and Other Cultural and Age-Related Risk Factors, Prevention Efforts, Adverse Health Effects, Treatment Options, and the Recovery Process

Along with Guidelines for Healthy Weight Control, a Glossary, and Directories of Additional Resources

Edited by Joyce Brennfleck Shannon. 560 pages. 2007. 978-0-7808-0948-2.

"Recommended for health science libraries that are open to the public, as well as hospital libraries. This book is a good resource for the consumer who is concerned about eating disorders." — *E-Streams, Mar '02*

"This volume is another convenient collection of excerpted articles. Recommended for school and public library patrons; lower-division undergraduates; and two-year technical program students."
— *Choice, Association of College & Research Libraries, Jan '02*

"Recommended reference source."
— *Booklist, American Library Association, Oct '01*

SEE ALSO *Diet & Nutrition Sourcebook, Digestive Diseases & Disorders Sourcebook, Gastrointestinal Diseases & Disorders Sourcebook*

Emergency Medical Services Sourcebook

Basic Consumer Health Information about Preventing, Preparing for, and Managing Emergency Situations, When and Who to Call for Help, What to Expect in the Emergency Room, the Emergency Medical Team, Patient Issues, and Current Topics in Emergency Medicine

Along with Statistical Data, a Glossary, and Sources of Additional Help and Information

Edited by Jenni Lynn Colson. 494 pages. 2002. 978-0-7808-0420-3.

"Handy and convenient for home, public, school, and college libraries. Recommended."
— *Choice, Association of College & Research Libraries, Apr '03*

"This reference can provide the consumer with answers to most questions about emergency care in the United States, or it will direct them to a resource where the answer can be found."
— *American Reference Books Annual, 2003*

"Recommended reference source."
— *Booklist, American Library Association, Feb '03*

Endocrine & Metabolic Disorders Sourcebook

Basic Information for the Layperson about Pancreatic and Insulin-Related Disorders Such as Pancreatitis, Diabetes, and Hypoglycemia; Adrenal Gland Disorders Such as Cushing's Syndrome, Addison's Disease, and Congenital Adrenal Hyperplasia; Pituitary Gland Disorders Such as Growth Hormone Deficiency, Acromegaly, and Pituitary Tumors; Thyroid Disorders Such as Hypothyroidism, Graves' Disease, Hashimoto's Disease, and Goiter; Hyperparathyroidism; and Other Diseases and Syndromes of Hormone Imbalance or Metabolic Dysfunction

Along with Reports on Current Research Initiatives

Edited by Linda M. Shin. 574 pages. 1998. 978-0-7808-0207-0.

"Omnigraphics has produced another needed resource for health information consumers."
— *American Reference Books Annual, 2000*

"Recommended reference source."
— *Booklist, American Library Association, Dec '98*

Environmental Health Sourcebook, 2nd Edition

Basic Consumer Health Information about the Environment and Its Effect on Human Health, Including the Effects of Air Pollution, Water Pollution, Hazardous Chemicals, Food Hazards, Radiation Hazards, Biological Agents, Household Hazards, Such as Radon, Asbestos, Carbon Monoxide, and Mold, and Information about Associated Diseases and Disorders, Including Cancer, Allergies, Respiratory Problems, and Skin Disorders

Along with Information about Environmental Concerns for Specific Populations, a Glossary of Related Terms, and Resources for Further Help and Information

Edited by Dawn D. Matthews. 673 pages. 2003. 978-0-7808-0632-0.

"This recently updated edition continues the level of quality and the reputation of the numerous other volumes in Omnigraphics' Health Reference Series."
— *American Reference Books Annual, 2004*

"An excellent updated edition."
— *The Bookwatch, Oct '03*

"Recommended reference source."
— *Booklist, American Library Association, Sep '98*

"This book will be a useful addition to anyone's library."
— *Choice Health Sciences Supplement, Association of College & Research Libraries, May '98*

". . . a good survey of numerous environmentally induced physical disorders . . . a useful addition to anyone's library."
— *Doody's Health Sciences Book Reviews, Jan '98*

Ethnic Diseases Sourcebook

Basic Consumer Health Information for Ethnic and Racial Minority Groups in the United States, Including General Health Indicators and Behaviors, Ethnic Diseases, Genetic Testing, the Impact of Chronic Diseases, Women's Health, Mental Health Issues, and Preventive Health Care Services

Along with a Glossary and a Listing of Additional Resources

Edited by Joyce Brennfleck Shannon. 664 pages. 2001. 978-0-7808-0336-7.

"Recommended for health sciences libraries where public health programs are a priority."
— *E-Streams, Jan '02*

"Not many books have been written on this topic to date, and the *Ethnic Diseases Sourcebook* is a strong addition to the list. It will be an important introductory resource for health consumers, students, health care

personnel, and social scientists. It is recommended for public, academic, and large hospital libraries."
— *American Reference Books Annual, 2002*

"Recommended reference source."
— *Booklist, American Library Association, Oct '01*

"Will prove valuable to any library seeking to maintain a current, comprehensive reference collection of health resources.... An excellent source of health information about genetic disorders which affect particular ethnic and racial minorities in the U.S."
— *The Bookwatch, Aug '01*

Eye Care Sourcebook, 2nd Edition

Basic Consumer Health Information about Eye Care and Eye Disorders, Including Facts about the Diagnosis, Prevention, and Treatment of Common Refractive Problems Such as Myopia, Hyperopia, Astigmatism, and Presbyopia, and Eye Diseases, Including Glaucoma, Cataract, Age-Related Macular Degeneration, and Diabetic Retinopathy

Along with a Section on Vision Correction and Refractive Surgeries, Including LASIK and LASEK, a Glossary, and Directories of Resources for Additional Help and Information

Edited by Amy L. Sutton. 543 pages. 2003. 978-0-7808-0635-1

"... a solid reference tool for eye care and a valuable addition to a collection."
— *American Reference Books Annual, 2004*

Family Planning Sourcebook

Basic Consumer Health Information about Planning for Pregnancy and Contraception, Including Traditional Methods, Barrier Methods, Hormonal Methods, Permanent Methods, Future Methods, Emergency Contraception, and Birth Control Choices for Women at Each Stage of Life

Along with Statistics, a Glossary, and Sources of Additional Information

Edited by Amy Marcaccio Keyzer. 520 pages. 2001. 978-0-7808-0379-4.

"Recommended for public, health, and undergraduate libraries as part of the circulating collection."
— *E-Streams, Mar '02*

"Information is presented in an unbiased, readable manner, and the sourcebook will certainly be a necessary addition to those public and high school libraries where Internet access is restricted or otherwise problematic." — *American Reference Books Annual, 2002*

"Recommended reference source."
— *Booklist, American Library Association, Oct '01*

"Will prove valuable to any library seeking to maintain a current, comprehensive reference collection of health resources.... Excellent reference."
— *The Bookwatch, Aug '01*

SEE ALSO Pregnancy & Birth Sourcebook

Fitness & Exercise Sourcebook, 3rd Edition

Basic Consumer Health Information about the Physical and Mental Benefits of Fitness, Including Cardiorespiratory Endurance, Muscular Strength, Muscular Endurance, and Flexibility, with Facts about Sports Nutrition and Exercise-Related Injuries and Tips about Physical Activity and Exercises for People of All Ages and for People with Health Concerns

Along with Advice on Selecting and Using Exercise Equipment, Maintaining Exercise Motivation, a Glossary of Related Terms, and a Directory of Resources for More Help and Information

Edited by Amy L. Sutton. 663 pages. 2007. 978-0-7808-0946-8.

"This work is recommended for all general reference collections."
— *American Reference Books Annual, 2002*

"Highly recommended for public, consumer, and school grades fourth through college." — *E-Streams, Nov '01*

"Recommended reference source."
— *Booklist, American Library Association, Oct '01*

"The information appears quite comprehensive and is considered reliable.... This second edition is a welcomed addition to the series."
— *Doody's Review Service, Sep '01*

Food Safety Sourcebook

Basic Consumer Health Information about the Safe Handling of Meat, Poultry, Seafood, Eggs, Fruit Juices, and Other Food Items, and Facts about Pesticides, Drinking Water, Food Safety Overseas, and the Onset, Duration, and Symptoms of Foodborne Illnesses, Including Types of Pathogenic Bacteria, Parasitic Protozoa, Worms, Viruses, and Natural Toxins

Along with the Role of the Consumer, the Food Handler, and the Government in Food Safety; a Glossary, and Resources for Additional Help and Information

Edited by Dawn D. Matthews. 339 pages. 1999. 978-0-7808-0326-8.

"This book is recommended for public libraries and universities with home economic and food science programs." — *E-Streams, Nov '00*

"Recommended reference source."
— *Booklist, American Library Association, May '00*

"This book takes the complex issues of food safety and foodborne pathogens and presents them in an easily understood manner. [It does] an excellent job of covering a large and often confusing topic."
— *American Reference Books Annual, 2000*

Forensic Medicine Sourcebook

Basic Consumer Information for the Layperson about Forensic Medicine, Including Crime Scene Investigation, Evidence Collection and Analysis, Expert Testimony, Computer-Aided Criminal Identification, Digital Imaging in the Courtroom, DNA Profiling, Accident Reconstruction, Autopsies, Ballistics, Drugs and Explosives Detection, Latent Fingerprints, Product Tampering, and Questioned Document Examination

Along with Statistical Data, a Glossary of Forensics Terminology, and Listings of Sources for Further Help and Information

Edited by Annemarie S. Muth. 574 pages. 1999. 978-0-7808-0232-2.

"Given the expected widespread interest in its content and its easy to read style, this book is recommended for most public and all college and university libraries."
— *E-Streams, Feb '01*

"Recommended for public libraries."
— *Reference & User Services Quarterly, American Library Association, Spring 2000*

"Recommended reference source."
— *Booklist, American Library Association, Feb '00*

"A wealth of information, useful statistics, references are up-to-date and extremely complete. This wonderful collection of data will help students who are interested in a career in any type of forensic field. It is a great resource for attorneys who need information about types of expert witnesses needed in a particular case. It also offers useful information for fiction and nonfiction writers whose work involves a crime. A fascinating compilation. All levels."
— *Choice, Association of College & Research Libraries, Jan '00*

"There are several items that make this book attractive to consumers who are seeking certain forensic data.... This is a useful current source for those seeking general forensic medical answers."
— *American Reference Books Annual, 2000*

■

Gastrointestinal Diseases & Disorders Sourcebook, 2nd Edition

Basic Consumer Health Information about the Upper and Lower Gastrointestinal (GI) Tract, Including the Esophagus, Stomach, Intestines, Rectum, Liver, and Pancreas, with Facts about Gastroesophageal Reflux Disease, Gastritis, Hernias, Ulcers, Celiac Disease, Diverticulitis, Irritable Bowel Syndrome, Hemorrhoids, Gastrointestinal Cancers, and Other Diseases and Disorders Related to the Digestive Process

Along with Information about Commonly Used Diagnostic and Surgical Procedures, Statistics, Reports on Current Research Initiatives and Clinical Trials, a Glossary, and Resources for Additional Help and Information

Edited by Sandra J. Judd. 681 pages. 2006. 978-0-7808-0798-3.

"... very readable form. The successful editorial work that brought this material together into a useful and understandable reference makes accessible to all readers information that can help them more effectively understand and obtain help for digestive tract problems."
— *Choice, Association of College & Research Libraries, Feb '97*

SEE ALSO *Diet & Nutrition Sourcebook, Digestive Diseases & Disorders, Eating Disorders Sourcebook*

■

Genetic Disorders Sourcebook, 3rd Edition

Basic Consumer Health Information about Hereditary Diseases and Disorders, Including Facts about the Human Genome, Genetic Inheritance Patterns, Disorders Associated with Specific Genes, Such as Sickle Cell Disease, Hemophilia, and Cystic Fibrosis, Chromosome Disorders, Such as Down Syndrome, Fragile X Syndrome, and Turner Syndrome, and Complex Diseases and Disorders Resulting from the Interaction of Environmental and Genetic Factors, Such as Allergies, Cancer, and Obesity

Along with Facts about Genetic Testing, Suggestions for Parents of Children with Special Needs, Reports on Current Research Initiatives, a Glossary of Genetic Terminology, and Resources for Additional Help and Information

Edited by Karen Bellenir. 777 pages. 2004. 978-0-7808-0742-6.

"This text is recommended for any library with an interest in providing consumer health resources."
— *E-Streams, Aug '05*

"This is a valuable resource for anyone wishing to have an understandable description of any of the topics or disorders included. The editor succeeds in making complex genetic issues understandable."
— *Doody's Book Review Service, May '05*

"A good acquisition for public libraries."
— *American Reference Books Annual, 2005*

"Excellent reference." — *The Bookwatch, Jan '05*

"Recommended reference source."
— *Booklist, American Library Association, Apr '01*

"Important pick for college-level health reference libraries." — *The Bookwatch, Mar '01*

■

Head Trauma Sourcebook

Basic Information for the Layperson about Open-Head and Closed-Head Injuries, Treatment Advances, Recovery, and Rehabilitation

Along with Reports on Current Research Initiatives

Edited by Karen Bellenir. 414 pages. 1997. 978-0-7808-0208-7.

Headache Sourcebook

Basic Consumer Health Information about Migraine, Tension, Cluster, Rebound and Other Types of Headaches, with Facts about the Cause and Prevention of Headaches, the Effects of Stress and the Environment, Headaches during Pregnancy and Menopause, and Childhood Headaches

Along with a Glossary and Other Resources for Additional Help and Information

Edited by Dawn D. Matthews. 362 pages. 2002. 978-0-7808-0337-4.

"Highly recommended for academic and medical reference collections." — *Library Bookwatch, Sep '02*

Healthy Aging Sourcebook

Basic Consumer Health Information about Maintaining Health through the Aging Process, Including Advice on Nutrition, Exercise, and Sleep, Help in Making Decisions about Midlife Issues and Retirement, and Guidance Concerning Practical and Informed Choices in Health Consumerism

Along with Data Concerning the Theories of Aging, Different Experiences in Aging by Minority Groups, and Facts about Aging Now and Aging in the Future; and Featuring a Glossary, a Guide to Consumer Help, Additional Suggested Reading, and Practical Resource Directory

Edited by Jenifer Swanson. 536 pages. 1999. 978-0-7808-0390-9.

"Recommended reference source."
— *Booklist, American Library Association, Feb '00*

SEE ALSO Physical & Mental Issues in Aging Sourcebook

Healthy Children Sourcebook

Basic Consumer Health Information about the Physical and Mental Development of Children between the Ages of 3 and 12, Including Routine Health Care, Preventative Health Services, Safety and First Aid, Healthy Sleep, Dental Care, Nutrition, and Fitness, and Featuring Parenting Tips on Such Topics as Bedwetting, Choosing Day Care, Monitoring TV and Other Media, and Establishing a Foundation for Substance Abuse Prevention

Along with a Glossary of Commonly Used Pediatric Terms and Resources for Additional Help and Information.

Edited by Chad T. Kimball. 647 pages. 2003. 978-0-7808-0247-6.

"It is hard to imagine that any other single resource exists that would provide such a comprehensive guide of timely information on health promotion and disease prevention for children aged 3 to 12."
— *American Reference Books Annual, 2004*

"The strengths of this book are many. It is clearly written, presented and structured."
— *Journal of the National Medical Association, 2004*

SEE ALSO Childhood Diseases & Disorders Sourcebook

Healthy Heart Sourcebook for Women

Basic Consumer Health Information about Cardiac Issues Specific to Women, Including Facts about Major Risk Factors and Prevention, Treatment and Control Strategies, and Important Dietary Issues

Along with a Special Section Regarding the Pros and Cons of Hormone Replacement Therapy and Its Impact on Heart Health, and Additional Help, Including Recipes, a Glossary, and a Directory of Resources

Edited by Dawn D. Matthews. 336 pages. 2000. 978-0-7808-0329-9.

"A good reference source and recommended for all public, academic, medical, and hospital libraries."
— *Medical Reference Services Quarterly, Summer '01*

"Because of the lack of information specific to women on this topic, this book is recommended for public libraries and consumer libraries."
— *American Reference Books Annual, 2001*

"Contains very important information about coronary artery disease that all women should know. The information is current and presented in an easy-to-read format. The book will make a good addition to any library." — *American Medical Writers Association Journal, Summer '00*

"Important, basic reference."
— *Reviewer's Bookwatch, Jul '00*

SEE ALSO Cardiovascular Diseases & Disorders Sourcebook, Women's Health Concerns Sourcebook

Hepatitis Sourcebook

Basic Consumer Health Information about Hepatitis A, Hepatitis B, Hepatitis C, and Other Forms of Hepatitis, Including Autoimmune Hepatitis, Alcoholic Hepatitis, Nonalcoholic Steatohepatitis, and Toxic Hepatitis, with Facts about Risk Factors, Screening Methods, Diagnostic Tests, and Treatment Options

Along with Information on Liver Health, Tips for People Living with Chronic Hepatitis, Reports on Current Research Initiatives, a Glossary of Terms Related to Hepatitis, and a Directory of Sources for Further Help and Information

Edited by Sandra J. Judd. 597 pages. 2005. 978-0-7808-0749-5.

"Highly recommended."
— *American Reference Books Annual, 2006*

Household Safety Sourcebook

Basic Consumer Health Information about Household Safety, Including Information about Poisons, Chemicals, Fire, and Water Hazards in the Home

Along with Advice about the Safe Use of Home Maintenance Equipment, Choosing Toys and Nursery Furniture, Holiday and Recreation Safety, a Glossary, and Resources for Further Help and Information

Edited by Dawn D. Matthews. 606 pages. 2002. 978-0-7808-0338-1.

"This work will be useful in public libraries with large consumer health and wellness departments."
— American Reference Books Annual, 2003

"As a sourcebook on household safety this book meets its mark. It is encyclopedic in scope and covers a wide range of safety issues that are commonly seen in the home." — E-Streams, Jul '02

Hypertension Sourcebook

Basic Consumer Health Information about the Causes, Diagnosis, and Treatment of High Blood Pressure, with Facts about Consequences, Complications, and Co-Occurring Disorders, Such as Coronary Heart Disease, Diabetes, Stroke, Kidney Disease, and Hypertensive Retinopathy, and Issues in Blood Pressure Control, Including Dietary Choices, Stress Management, and Medications

Along with Reports on Current Research Initiatives and Clinical Trials, a Glossary, and Resources for Additional Help and Information

Edited by Dawn D. Matthews and Karen Bellenir. 613 pages. 2004. 978-0-7808-0674-0.

"Academic, public, and medical libraries will want to add the Hypertension Sourcebook to their collections."
— E-Streams, Aug '05

"The strength of this source is the wide range of information given about hypertension."
— American Reference Books Annual, 2005

Immune System Disorders Sourcebook, 2nd Edition

Basic Consumer Health Information about Disorders of the Immune System, Including Immune System Function and Response, Diagnosis of Immune Disorders, Information about Inherited Immune Disease, Acquired Immune Disease, and Autoimmune Diseases, Including Primary Immune Deficiency, Acquired Immunodeficiency Syndrome (AIDS), Lupus, Multiple Sclerosis, Type 1 Diabetes, Rheumatoid Arthritis, and Graves' Disease

Along with Treatments, Tips for Coping with Immune Disorders, a Glossary, and a Directory of Additional Resources.

Edited by Joyce Brennfleck Shannon. 671 pages. 2005. 978-0-7808-0748-8.

"Highly recommended for academic and public libraries." — American Reference Books Annual, 2006

"The updated second edition is a 'must' for any consumer health library seeking a solid resource covering

the treatments, symptoms, and options for immune disorder sufferers.... An excellent guide."
— MBR Bookwatch, Jan '06

Infant & Toddler Health Sourcebook

Basic Consumer Health Information about the Physical and Mental Development of Newborns, Infants, and Toddlers, Including Neonatal Concerns, Nutrition Recommendations, Immunization Schedules, Common Pediatric Disorders, Assessments and Milestones, Safety Tips, and Advice for Parents and Other Caregivers

Along with a Glossary of Terms and Resource Listings for Additional Help

Edited by Jenifer Swanson. 585 pages. 2000. 978-0-7808-0246-9.

"As a reference for the general public, this would be useful in any library." — E-Streams, May '01

"Recommended reference source."
— Booklist, American Library Association, Feb '01

"This is a good source for general use."
— American Reference Books Annual, 2001

Infectious Diseases Sourcebook

Basic Consumer Health Information about Non-Contagious Bacterial, Viral, Prion, Fungal, and Parasitic Diseases Spread by Food and Water, Insects and Animals, or Environmental Contact, Including Botulism, E. Coli, Encephalitis, Legionnaires' Disease, Lyme Disease, Malaria, Plague, Rabies, Salmonella, Tetanus, and Others, and Facts about Newly Emerging Diseases, Such as Hantavirus, Mad Cow Disease, Monkeypox, and West Nile Virus

Along with Information about Preventing Disease Transmission, the Threat of Bioterrorism, and Current Research Initiatives, with a Glossary and Directory of Resources for More Information

Edited by Karen Bellenir. 634 pages. 2004. 978-0-7808-0675-7.

"This reference continues the excellent tradition of the Health Reference Series in consolidating a wealth of information on a selected topic into a format that is easy to use and accessible to the general public."
— American Reference Books Annual, 2005

"Recommended for public and academic libraries."
— E-Streams, Jan '05

Injury & Trauma Sourcebook

Basic Consumer Health Information about the Impact of Injury, the Diagnosis and Treatment of Common and Traumatic Injuries, Emergency Care, and Specific Injuries Related to Home, Community, Workplace, Transportation, and Recreation

Along with Guidelines for Injury Prevention, a Glossary, and a Directory of Additional Resources

Edited by Joyce Brennfleck Shannon. 696 pages. 2002. 978-0-7808-0421-0.

"This publication is the most comprehensive work of its kind about injury and trauma."
— *American Reference Books Annual, 2003*

"This sourcebook provides concise, easily readable, basic health information about injuries. . . . This book is well organized and an easy to use reference resource suitable for hospital, health sciences and public libraries with consumer health collections."
— *E-Streams, Nov '02*

"Practitioners should be aware of guides such as this in order to facilitate their use by patients and their families."
— *Doody's Health Sciences Book Review Journal, Sep-Oct '02*

"Recommended reference source."
— *Booklist, American Library Association, Sep '02*

"Highly recommended for academic and medical reference collections."
— *Library Bookwatch, Sep '02*

Kidney & Urinary Tract Diseases & Disorders Sourcebook

SEE Urinary Tract & Kidney Diseases & Disorders Sourcebook, 2nd Edition

---

Learning Disabilities Sourcebook, 2nd Edition

Basic Consumer Health Information about Learning Disabilities, Including Dyslexia, Developmental Speech and Language Disabilities, Non-Verbal Learning Disorders, Developmental Arithmetic Disorder, Developmental Writing Disorder, and Other Conditions That Impede Learning Such as Attention Deficit/ Hyperactivity Disorder, Brain Injury, Hearing Impairment, Klinefelter Syndrome, Dyspraxia, and Tourette's Syndrome

Along with Facts about Educational Issues and Assistive Technology, Coping Strategies, a Glossary of Related Terms, and Resources for Further Help and Information

Edited by Dawn D. Matthews. 621 pages. 2003. 978-0-7808-0626-9.

"The second edition of Learning Disabilities Sourcebook far surpasses the earlier edition in that it is more focused on information that will be useful as a consumer health resource."
— *American Reference Books Annual, 2004*

"Teachers as well as consumers will find this an essential guide to understanding various syndromes and their latest treatments. [An] invaluable reference for public and school library collections alike."
— *Library Bookwatch, Apr '03*

Named "Outstanding Reference Book of 1999."
— *New York Public Library, Feb 2000*

"An excellent candidate for inclusion in a public library reference section. It's a great source of information. Teachers will also find the book useful. Definitely worth reading."
— *Journal of Adolescent & Adult Literacy, Feb 2000*

"Readable . . . provides a solid base of information regarding successful techniques used with individuals who have learning disabilities, as well as practical suggestions for educators and family members. Clear language, concise descriptions, and pertinent information for contacting multiple resources add to the strength of this book as a useful tool."
— *Choice, Association of College & Research Libraries, Feb '99*

"Recommended reference source."
— *Booklist, American Library Association, Sep '98*

"A useful resource for libraries and for those who don't have the time to identify and locate the individual publications."
— *Disability Resources Monthly, Sep '98*

Leukemia Sourcebook

Basic Consumer Health Information about Adult and Childhood Leukemias, Including Acute Lymphocytic Leukemia (ALL), Chronic Lymphocytic Leukemia (CLL), Acute Myelogenous Leukemia (AML), Chronic Myelogenous Leukemia (CML), and Hairy Cell Leukemia, and Treatments Such as Chemotherapy, Radiation Therapy, Peripheral Blood Stem Cell and Marrow Transplantation, and Immunotherapy

Along with Tips for Life During and After Treatment, a Glossary, and Directories of Additional Resources

Edited by Joyce Brennfleck Shannon. 587 pages. 2003. 0-7808-0627-6.

"Unlike other medical books for the layperson, . . . the language does not talk down to the reader. . . . This volume is highly recommended for all libraries."
— *American Reference Books Annual, 2004*

". . . a fine title which ranges from diagnosis to alternative treatments, staging, and tips for life during and after diagnosis."
— *The Bookwatch, Dec '03*

Liver Disorders Sourcebook

Basic Consumer Health Information about the Liver and How It Works; Liver Diseases, Including Cancer, Cirrhosis, Hepatitis, and Toxic and Drug Related Diseases; Tips for Maintaining a Healthy Liver; Laboratory Tests, Radiology Tests, and Facts about Liver Transplantation

Along with a Section on Support Groups, a Glossary, and Resource Listings

Edited by Joyce Brennfleck Shannon. 591 pages. 2000. 978-0-7808-0383-1.

"A valuable resource."
— *American Reference Books Annual, 2001*

"This title is recommended for health sciences and public libraries with consumer health collections."
— *E-Streams, Oct '00*

Lung Disorders Sourcebook

Basic Consumer Health Information about Emphysema, Pneumonia, Tuberculosis, Asthma, Cystic Fibrosis, and Other Lung Disorders, Including Facts about Diagnostic Procedures, Treatment Strategies, Disease Prevention Efforts, and Such Risk Factors as Smoking, Air Pollution, and Exposure to Asbestos, Radon, and Other Agents

Along with a Glossary and Resources for Additional Help and Information

Edited by Dawn D. Matthews. 678 pages. 2002. 978-0-7808-0339-8.

"This title is a great addition for public and school libraries because it provides concise health information on the lungs."
— *American Reference Books Annual, 2003*

"Highly recommended for academic and medical reference collections." — *Library Bookwatch, Sep '02*

SEE ALSO *Respiratory Diseases & Disorders Sourcebook*

Medical Tests Sourcebook, 2nd Edition

Basic Consumer Health Information about Medical Tests, Including Age-Specific Health Tests, Important Health Screenings and Exams, Home-Use Tests, Blood and Specimen Tests, Electrical Tests, Scope Tests, Genetic Testing, and Imaging Tests, Such as X-Rays, Ultrasound, Computed Tomography, Magnetic Resonance Imaging, Angiography, and Nuclear Medicine

Along with a Glossary and Directory of Additional Resources

Edited by Joyce Brennfleck Shannon. 654 pages. 2004. 978-0-7808-0670-2.

"Recommended for hospital and health sciences libraries with consumer health collections."
— *E-Streams, Mar '00*

"This is an overall excellent reference with a wealth of general knowledge that may aid those who are reluctant to get vital tests performed."
— *Today's Librarian, Jan '00*

"A valuable reference guide."
— *American Reference Books Annual, 2000*

Men's Health Concerns Sourcebook, 2nd Edition

Basic Consumer Health Information about the Medical and Mental Concerns of Men, Including Theories about the Shorter Male Lifespan, the Leading Causes of Death and Disability, Physical Concerns of Special Significance to Men, Reproductive and Sexual Concerns, Sexually Transmitted Diseases, Men's Mental and Emotional Health, and Lifestyle Choices That Affect Wellness, Such as Nutrition, Fitness, and Substance Use

Along with a Glossary of Related Terms and a Directory of Organizational Resources in Men's Health

Edited by Robert Aquinas McNally. 644 pages. 2004. 978-0-7808-0671-9.

"A very accessible reference for non-specialist general readers and consumers." — *The Bookwatch, Jun '04*

"This comprehensive resource and the series are highly recommended."
— *American Reference Books Annual, 2000*

"Recommended reference source."
— *Booklist, American Library Association, Dec '98*

Mental Health Disorders Sourcebook, 3rd Edition

Basic Consumer Health Information about Mental and Emotional Health and Mental Illness, Including Facts about Depression, Bipolar Disorder, and Other Mood Disorders, Phobias, Post-Traumatic Stress Disorder (PTSD), Obsessive-Compulsive Disorder, and Other Anxiety Disorders, Impulse Control Disorders, Eating Disorders, Personality Disorders, and Psychotic Disorders, Including Schizophrenia and Dissociative Disorders

Along with Statistical Information, a Special Section Concerning Mental Health Issues in Children and Adolescents, a Glossary, and Directories of Resources for Additional Help and Information

Edited by Karen Bellenir. 661 pages. 2005. 978-0-7808-0747-1.

"Recommended for public libraries and academic libraries with an undergraduate program in psychology."
— *American Reference Books Annual, 2006*

"Recommended reference source."
— *Booklist, American Library Association, Jun '00*

Mental Retardation Sourcebook

Basic Consumer Health Information about Mental Retardation and Its Causes, Including Down Syndrome, Fetal Alcohol Syndrome, Fragile X Syndrome, Genetic Conditions, Injury, and Environmental Sources

Along with Preventive Strategies, Parenting Issues, Educational Implications, Health Care Needs, Employment and Economic Matters, Legal Issues, a Glossary, and a Resource Listing for Additional Help and Information

Edited by Joyce Brennfleck Shannon. 642 pages. 2000. 978-0-7808-0377-0.

"Public libraries will find the book useful for reference and as a beginning research point for students, parents, and caregivers."
— *American Reference Books Annual, 2001*

"The strength of this work is that it compiles many basic fact sheets and addresses for further information in one volume. It is intended and suitable for the general public. This sourcebook is relevant to any collection providing health information to the general public."
— E-Streams, Nov '00

"From preventing retardation to parenting and family challenges, this covers health, social and legal issues and will prove an invaluable overview."
— Reviewer's Bookwatch, Jul '00

Movement Disorders Sourcebook

Basic Consumer Health Information about Neurological Movement Disorders, Including Essential Tremor, Parkinson's Disease, Dystonia, Cerebral Palsy, Huntington's Disease, Myasthenia Gravis, Multiple Sclerosis, and Other Early-Onset and Adult-Onset Movement Disorders, Their Symptoms and Causes, Diagnostic Tests, and Treatments

Along with Mobility and Assistive Technology Information, a Glossary, and a Directory of Additional Resources

Edited by Joyce Brennfleck Shannon. 655 pages. 2003. 978-0-7808-0628-3.

"... a good resource for consumers and recommended for public, community college and undergraduate libraries." — *American Reference Books Annual, 2004*

Muscular Dystrophy Sourcebook

Basic Consumer Health Information about Congenital, Childhood-Onset, and Adult-Onset Forms of Muscular Dystrophy, Such as Duchenne, Becker, Emery-Dreifuss, Distal, Limb-Girdle, Facioscapulohumeral (FSHD), Myotonic, and Ophthalmoplegic Muscular Dystrophies, Including Facts about Diagnostic Tests, Medical and Physical Therapies, Management of Co-Occurring Conditions, and Parenting Guidelines

Along with Practical Tips for Home Care, a Glossary, and Directories of Additional Resources

Edited by Joyce Brennfleck Shannon. 577 pages. 2004. 978-0-7808-0676-4.

"This book is highly recommended for public and academic libraries as well as health care offices that support the information needs of patients and their families."
— E-Streams, Apr '05

"Excellent reference." — The Bookwatch, Jan '05

Obesity Sourcebook

Basic Consumer Health Information about   Diseases and Other Problems Associated with Obesity, and Including Facts about Risk Factors, Prevention Issues, and Management Approaches

Along with Statistical and Demographic Data, Information about Special Populations, Research Updates, a Glossary, and Source Listings for Further Help and Information

Edited by Wilma Caldwell and Chad T. Kimball. 376 pages. 2001. 978-0-7808-0333-6.

"The book synthesizes the reliable medical literature on obesity into one easy-to-read and useful resource for the general public."
— American Reference Books Annual, 2002

"This is a very useful resource book for the lay public."
— Doody's Review Service, Nov '01

"Well suited for the health reference collection of a public library or an academic health science library that serves the general population." — E-Streams, Sep '01

"Recommended reference source."
— Booklist, American Library Association, Apr '01

"Recommended pick both for specialty health library collections and any general consumer health reference collection." — The Bookwatch, Apr '01

Oral Health Sourcebook

SEE *Dental Care & Oral Health Sourcebook, 2nd Edition*

Osteoporosis Sourcebook

Basic Consumer Health Information about Primary and Secondary Osteoporosis and Juvenile Osteoporosis and Related Conditions, Including Fibrous Dysplasia, Gaucher Disease, Hyperthyroidism, Hypophosphatasia, Myeloma, Osteopetrosis, Osteogenesis Imperfecta, and Paget's Disease

Along with Information about Risk Factors, Treatments, Traditional and Non-Traditional Pain Management, a Glossary of Related Terms, and a Directory of Resources

Edited by Allan R. Cook. 584 pages. 2001. 978-0-7808-0239-1.

"This would be a book to be kept in a staff or patient library. The targeted audience is the layperson, but the therapist who needs a quick bit of information on a particular topic will also find the book useful."
— Physical Therapy, Jan '02

"This resource is recommended as a great reference source for public, health, and academic libraries, and is another triumph for the editors of Omnigraphics."
— American Reference Books Annual, 2002

"Recommended for all public libraries and general health collections, especially those supporting patient education or consumer health programs."
— E-Streams, Nov '01

"Will prove valuable to any library seeking to maintain a current, comprehensive reference collection of health resources. ... From prevention to treatment and associated conditions, this provides an excellent survey."
— The Bookwatch, Aug '01

Pain Sourcebook, 2nd Edition

Basic Consumer Health Information about Specific Forms of Acute and Chronic Pain, Including Muscle and Skeletal Pain, Nerve Pain, Cancer Pain, and Disorders Characterized by Pain, Such as Fibromyalgia, Shingles, Angina, Arthritis, and Headaches

Along with Information about Pain Medications and Management Techniques, Complementary and Alternative Pain Relief Options, Tips for People Living with Chronic Pain, a Glossary, and a Directory of Sources for Further Information

Edited by Karen Bellenir. 670 pages. 2002. 978-0-7808-0612-2.

Pediatric Cancer Sourcebook

Basic Consumer Health Information about Leukemias, Brain Tumors, Sarcomas, Lymphomas, and Other Cancers in Infants, Children, and Adolescents, Including Descriptions of Cancers, Treatments, and Coping Strategies

Along with Suggestions for Parents, Caregivers, and Concerned Relatives, a Glossary of Cancer Terms, and Resource Listings

Edited by Edward J. Prucha. 587 pages. 1999. 978-0-7808-0245-2.

Physical & Mental Issues in Aging Sourcebook

Basic Consumer Health Information on Physical and Mental Disorders Associated with the Aging Process, Including Concerns about Cardiovascular Disease, Pulmonary Disease, Oral Health, Digestive Disorders, Musculoskeletal and Skin Disorders, Metabolic Changes, Sexual and Reproductive Issues, and Changes in Vision, Hearing, and Other Senses

Along with Data about Longevity and Causes of Death, Information on Acute and Chronic Pain, Descriptions of Mental Concerns, a Glossary of Terms, and Resource Listings for Additional Help

Edited by Jenifer Swanson. 660 pages. 1999. 978-0-7808-0233-9.

Podiatry Sourcebook, 2nd Edition

Basic Consumer Health Information about Disorders, Diseases, Deformities, and Injuries that Affect the Foot and Ankle, Including Sprains, Corns, Calluses, Bunions, Plantar Warts, Plantar Fasciitis, Neuromas, Clubfoot, Flat Feet, Achilles Tendonitis, and Much More

Along with Information about Selecting a Foot Care Specialist, Foot Fitness, Shoes and Socks, Diagnostic Tests and Corrective Procedures, Financial Assistance for Corrective Devices, a Glossary of Related Terms, and a Directory of Resources for Additional Help and Information

Edited by Ivy L. Alexander. 543 pages. 2007. 978-0-7808-0944-4.

Pregnancy & Birth Sourcebook, 2nd Edition

Basic Consumer Health Information about Conception and Pregnancy, Including Facts about Fertility, Infertility, Pregnancy Symptoms and Complications, Fetal Growth and Development, Labor, Delivery, and the Postpartum Period, as Well as Information about Maintaining Health and Wellness during Pregnancy and Caring for a Newborn

Along with Information about Public Health Assistance for Low-Income Pregnant Women, a Glossary, and Directories of Agencies and Organizations Providing Help and Support

Edited by Amy L. Sutton. 626 pages. 2004. 978-0-7808-0672-6.

"Will appeal to public and school reference collections strong in medicine and women's health. . . . Deserves a spot on any medical reference shelf."
— *The Bookwatch, Jul '04*

"A well-organized handbook. Recommended."
— *Choice, Association of College & Research Libraries, Apr '98*

"Recommended reference source."
— *Booklist, American Library Association, Mar '98*

"Recommended for public libraries."
— *American Reference Books Annual, 1998*

SEE ALSO Breastfeeding Sourcebook, Congenital Disorders Sourcebook, Family Planning Sourcebook

Prostate Cancer Sourcebook

Basic Consumer Health Information about Prostate Cancer, Including Information about the Associated Risk Factors, Detection, Diagnosis, and Treatment of Prostate Cancer

Along with Information on Non-Malignant Prostate Conditions, and Featuring a Section Listing Support and Treatment Centers and a Glossary of Related Terms

Edited by Dawn D. Matthews. 358 pages. 2001. 978-0-7808-0324-4.

"Recommended reference source."
— *Booklist, American Library Association, Jan '02*

"A valuable resource for health care consumers seeking information on the subject. . . . All text is written in a clear, easy-to-understand language that avoids technical jargon. Any library that collects consumer health resources would strengthen their collection with the addition of the Prostate Cancer Sourcebook."
— *American Reference Books Annual, 2002*

SEE ALSO Men's Health Concerns Sourcebook

Prostate & Urological Disorders Sourcebook

Basic Consumer Health Information about Urogenital and Sexual Disorders in Men, Including Prostate and Other Andrological Cancers, Prostatitis, Benign Prostatic Hyperplasia, Testicular and Penile Trauma,

Cryptorchidism, Peyronie Disease, Erectile Dysfunction, and Male Factor Infertility, and Facts about Commonly Used Tests and Procedures, Such as Prostatectomy, Vasectomy, Vasectomy Reversal, Penile Implants, and Semen Analysis

Along with a Glossary of Andrological Terms and a Directory of Resources for Additional Information

Edited by Karen Bellenir. 631 pages. 2005. 978-0-7808-0797-6.

Reconstructive & Cosmetic Surgery Sourcebook

Basic Consumer Health Information on Cosmetic and Reconstructive Plastic Surgery, Including Statistical Information about Different Surgical Procedures, Things to Consider Prior to Surgery, Plastic Surgery Techniques and Tools, Emotional and Psychological Considerations, and Procedure-Specific Information

Along with a Glossary of Terms and a Listing of Resources for Additional Help and Information

Edited by M. Lisa Weatherford. 374 pages. 2001. 978-0-7808-0214-8.

"An excellent reference that addresses cosmetic and medically necessary reconstructive surgeries. . . . The style of the prose is calm and reassuring, discussing the many positive outcomes now available due to advances in surgical techniques."
— *American Reference Books Annual, 2002*

"Recommended for health science libraries that are open to the public, as well as hospital libraries that are open to the patients. This book is a good resource for the consumer interested in plastic surgery."
— *E-Streams, Dec '01*

"Recommended reference source."
— *Booklist, American Library Association, Jul '01*

Rehabilitation Sourcebook

Basic Consumer Health Information about Rehabilitation for People Recovering from Heart Surgery, Spinal Cord Injury, Stroke, Orthopedic Impairments, Amputation, Pulmonary Impairments, Traumatic Injury, and More, Including Physical Therapy, Occupational Therapy, Speech/Language Therapy, Massage Therapy, Dance Therapy, Art Therapy, and Recreational Therapy

Along with Information on Assistive and Adaptive Devices, a Glossary, and Resources for Additional Help and Information

Edited by Dawn D. Matthews. 531 pages. 1999. 978-0-7808-0236-0.

"This is an excellent resource for public library reference and health collections."
— *American Reference Books Annual, 2001*

"Recommended reference source."
— *Booklist, American Library Association, May '00*

Respiratory Diseases & Disorders Sourcebook

Basic Information about Respiratory Diseases and Disorders, Including Asthma, Cystic Fibrosis, Pneumonia, the Common Cold, Influenza, and Others, Featuring Facts about the Respiratory System, Statistical and Demographic Data, Treatments, Self-Help Management Suggestions, and Current Research Initiatives

Edited by Allan R. Cook and Peter D. Dresser. 771 pages. 1995. 978-0-7808-0037-3.

"Designed for the layperson and for patients and their families coping with respiratory illness. . . . an extensive array of information on diagnosis, treatment, management, and prevention of respiratory illnesses for the general reader." — *Choice, Association of College & Research Libraries, Jun '96*

"A highly recommended text for all collections. It is a comforting reminder of the power of knowledge that good books carry between their covers." — *Academic Library Book Review, Spring '96*

"A comprehensive collection of authoritative information presented in a nontechnical, humanitarian style for patients, families, and caregivers." — *Association of Operating Room Nurses, Sep/Oct '95*

SEE ALSO *Lung Disorders Sourcebook*

Sexually Transmitted Diseases Sourcebook, 3rd Edition

Basic Consumer Health Information about Chlamydial Infections, Gonorrhea, Hepatitis, Herpes, HIV/AIDS, Human Papillomavirus, Pubic Lice, Scabies, Syphilis, Trichomoniasis, Vaginal Infections, and Other Sexually Transmitted Diseases, Including Facts about Risk Factors, Symptoms, Diagnosis, Treatment, and the Prevention of Sexually Transmitted Infections

Along with Updates on Current Research Initiatives, a Glossary of Related Terms, and Resources for Additional Help and Information

Edited by Amy L. Sutton. 629 pages. 2006. 978-0-7808-0824-9.

"Recommended for consumer health collections in public libraries, and secondary school and community college libraries." — *American Reference Books Annual, 2002*

"Every school and public library should have a copy of this comprehensive and user-friendly reference book." — *Choice, Association of College & Research Libraries, Sep '01*

"This is a highly recommended book. This is an especially important book for all school and public libraries." — *AIDS Book Review Journal, Jul-Aug '01*

"Recommended reference source." — *Booklist, American Library Association, Apr '01*

Sleep Disorders Sourcebook, 2nd Edition

Basic Consumer Health Information about Sleep and Sleep Disorders, Including Insomnia, Sleep Apnea, Restless Legs Syndrome, Narcolepsy, Parasomnias, and Other Health Problems That Affect Sleep, Plus Facts about Diagnostic Procedures, Treatment Strategies, Sleep Medications, and Tips for Improving Sleep Quality

Along with a Glossary of Related Terms and Resources for Additional Help and Information

Edited by Amy L. Sutton. 567 pages. 2005. 978-0-7808-0743-3.

"This book will be useful for just about everybody, especially the 40 million Americans with sleep disorders." — *American Reference Books Annual, 2006*

"Recommended for public libraries and libraries supporting health care professionals." — *E-Streams, Sep '05*

". . . key medical library acquisition." — *The Bookwatch, Jun '05*

Smoking Concerns Sourcebook

Basic Consumer Health Information about Nicotine Addiction and Smoking Cessation, Featuring Facts about the Health Effects of Tobacco Use, Including Lung and Other Cancers, Heart Disease, Stroke, and Respiratory Disorders, Such as Emphysema and Chronic Bronchitis

Along with Information about Smoking Prevention Programs, Suggestions for Achieving and Maintaining a Smoke-Free Lifestyle, Statistics about Tobacco Use, Reports on Current Research Initiatives, a Glossary of Related Terms, and Directories of Resources for Additional Help and Information

Edited by Karen Bellenir. 621 pages. 2004. 978-0-7808-0323-7.

"Provides everything needed for the student or general reader seeking practical details on the effects of tobacco use." — *The Bookwatch, Mar '05*

"Public libraries and consumer health care libraries will find this work useful." — *American Reference Books Annual, 2005*

Sports Injuries Sourcebook, 2nd Edition

Basic Consumer Health Information about the Diagnosis, Treatment, and Rehabilitation of Common Sports-Related Injuries in Children and Adults

Along with Suggestions for Conditioning and Training, Information and Prevention Tips for Injuries Frequently Associated with Specific Sports and Special Populations, a Glossary, and a Directory of Additional Resources

Edited by Joyce Brennfleck Shannon. 614 pages. 2002. 978-0-7808-0604-7.

Stress-Related Disorders Sourcebook

Basic Consumer Health Information about Stress and Stress-Related Disorders, Including Stress Origins and Signals, Environmental Stress at Work and Home, Mental and Emotional Stress Associated with Depression, Post-Traumatic Stress Disorder, Panic Disorder, Suicide, and the Physical Effects of Stress on the Cardiovascular, Immune, and Nervous Systems

Along with Stress Management Techniques, a Glossary, and a Listing of Additional Resources

Edited by Joyce Brennfleck Shannon. 610 pages. 2002. 978-0-7808-0560-6.

Stroke Sourcebook

Basic Consumer Health Information about Stroke, Including Ischemic, Hemorrhagic, Transient Ischemic Attack (TIA), and Pediatric Stroke, Stroke Triggers and Risks, Diagnostic Tests, Treatments, and Rehabilitation Information

Along with Stroke Prevention Guidelines, Legal and Financial Information, a Glossary, and a Directory of Additional Resources

Edited by Joyce Brennfleck Shannon. 606 pages. 2003. 978-0-7808-0630-6.

Surgery Sourcebook

Basic Consumer Health Information about Inpatient and Outpatient Surgeries, Including Cardiac, Vascular, Orthopedic, Ocular, Reconstructive, Cosmetic, Gynecologic, and Ear, Nose, and Throat Procedures and More

Along with Information about Operating Room Policies and Instruments, Laser Surgery Techniques, Hos-

pital Errors, Statistical Data, a Glossary, and Listings of Sources for Further Help and Information

Edited by Annemarie S. Muth and Karen Bellenir. 596 pages. 2002. 978-0-7808-0380-0.

Thyroid Disorders Sourcebook

Basic Consumer Health Information about Disorders of the Thyroid and Parathyroid Glands, Including Hypothyroidism, Hyperthyroidism, Graves Disease, Hashimoto Thyroiditis, Thyroid Cancer, and Parathyroid Disorders, Featuring Facts about Symptoms, Risk Factors, Tests, and Treatments

Along with Information about the Effects of Thyroid Imbalance on Other Body Systems, Environmental Factors That Affect the Thyroid Gland, a Glossary, and a Directory of Additional Resources

Edited by Joyce Brennfleck Shannon. 599 pages. 2005. 978-0-7808-0745-7.

Transplantation Sourcebook

Basic Consumer Health Information about Organ and Tissue Transplantation, Including Physical and Financial Preparations, Procedures and Issues Relating to Specific Solid Organ and Tissue Transplants, Rehabilitation, Pediatric Transplant Information, the Future of Transplantation, and Organ and Tissue Donation

Along with a Glossary and Listings of Additional Resources

Edited by Joyce Brennfleck Shannon. 628 pages. 2002. 978-0-7808-0322-0.

Traveler's Health Sourcebook

Basic Consumer Health Information for Travelers, Including Physical and Medical Preparations, Transportation Health and Safety, Essential Information about Food and Water, Sun Exposure, Insect and Snake Bites, Camping and Wilderness Medicine, and Travel with Physical or Medical Disabilities

Along with International Travel Tips, Vaccination Recommendations, Geographical Health Issues, Disease Risks, a Glossary, and a Listing of Additional Resources

Edited by Joyce Brennfleck Shannon. 613 pages. 2000. 978-0-7808-0384-8.

"Recommended reference source."
— *Booklist, American Library Association. Feb '01*

"This book is recommended for any public library, any travel collection, and especially any collection for the physically disabled."
— *American Reference Books Annual, 2001*

SEE ALSO *Worldwide Health Sourcebook*

Urinary Tract & Kidney Diseases & Disorders Sourcebook, 2nd Edition

Basic Consumer Health Information about the Urinary System, Including the Bladder, Urethra, Ureters, and Kidneys, with Facts about Urinary Tract Infections, Incontinence, Congenital Disorders, Kidney Stones, Cancers of the Urinary Tract and Kidneys, Kidney Failure, Dialysis, and Kidney Transplantation

Along with Statistical and Demographic Information, Reports on Current Research in Kidney and Urologic Health, a Summary of Commonly Used Diagnostic Tests, a Glossary of Related Terms, and a Directory of Resources for Additional Help and Information

Edited by Ivy L. Alexander. 649 pages. 2005. 978-0-7808-0750-1.

"A good choice for a consumer health information library or for a medical library needing information to refer to their patients."
— *American Reference Books Annual, 2006*

Vegetarian Sourcebook

Basic Consumer Health Information about Vegetarian Diets, Lifestyle, and Philosophy, Including Definitions of Vegetarianism and Veganism, Tips about Adopting Vegetarianism, Creating a Vegetarian Pantry, and Meeting Nutritional Needs of Vegetarians, with Facts Regarding Vegetarianism's Effect on Pregnant and Lactating Women, Children, Athletes, and Senior Citizens

Along with a Glossary of Commonly Used Vegetarian Terms and Resources for Additional Help and Information

Edited by Chad T. Kimball. 360 pages. 2002. 978-0-7808-0439-5.

"Organizes into one concise volume the answers to the most common questions concerning vegetarian diets and lifestyles. This title is recommended for public and secondary school libraries." — *E-Streams, Apr '03*

"Invaluable reference for public and school library collections alike." — *Library Bookwatch, Apr '03*

"The articles in this volume are easy to read and come from authoritative sources. The book does not necessarily support the vegetarian diet but instead provides the pros and cons of this important decision. The Vegetarian Sourcebook is recommended for public libraries and consumer health libraries."
— *American Reference Books Annual, 2003*

SEE ALSO *Diet & Nutrition Sourcebook*

Women's Health Concerns Sourcebook, 2nd Edition

Basic Consumer Health Information about the Medical and Mental Concerns of Women, Including Maintaining Health and Wellness, Gynecological Concerns, Breast Health, Sexuality and Reproductive Issues, Menopause, Cancer in Women, Leading Causes of Death and Disability among Women, Physical Concerns of Special Significance to Women, and Women's Mental and Emotional Health

Along with a Glossary of Related Terms and Directories of Resources for Additional Help and Information

Edited by Amy L. Sutton. 746 pages. 2004. 978-0-7808-0673-3.

"This is a useful reference book, which makes the reader knowledgeable about several issues that concern women's health. It is recommended for public libraries and home library collections." — *E-Streams, May '05*

"A useful addition to public and consumer health library collections."
— *American Reference Books Annual, 2005*

"A highly recommended title."
— *The Bookwatch, May '04*

"Handy compilation. There is an impressive range of diseases, devices, disorders, procedures, and other physical and emotional issues covered . . . well organized, illustrated, and indexed." — *Choice, Association of College & Research Libraries, Jan '98*

SEE ALSO *Breast Cancer Sourcebook, Cancer Sourcebook for Women, Healthy Heart Sourcebook for Women, Osteoporosis Sourcebook*

Workplace Health & Safety Sourcebook

Basic Consumer Health Information about Workplace Health and Safety, Including the Effect of Workplace Hazards on the Lungs, Skin, Heart, Ears, Eyes, Brain, Reproductive Organs, Musculoskeletal System, and Other Organs and Body Parts

Along with Information about Occupational Cancer, Personal Protective Equipment, Toxic and Hazardous

Chemicals, Child Labor, Stress, and Workplace Violence

Edited by Chad T. Kimball. 626 pages. 2000. 978-0-7808-0231-5.

"As a reference for the general public, this would be useful in any library." — *E-Streams, Jun '01*

"Provides helpful information for primary care physicians and other caregivers interested in occupational medicine. . . . General readers; professionals."
— *Choice, Association of College & Research Libraries, May '01*

"Recommended reference source."
— *Booklist, American Library Association, Feb '01*

"Highly recommended." — *The Bookwatch, Jan '01*

Worldwide Health Sourcebook

Basic Information about Global Health Issues, Including Malnutrition, Reproductive Health, Disease Dispersion and Prevention, Emerging Diseases, Risky Health Behaviors, and the Leading Causes of Death

Along with Global Health Concerns for Children, Women, and the Elderly, Mental Health Issues, Research and Technology Advancements, and Economic, Environmental, and Political Health Implications, a Glossary, and a Resource Listing for Additional Help and Information

Edited by Joyce Brennfleck Shannon. 614 pages. 2001. 978-0-7808-0330-5.

"Named an Outstanding Academic Title."
— *Choice, Association of College & Research Libraries, Jan '02*

"Yet another handy but also unique compilation in the extensive Health Reference Series, this is a useful work because many of the international publications reprinted or excerpted are not readily available. Highly recommended." — *Choice, Association of College & Research Libraries, Nov '01*

"Recommended reference source."
— *Booklist, American Library Association, Oct '01*

***SEE ALSO** Traveler's Health Sourcebook*

Teen Health Series

Helping Young Adults Understand, Manage, and Avoid Serious Illness

List price $65 per volume. **School and library price $58 per volume.**

Alcohol Information for Teens
Health Tips about Alcohol and Alcoholism

Including Facts about Underage Drinking, Preventing Teen Alcohol Use, Alcohol's Effects on the Brain and the Body, Alcohol Abuse Treatment, Help for Children of Alcoholics, and More

Edited by Joyce Brennfleck Shannon. 370 pages. 2005. 978-0-7808-0741-9.

"Boxed facts and tips add visual interest to the well-researched and clearly written text."
— *Curriculum Connection, Apr '06*

Allergy Information for Teens
Health Tips about Allergic Reactions Such as Anaphylaxis, Respiratory Problems, and Rashes

Including Facts about Identifying and Managing Allergies to Food, Pollen, Mold, Animals, Chemicals, Drugs, and Other Substances

Edited by Karen Bellenir. 410 pages. 2006. 978-0-7808-0799-0.

Asthma Information for Teens
Health Tips about Managing Asthma and Related Concerns

Including Facts about Asthma Causes, Triggers, Symptoms, Diagnosis, and Treatment

Edited by Karen Bellenir. 386 pages. 2005. 978-0-7808-0770-9.

"Highly recommended for medical libraries, public school libraries, and public libraries."
— *American Reference Books Annual, 2006*

"It is so clearly written and well organized that even hesitant readers will be able to find the facts they need, whether for reports or personal information. . . . A succinct but complete resource."
— *School Library Journal, Sep '05*

Body Information for Teens
Health Tips about Maintaining Well-Being for a Lifetime

Including Facts about the Development and Functioning of the Body's Systems, Organs, and Structures and the Health Impact of Lifestyle Choices

Edited by Sandra Augustyn Lawton. 440 pages. 2007. 978-0-7808-0443-2.

Cancer Information for Teens
Health Tips about Cancer Awareness, Prevention, Diagnosis, and Treatment

Including Facts about Frequently Occurring Cancers, Cancer Risk Factors, and Coping Strategies for Teens Fighting Cancer or Dealing with Cancer in Friends or Family Members

Edited by Wilma R. Caldwell. 428 pages. 2004. 978-0-7808-0678-8.

"Recommended for school libraries, or consumer libraries that see a lot of use by teens."
— *E-Streams, May 2005*

"A valuable educational tool."
— *American Reference Books Annual, 2005*

"Young adults and their parents alike will find this new addition to the *Teen Health Series* an important reference to cancer in teens."
— *Children's Bookwatch, Feb '05*

Complementary and Alternative Medicine Information for Teens
Health Tips about Non-Traditional and Non-Western Medical Practices

Including Information about Acupuncture, Chiropractic Medicine, Dietary and Herbal Supplements, Hypnosis, Massage Therapy, Prayer and Spirituality, Reflexology, Yoga, and More

Edited by Sandra Augustyn Lawton. 405 pages. 2006. 978-0-7808-0966-6.

Diabetes Information for Teens
Health Tips about Managing Diabetes and Preventing Related Complications

Including Information about Insulin, Glucose Control, Healthy Eating, Physical Activity, and Learning to Live with Diabetes

Edited by Sandra Augustyn Lawton. 410 pages. 2006. 978-0-7808-0811-9.

541

Diet Information for Teens, 2nd Edition

Health Tips about Diet and Nutrition

Including Facts about Dietary Guidelines, Food Groups, Nutrients, Healthy Meals, Snacks, Weight Control, Medical Concerns Related to Diet, and More

Edited by Karen Bellenir. 432 pages. 2006. 978-0-7808-0820-1.

"Full of helpful insights and facts throughout the book. . . . An excellent resource to be placed in public libraries or even in personal collections."
— *American Reference Books Annual, 2002*

"Recommended for middle and high school libraries and media centers as well as academic libraries that educate future teachers of teenagers. It is also a suitable addition to health science libraries that serve patrons who are interested in teen health promotion and education."
— *E-Streams, Oct '01*

"This comprehensive book would be beneficial to collections that need information about nutrition, dietary guidelines, meal planning, and weight control. . . . This reference is so easy to use that its purchase is recommended."
— *The Book Report, Sep-Oct '01*

"This book is written in an easy to understand format describing issues that many teens face every day, and then provides thoughtful explanations so that teens can make informed decisions. This is an interesting book that provides important facts and information for today's teens."
— *Doody's Health Sciences Book Review Journal, Jul-Aug '01*

"A comprehensive compendium of diet and nutrition. The information is presented in a straightforward, plain-spoken manner. This title will be useful to those working on reports on a variety of topics, as well as to general readers concerned about their dietary health."
— *School Library Journal, Jun '01*

Drug Information for Teens, 2nd Edition

Health Tips about the Physical and Mental Effects of Substance Abuse

Including Information about Marijuana, Inhalants, Club Drugs, Stimulants, Hallucinogens, Opiates, Prescription and Over-the-Counter Drugs, Herbal Products, Tobacco, Alcohol, and More

Edited by Sandra Augustyn Lawton. 468 pages. 2006. 978-0-7808-0862-1.

"A clearly written resource for general readers and researchers alike."
— *School Library Journal*

"This book is well-balanced. . . . a must for public and school libraries."
— *VOYA: Voice of Youth Advocates, Dec '03*

"The chapters are quick to make a connection to their teenage reading audience. The prose is straightforward and the book lends itself to spot reading. It should be useful both for practical information and for research, and it is suitable for public and school libraries."
— *American Reference Books Annual, 2003*

"Recommended reference source."
— *Booklist, American Library Association, Feb '03*

"This is an excellent resource for teens and their parents. Education about drugs and substances is key to discouraging teen drug abuse and this book provides this much needed information in a way that is interesting and factual."
— *Doody's Review Service, Dec '02*

Eating Disorders Information for Teens

Health Tips about Anorexia, Bulimia, Binge Eating, and Other Eating Disorders

Including Information on the Causes, Prevention, and Treatment of Eating Disorders, and Such Other Issues as Maintaining Healthy Eating and Exercise Habits

Edited by Sandra Augustyn Lawton. 337 pages. 2005. 978-0-7808-0783-9.

"An excellent resource for teens and those who work with them."
— *VOYA: Voice of Youth Advocates, Apr '06*

"A welcome addition to high school and undergraduate libraries." — *American Reference Books Annual, 2006*

"This book covers the topic in a lucid manner but delves deeper into every aspect of an eating disorder. A solid addition for any nonfiction or reference collection."
— *School Library Journal, Dec '05*

Fitness Information for Teens

Health Tips about Exercise, Physical Well-Being, and Health Maintenance

Including Facts about Aerobic and Anaerobic Conditioning, Stretching, Body Shape and Body Image, Sports Training, Nutrition, and Activities for Non-Athletes

Edited by Karen Bellenir. 425 pages. 2004. 978-0-7808-0679-5.

"Another excellent offering from Omnigraphics in their *Teen Health Series*. . . . This book will be a great addition to any public, junior high, senior high, or secondary school library."
— *American Reference Books Annual, 2005*

Learning Disabilities Information for Teens

Health Tips about Academic Skills Disorders and Other Disabilities That Affect Learning

Including Information about Common Signs of Learning Disabilities, School Issues, Learning to Live with a Learning Disability, and Other Related Issues

Edited by Sandra Augustyn Lawton. 337 pages. 2005. 978 0 7808 0796 9.

"This book provides a wealth of information for any reader interested in the signs, causes, and consequences

of learning disabilities, as well as related legal rights and educational interventions. . . . Public and academic libraries should want this title for both students and general readers."
— *American Reference Books Annual, 2006*

■

Mental Health Information for Teens, 2nd Edition

Health Tips about Mental Wellness and Mental Illness

Including Facts about Mental and Emotional Health, Depression and Other Mood Disorders, Anxiety Disorders, Behavior Disorders, Self-Injury, Psychosis, Schizophrenia, and More

Edited by Karen Bellenir. 400 pages. 2006. 978-0-7808-0863-8.

"In both language and approach, this user-friendly entry in the *Teen Health Series* is on target for teens needing information on mental health concerns."
— *Booklist, American Library Association, Jan '02*

"Readers will find the material accessible and informative, with the shaded notes, facts, and embedded glossary insets adding appropriately to the already interesting and succinct presentation."
— *School Library Journal, Jan '02*

"This title is highly recommended for any library that serves adolescents and parents/caregivers of adolescents."
— *E-Streams, Jan '02*

"Recommended for high school libraries and young adult collections in public libraries. Both health professionals and teenagers will find this book useful."
— *American Reference Books Annual, 2002*

"This is a nice book written to enlighten the society, primarily teenagers, about common teen mental health issues. It is highly recommended to teachers and parents as well as adolescents."
— *Doody's Review Service, Dec '01*

■

Sexual Health Information for Teens

Health Tips about Sexual Development, Human Reproduction, and Sexually Transmitted Diseases

Including Facts about Puberty, Reproductive Health, Chlamydia, Human Papillomavirus, Pelvic Inflammatory Disease, Herpes, AIDS, Contraception, Pregnancy, and More

Edited by Deborah A. Stanley. 391 pages. 2003. 978-0-7808-0445-6.

"This work should be included in all high school libraries and many larger public libraries. . . . highly recommended."
— *American Reference Books Annual, 2004*

"*Sexual Health* approaches its subject with appropriate seriousness and offers easily accessible advice and information." — *School Library Journal, Feb '04*

Skin Health Information for Teens

Health Tips about Dermatological Concerns and Skin Cancer Risks

Including Facts about Acne, Warts, Hives, and Other Conditions and Lifestyle Choices, Such as Tanning, Tattooing, and Piercing, That Affect the Skin, Nails, Scalp, and Hair

Edited by Robert Aquinas McNally. 429 pages. 2003. 978-0-7808-0446-3.

"This volume, as with others in the series, will be a useful addition to school and public library collections." — *American Reference Books Annual, 2004*

"There is no doubt that this reference tool is valuable."
— *VOYA: Voice of Youth Advocates, Feb '04*

"This volume serves as a one-stop source and should be a necessity for any health collection."
— *Library Media Connection*

■

Sports Injuries Information for Teens

Health Tips about Sports Injuries and Injury Protection

Including Facts about Specific Injuries, Emergency Treatment, Rehabilitation, Sports Safety, Competition Stress, Fitness, Sports Nutrition, Steroid Risks, and More

Edited by Joyce Brennfleck Shannon. 405 pages. 2003. 978-0-7808-0447-0.

"This work will be useful in the young adult collections of public libraries as well as high school libraries."
— *American Reference Books Annual, 2004*

■

Suicide Information for Teens

Health Tips about Suicide Causes and Prevention

Including Facts about Depression, Risk Factors, Getting Help, Survivor Support, and More

Edited by Joyce Brennfleck Shannon. 368 pages. 2005. 978-0-7808-0737-2.

■

Tobacco Information for Teens

Health Tips about the Hazards of Using Cigarettes, Smokeless Tobacco, and Other Nicotine Products

Including Facts about Nicotine Addiction, Immediate and Long-Term Health Effects of Tobacco Use, Related Cancers, Smoking Cessation, Tobacco Use Prevention, and Tobacco Use Statistics

Edited by Karen Bellenir. 440 pages. 2007. 978-0-7808-0976-5.

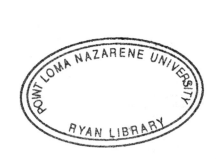

Health Reference Series